Recent Results in Cancer Research 139

C. Garbe S. Schmitz
C.E. Orfanos (Eds.)

Skin Cancer: Basic Science, Clinical Research and Treatment

With 85 Figures and 72 Tables

Springer-Verlag
Berlin Heidelberg New York
London Paris Tokyo
Hong Kong Barcelona
Budapest

Prof. Dr. med. Claus Garbe
Dr. med. Stefan Schmitz
Prof. Dr. med. Prof. h.c. Constantin E. Orfanos

Freie Universität Berlin
University Department of Dermatology
Medical Centre Benjamin Franklin
Hindenburgdamm 30
12200 Berlin, Germany

ISBN-13: 978-3-642-78773-7 e-ISBN-13: 978-3-642-78771-3
DOI: 10.1007/978-3-642-78771-3

Library of Congress Cataloging-in-Publication Data. Skin Cancer: basic science, clinical research, and treatment/C. Garbe, S. Schmitz, C.E. Orfanos (eds.). p. cm. – (Recent results in cancer research; 139) Includes bibliographical references and index.

Cancer – Congresses. I. Garbe, C. (Claus), 1951– . II. Schmitz, S. (Stefan), 1960– . III. Orfanos, C.E. (Constantin E.) IV. Series. [DNLM: 1. Skin Neoplasms – congresses. W1 RE106P v. 139 1995] RC261.R35 vol. 139 [RC280.S5] 616.99'4 s – dc20 [616.99'477] DNLM/DLC for Library of Congress 94-36423

Softcover reprint of the hardcover 1st edition 1995

Typesetting: Best-set Typesetter Ltd., Hong Kong

SPIN: 10127896 19/3130/SPS – 5 4 3 2 1 0 – Printed on acid-free paper

Preface

In the past two decades, considerable interest in skin cancer has developed in the public and scientific communities. There may have been several reasons for this:

- The rise in the global incidence of cutaneous cancers
- New molecular biology techniques resulting in a better understanding of pathogenesis and improved diagnostic procedures
- The advent of new pathological entities, e.g., the endemic form of Kaposi's sarcoma
- A constantly increasing range of therapeutic modalities, providing even more efficacious treatment and management of skin cancers

As N.E. Fusenig describes in the first chapter of this volume, basic research is only beginning to unravel the complex mechanism involved in cellular dedifferentiation and tumor progression. Progress is dearly needed, especially in dermato-oncology, where the rise in the incidence of epithelial tumors has inflated the overall skin cancer incidence. The incidence of tumors of the skin exceeds that of all other neoplasias in humans, with recreational sun exposure being a suspected primary cause. Several studies on the effects of UV radiation have been included at the beginning of this volume. Even the role of long wavelength UV (UVA) has become a focus of research activities. The main concern is that the low carcinogenicity of UVA, in comparison to UVB, may be outweighed and exceeded in its effects by increased UVA exposure, e.g., in tanning parlors, and possibly also by using UVB sunscreens, thus prolonging the time for UV erythema to develop. Interestingly, the recent increase in epithelial skin cancers is not confined exclusively to whites, but rather it is a global phenomenon, as indicated by the Japanese data presented.

A marked increase in incidence has been recorded for malignant melanoma in the past four decades. Melanoma research attracted most of the attention during the conference as melanoma is the tumor with the highest mortality of all skin tumors. Basic molecular research and studies on the properties of metastasizing melanoma cells were key issues, as reflected by the respective selection of articles. In addition, some promising approaches in immunotargeting and cytokine research were included. The interaction of melanoma cells with immunocompetent cells and the role of cellular surface molecules were further topics. The increased incidence of melanoma has coincided with increased publicity, which raised such issues as prevention and early diagnosis, represented in this volume in particular by US studies.

The research on cutaneous lymphomas has been dominated by developments in molecular biology, mainly resulting in refined diagnostic procedures. Today northern blotting and polymerase chain reaction have become major supplements to routine immunohistochemical techniques. The application of the newer techniques goes beyond the study of T-cell lymphomas, as described in one article, where oncogenes in B-cell lymphomas have been analyzed.

Much attention has been devoted to HIV-associated Kaposi's sarcoma by the medical community and the public during the past decade. A large follow-up study of Kaposi patients is presented which comprises over 10 years of therapeutic experience in Berlin, Germany. A detailed discussion of various etiologic theories is included. A report of the clinical research on basal cell carcinomas and adnexal tumors concludes the tumor section.

The last part of the volume contains articles dealing with treatment and management of skin tumors, again, malignant melanoma being the main focus of interest. Current debates on melanoma treatment are covered in detail, i.e., excisional margins, elective lymphadenectomy, systemic treatment. The scope of the therapeutic approaches ranges from vaccination therapy, and the use of cytokines to the combination of the latter with chemotherapeutic agents, with reference to the state of the art in the treatment of T-cell lymphomas and the Kaposi's sarcoma. Two relatively new therapeutic modalities are the application of extracorporeal photopheresis for treatment of T-cell lymphomas and the application of lasers, especially for photodynamic therapy. The therapeutic section of the volume thus provides a concise review of treatment of skin cancer.

Overall a selection of articles is presented which represent the major scientific and clinical debates being conducted in the field. We hope that this volume will prove useful to all readers interested in skin oncology.

Berlin, November 1994 The Editors

Contents

*List of Contributors**

* The address of the principal author is given on the first page of each contribution.
[1] Page on which contribution begins.

Kroumpouzos, G. *123*
Krüger-Krasagakes, S. *155*
Krüse-Wolters, M. *57*
Landthaler, M. *195, 417*
Leigh, I.M. *69*
Marghoob, A.A. *87*
Mielke, V. *403*
Möhler, T. *383*
Möller, K. *31*
Müller-Eckhardt, G. *297*
Nagano, T. *263*
Nakamura, T. *263*
Naruse, K. *263*
Neri, A. *249*
Orfanos, C.E. *43, 123, 169, 275, 409*
Otte, H.G. *391*
Owsianowski, M. *409*
Petres, J. *297, 323*
Pilch, H. *137*
Quax, P.H.A. *105*
Ramaker, J. *409*
Reichert, U. *183*
Rigel, D.S. *87*
Rompel, R. *297, 323*
Roscetti, E. *249*
Ruiter, D.J. *57, 105*
Rülke, D. *303*
Rünger, T.M. *31*
Salopek, T.G. *87*
Santinami, M. *317*
Schadendorf, D. *183*
Scheibenbogen, C. *383*
Schiffner, R. *195*
Schmitz, S. *43*
Schrier, P. *57*
Slade, J. *87*
Stadler, R. *391*
Staib, G. *239, 403*
Stark, H.-J. *1*
Sterry, W. *239, 403*
Stolz, W. *195*
Suzuki, T. *263*
Szeimies, R.-M. *417*
Teichelmann, K. *323*
Thiel, E. *371*
Tilgen, W. *383*
Tomakidi, P. *1*
Trecca, D. *249*
Vacca, A. *57*
van der Flier, S. *57*
van Elsas, A. *57*
van Muijen, G.N.P. *105*
Verheijen, J.H. *105*
Vogt, T. *195*
Wadabayashi, N. *263*
Wadler, S. *371*
Watanabe, S. *263*
Weiss, J. *137*
Wölfer, U. *275*
Wollina, U. *303*
Worm, M. *183*
Wulff, A. *43*
Zerp, S. *57*
Zouboulis, Ch.C. *169*

I. Carcinogenesis

Differentiation and Tumor Progression

N.E. Fusenig, D. Breitkreutz, P. Boukamp, P. Tomakidi, and H.-J. Stark

Division of Carcinogenesis and Differentiation, German Cancer Research Center, 69120 Heidelberg, Germany

Abstract

Clinical and experimental experience indicate that differentiation and malignancy are inversely correlated. However, more recent experimental studies using mouse and human keratinocyte systems have demonstrated that complete or even substantial loss in overall epithelial differentiation is not a prerequisite for malignant growth of cancer cells. Major defects in differentiation are also not a prerequisite for premalignant stages, in particular for cell immortalization, which is considered an early and essential step in the transformation process. Moreover, progressive dedifferentiation, often associated with advanced tumor stages, is also found in immortalized cell lines which are, however, nontumorigenic. On the other hand, malignant cell lines may have maintained a high degree of their normal differentiation program and sensitivity to differentiation modulators. However, to date no transformed keratinocyte cell lines with completely normal differentiation have been observed. Since epidermal keratinization is a very complex process involving many different parameters and is fully expressed only under in vivo conditions, an exact and quantitative comparison of such ill-defined phenomena (differentiation and malignancy) is still problematic.

Obviously, both phenomena are under separate control and not causally linked. Nevertheless, a better understanding of factors and mechanisms regulating differentiation and of their disturbance in carcinogenesis would offer new possibilities to design novel tumor therapeutic strategies in the field of differentiation therapy.

Introduction

Malignancy is a collective term for a number of disturbances in the regulation of cellular proliferation and differentiation in multicellular organisms.

Recent Results in Cancer Research, Vol. 139

Due to this complexity, also reflected in the high degree of phenotypic and genetic heterogeneity in malignant tumors, our understanding of the essential biological parameters characterizing malignancy is still incomplete. Histopathologic observations have revealed that defects in the differentiation program are a common phenotypic feature of tumor cells. However, the significance of these alterations as causal factors for the carcinogenesis process is still unclear.

Most malignant epithelial tumors arise in self-renewing tissues lining the inner or outer surface of the body, such as the skin. In addition to cellular proliferation, by which these tissues continuously replace the loss of cells from the surface, there is a highly regulated way of maturation of the self-renewing precursor cells to committed cells, which eventually acquire specialized functions leading in skin to the formation of a stratum corneum. In these tissues, the rules of cell replacement seem to be arranged in such a way that variants with disregulated proliferation, i.e., potential tumor cells, are suppressed. This is achieved partly by the close relationship between tissue architecture and terminal differentiation as well as by control mechanisms acting in different ways in cell–cell interactions. In malignancy this highly regulated process of terminal differentiation is disturbed. In fact, alterations in tissue-specific differentiation visible at the histologic level are major parameters for the diagnosis of neoplastic changes and provide the basis for their classification.

Differentiation and Malignancy

It is now widely accepted that cancer develops as a progressive, multistage process in which cells pass through different stages of phenotypic and genetic alterations, gradually acquiring the phenotype which is usually associated with malignancy. Furthermore, tumor cells progress to cell populations with increased malignant potential and this often coincides with further decrease or a total loss of differentiation features. For squamous cell carcinomas (SCC), a "grading theory" based on empirical histopathologic and clinical observations was originally formulated by Broders (1932). This hypothesis has been substantiated by experimental data obtained from carcinogenesis studies in animal tissues revealing an inverse relationship between the grade of tumor differentiation and the metastatic capacity of a particular tumor (for review see Gabbert et al. 1985; Eccles 1983). However, although according to histopathology the most aggressive carcinomas are usually the least differentiated, there are highly differentiated SCC (such as the verrucous carcinomas of the skin or the so-called de novo cutaneous SCC) which may express a high degree of differentiation but are nevertheless highly malignant (Schwartz 1988).

The oversimplifying reason most frequently given to explain this higher degree of malignancy is that the activity of poorly differentiated tumors would be more proliferative. However, this explanation is contradicted by many observations demonstrating that proliferation in benign tumors may be as high as in malignant tumors. In addition, there is experimental evidence that highly invasive undifferentiated carcinomas display a significantly lower proliferative activity than the far less invasive differentiated carcinomas (Gabbert et al. 1985). Thus, the influence of tumor differentiation on the process of invasion and metastasis cannot be satisfactorily explained by higher tumor cell proliferation alone, but has to be understood in the context of tissue homeostasis, which is maintained by the balance between cell renewal and cell loss.

Proliferation and differentiation of normal cells are usually controlled by well-balanced feedback mechanisms involving different signal transduction pathways. The controlled interactions of these regulating mechanisms warrant the homeostatic balance between cell proliferation and terminal differentiation and by this the constancy of tissue mass and architecture. Permanent uncoupling of this normal balance by genetic or epigenetic mechanisms is thought to be a critical step in the generation and further progression of malignant cells. It has been hypothesized that preneoplastic cells gain a clonal growth advantage over normal cells by the acquisition of a selective resistance to inducers of differentiation (Rheinwald and Beckett 1980; Harris 1987; Parkinson 1985; Wille et al. 1982). Although these and other data strongly support the hypothesis that uncoupling of differentiation and proliferation pathways are involved in the generation of neoplasms, aberrations in the differentiation pathway per se are insufficient to cause malignancy.

On the other hand it is well known that many tumors exhibit pronounced morphological heterogeneity visible as cellular pleomorphism and variable degrees of tissue differentiation in different parts of the same tumor. Such phenotypic changes occurring during tumor progression are usually associated with increased genomic instability of cancer cells apparent by the accumulation of karyotypic aberrations. Thus, it was hypothesized that alterations in differentiation capacity at later tumor stages are secondary effects, i.e., rather the consequence of the genetic instability of the neoplastic cells than unrelated to the very transformation process itself (Heim et al. 1988). At present, it is not possible to decide whether tumor cells bear genetic defects in their proper differentiation programs or exhibit incomplete expression due to alterations or defects in their response to external differentiation signals.

Most tumor cells, however, maintain a certain, although mostly low degree of tissue-specific differentiation visualized by morphologic and or biochemical criteria at the tissue and single cell level (i.e., intermediate filaments, enzymes, endo- or exocrine activity) as well as basic features of tissue architecture, which are successfully used for the diagnosis of tissue origin and subtype of tumors (Osborn and Weber 1983; Moll et al. 1984; Morgan et al. 1987). This maintained, although often rudimentary differentiation capacity of tumor cells has attracted much attention as a possible target for new therapeutic concepts known as "differentiation therapy." In this context it has been shown that many tumor cells still respond to a certain degree to external differentiation signals which, at least in experimental systems, can be successfully used as therapeutic tools. However, our still limited knowledge about the nature of these differentiation signals and their mechanism of action in regulating differentiation has so far limited these attempts. In this context it became evident that a better understanding of the differentiation control of normal cells would help to identify alterations occurring in tumor cells and thus greatly improve our chances for more effective differentiation-inducing tumor therapy.

Expression of the Differentiated Phenotype in Carcinoma Cell Lines

Progress in our understanding of the differentiated state and differentiation potential of neoplastic human epithelia has improved considerably with the availability of cultured tumor cells providing enough material of suitable homogeneity. Although it is still difficult to grow cells of many human malignancies in vitro, cell lines have been established from most frequent human carcinomas. However, the use of these cell lines is restricted due to their antiquity, highly selective nature, and sometimes questionable phenotypic relation to the tumor from which they were originally derived. Moreover, these cultured tumor cells frequently display phenotypic instability during prolonged propagation in vitro due to their genetic instability and also depending on variations in culture conditions and handling of cells. Nevertheless, they are at present the most frequently used in vitro models for studying human tumor cells.

Thus, carcinoma cell lines derived from different tissues and organ sites have been classified by various investigators according to different criteria, including morphology, karyotype, growth kinetics in vitro, and tumorigenicity, but only to a limited extent by functional criteria related to differentiation (for review see Fusenig et al. 1991b).

It has been demonstrated in many cases that such cell lines derived from primary tumors of human carcinomas have maintained to certain extent the degree of differentiation of the original tumor. This, however, is best demonstrated in experimental tumors obtained after their subcutaneous transplantation to suitable hosts, indicating the important role of environmental conditions for the expression of differentiation features. Further studies using more in vivo-like culture models and in vivo systems, which allow the development of three-dimensional tissues, could demonstrate large similarities between the original tumor or tissue and the structures formed under these experimental conditions (Wu and Rheinwald 1981; Boukamp et al. 1982, 1985; Tilgen et al. 1983; Easty et al. 1986).

When such tumor-derived cell lines were studied over many passages in vitro, a remarkable stability of their phenotypic traits was observed, indicating that they represent reliable models to study the significance of the degree of differentiation for the malignant phenotype (Tilgen et al. 1983; Boukamp et al. 1985; Easty et al. 1986; Auersperg et al. 1989).

Differentiation Parameters and Models for Squamous Epithelia

Differentiation of squamous epithelial tissues is a complex process of well-regulated expression of specific functional products closely associated with cell polarization and structural organization of the tissue as best studied in the skin (for review see Bowden et al. 1987 and Fuchs 1990). This differentiation process is obviously regulated by intrinsic programs of the epithelial cells, but strongly influenced by external regulatory factors contributed by the local environment, as demonstrated by transplantation studies with isolated and recombined epithelial and mesenchymal tissue components of various body sites (for review see Fusenig et al. 1991a; Fusenig 1994). As a consequence, isolated epithelial cell – either from normal or malignant tissues – express under conventional culture conditions in vitro only an incomplete or alternative differentiation program; some differentiation products are either not synthesized or their expression is not (or poorly) uncoordinated with other parameters which are usually tightly linked in the tissue (Boukamp et al. 1985; Breitkreutz et al. 1986, 1989, 1991a,b; Fusenig et al. 1991b).

Therefore, in order to provide appropriate conditions for the expression of the differentiation pattern, improved culture models have been developed to allow tissue-specific organization and differentiation of both normal and tumor cells. This is realized in organotypic cultures where epithelial cells are cultured on an extracellular matrix in the presence of mesenchymal cells. Usually multicellular structures develop resembling more closely the histology of the normal tissue or primary tumors than observed in conventional cultures. In these coculture systems, a detailed analysis of the structural organization and associated expression of differentiation products is feasible under more physiologic, but still rather defined conditions (Boukamp et al. 1990b; Hornung et al. 1987; Ryle et al. 1989; Fusenig et al. 1983, 1991a; Mackenzie et al. 1993; McCance et al. 1988; Coulomb et al. 1989).

However, from these studies it became evident that both tumor and normal epithelia expressed their full differentiation potential only under in vivo conditions when growing in their natural environment, i.e., for skin keratinocytes as surface transplants. In particular, this device is considered a more physiologic environment for surface epithelia than when cells are injected subcutaneously, i.e., into a foreign mesenchyma. In surface transplants, the tumor cells also expressed more readily their respective tumorigenic growth potential as well as their individual differentiation program as compared to heterotransplants after subcutaneous injection (Boukamp et al. 1985, 1990b; Knight et al. 1984; Fusenig et al. 1991a,b).

Differentiation Characteristics of Epithelial Skin Tumors

The assessment of the role of differentiation or loss of differentiation in the carcinogenesis process is complicated among other things by the phenotypic heterogeneity of tumors, as mentioned above, and by the complex and multifacetted image of differentiation. As far as tumor diagnosis is concerned, morphologic alterations in the histologic picture are the major or often only parameters to describe the degree of differentiation. Recent developments in the identification and analysis of various differentiation parameters at the cellular and molecular level have greatly improved our understanding of the complex differentiation process. Moreover, this improved knowledge has provided many tools for the detailed diagnosis of the state of differentiation as well as the defects in its performance in many diseased states. Such studies using specific antibodies and more recently antisense RNA probes have greatly broadened our view of the many variations in tumor cell differentiation as such and within the same tumor. They have also demonstrated that the diagnosis of the "degree of differentiation" depends largely on the type and number of parameters analyzed. Moreover, such parameters, which are linked and coexpressed in normal tissue, often become dissociated in their sequence of appearance or even independently lost. In addition, new differentiation markers (atypical in the tissue of origin) may be expressed in tumor cells, but it may be questionable whether and how they contribute to the differentiated (or dedifferentiated) state of a given tumor. Thus, due to the increasing complexity of the multifacetted picture of the general term differentiation, it is increasingly problematic to determine the degree of differentiation of a given tumor and to relate this to its clinical or biological state of progression.

The state of differentiation of given skin carcinoma is characterized by its specific stuctural organization and the expression of a characteristic ensemble of proteins. In the epidermis, one of the best-known and -studied examples of stratified epithelia, the intimate link between structural organization and spatial expression of specific differentiation products is particularly well documented. Cell maturation is characterized by the appearance of several differentiation products strictly linked to different cell layers and often visible as specific structural differentiation markers (for review see Bowden et al. 1987).

The major differentiation products of the epidermis are the keratins, the epithelial representatives of the intermediate filament proteins. As obligatory heterodimers (composed of one member of the acidic and the basic subfamily), the keratins are the building blocks of tonofilaments and show a characteristic distribution in stratified epithelia (Moll et al. 1982; Steinert and Roop 1988). While the keratins 5 and 14 are expressed in the proliferating basal cells, differentiating cells are characterized by K1 and K10 (analogous to K4 and K13 in internal, noncornified squamous epithelia). Upon skin irritation or wounding, K6, K16, and K17 are induced, which are common in hyperproliferative, wounded, or otherwise modified stratified epithelia such as outer root sheath of hair follicle. On the other hand, K7, K8, K18, and K19 are normally only found in simple, nonstratified epithelia (for review see Bowden et al. 1987), but can be aberrantly expressed in tumors together with K19 common in many transitional epithelia.

In epithelial skin tumors, the keratin distribution is characteristic of the tissue of origin, but also of the specific tumor type, clearly distinguishing basal cell carcinomas and SCC. However, in most tumors the keratin pattern of the tissue of origin is substantially modified. While characteristic ones of the normal epithelium are often lost, additional keratins might be present. However, no tumor-specific keratins have been found so far in human epithelial tumors which might serve as diagnostic markers (Moll et al. 1984, 1988; Breitkreutz et al. 1981; Morgan et al. 1987), although simple epithelial keratins (K8, 18) seem to be more frequent in advanced malignancies (Markey et al. 1991). Comparable to normal epidermis, keratin expression of tumor cells changes when cells are transferred to in vitro conditions, where they might even express a broader spectrum of keratins (Breitkreutz et al. 1981, 1991a,b; Tilgen et al. 1983). Usually some of the tissue-specific keratins are reduced under in vitro conditions, while keratins of the hyperproliferative and simple epithelial type are more expressed. Following transplantation or reinjection into animals, the keratin patterns expressed under in vitro conditions "renormalize" again, approaching those seen in the tumor biopsies (e.g., Tilgen et al. 1983; Breitkreutz et al. 1991 a,b).

Most human SCC analyzed so far have (to a large extent or completely) lost the expression of the differentiation-specific keratins K1 and K10, although some areas of established tumors may be found positive when tested with specific antibodies, indicating tumor heterogeneity in their differentiation potential (Markey et al. 1991).

Another late differentiation marker specific for squamous epithelia is the formation of cornified cells (corneocytes), the so-called cornified envelopes, and the synthesis of its major biochemical substrate involucrin (Rice and Green 1979; Rheinwald and Beckett 1980; Levitt et al. 1990). A survey of a wide variety of normal and neoplastic tissues has demonstrated involucrin to be a specific marker for squamous differentiation and its presence in those normal and neoplastic tissues showed a positive correlation with morphologic criteria of squamous differentiation. Thus, cornification and appearance of horn cells is usually the differentiation marker most easily observed and used in histopathologic diagnosis of SCC.

Differentiation and Carcinogenesis

In general, it has been difficult to study the central or causal role of alterations in the differentiation program for the development of malignancy and its progression based only on work with clinically established tumors with mostly unknown etiology, latency period, and state of development. Although disturbances of normal tissue differentiation are often detected in premalignant lesions (dysplasias), their causal role for these preneoplastic changes and even more for progression to malignancy can only be identified in experimental systems.

The role of altered differentiation in the process of tumorigenesis has been studied in animal experiments, mostly on mouse skin (Kartasowa et al. 1992; Stoler et al. 1993; Roop et al. 1988; Nischt et al. 1988). However, a dramatic loss of differentiation suggested by the initial studies on mouse keratinocytes (Yuspa et al. 1985) was apparently not obligatory for the development of a fully malignant phenotype (Breitkreutz et al. 1986; Tennenbaum et al. 1992). More recently corresponding investigations in vitro have been performend also with human epithelial cells. Although in vitro transformation of human cells is very difficult to achieve (in contrast to rodent cells), several model systems have been established in which the multistep process of carcinogenesis could be studied (for review see Fusenig et al. 1989).

As a first stage of transformation, human cells were immortalized to nontumorigenic, but permanently growing cell lines by oncogenes of DNA tumor viruses such as the T antigen of Simian virus 40 (SV40) and the E-6 and E-7 oncogenes of some human papillomaviruses (HPV; for review seen Chang 1986; Fusenig et al. 1987; Dürst et al. 1987). These immortalized cell lines exhibit various alterations in their differention potential, ranging from highly differentiated to "undifferentiated," allowing no definite conclusion as to the causal relation of differentiation loss and transformation per se. In addition, considerable differences were observed when SV40-immortalized keratinocyte cell lines were tested for morphologic and biochemical differentiation criteria under in vitro or in vivo conditions (Bernard et al. 1985; Banks-Schlegel and Howley 1983; Chang 1986). Less pronounced changes in the differentiation program have been found in cell lines immortalized by HPV DNA (Dürst et al. 1987; McCance et al. 1988) when tested in vitro as well as in vivo (Woodworth et al. 1988; Breitkreutz et al. 1991b).

A model system particularly well suited for studying the relationship of differentiation and carcinogenesis has been established in our laboratory with the development of a spontaneously immortalized keratinocyte cell line derived from adult human skin (Boukamp et al. 1988). Both this HaCaT cell line as well as derived *ras* oncogene-transfected tumorigenic benign and malignant cell clones maintained a high degree of morphologic and biochemical differentiation (Boukamp et al. 1990b; Ryle et al. 1989; Breitkreutz et al. 1991a,b). Using these HaCaT cell lines and Various descendants with altered differentiation and different states of transformation, the causal relationship of these phenomena has been studied. It was of particular interest to identify whether tumor cells had completely lost their sensitivity towards differentiation-inducing conditions or to what degree this response was only reduced and could be stimulated under experimental conditions.

Differentiation and Immortalization

Although it is still a matter of debate whether all malignant cells are necessarily immortal and which clinical lesions can be considered as biological correlates to in vitro immortalized cells, it is the general experience that immortalization is a prerequisite for successful tumorigenic transformation in vitro (Fusenig et al. 1989, 1991b). This process usually involves several steps including, among others, inactivation of senescence genes. The established cell lines are mostly aneuploid with many structural chromosomal alterations, In the case of the HaCaT cell line, it is hypothesized that (typically UV induced) mutations in the p53 gene (leading to increased frequency of genetic aberrations) and specific culture conditions (elevated temperature) have been the major factors to enhance chromosomal alterations, leading eventually to the loss of chromosomes carrying putative senescence genes (Boukamp et al. 1993). Most probably the initial as well as the consecutive chromosomal alterations are the consequence of un- or misrepaired random DNA damages. It is quite conceivable that these changes could also have involved structural or regulatory genes essential for the differentiation process. Although no detailed studies exist, it is interesting to note that the cell lines with highest genetic instability and chromosomal alterations (e.g., SV40-transformed ones) usually exhibit severe alterations in differentiation. This would imply that defects in differentiation in such genetically altered cell lines are consequences of the higher rate of genomic aberrations involving structural or regulatory differentiation genes and not causal for the transformation process. Since all the immortalized human cell lines are initially nontumorigenic, irrespective of their state of differentiation, this suggests that the degree of differentiation is of no rate-limiting importance for the progression to tumorigenicity.

These as well as other studies have clearly demonstrated that immortalization is not intimately linked to the loss of differentiation, but that permanently growing cells can maintain the ability to terminally differentiation under in vitro and in vivo conditions. This is particularly evident in the case of the spontaneously immortalized HaCaT cell line, which is a highly differentiated keratinocyte cell line (Boukamp et al. 1988). These cells form epithelia in surface transplants on nude mice very similar, although not identical, to normal epidermis with a parakeratotic stratum corneum, but show altered expression of differentiation-specific keratins. The differentiation-specific keratins K1 and K10 are expressed, as in epidermis, but their onset of expression and localization are altered: K1 is atypically visible throughout the whole epidermis, including the (normally K1-free) basal layer, and thus dissociated from K10 (Breitkreutz et al. 1991a). In contrast to normal keratinocytes, HaCaT cells also express these keratins under normal culture conditions, possibly indicating altered sensitivity to negatively regulating factors such as vitamin A (Ryle et al. 1989; Breitkreutz et al. 1991a,b, 1993a). At the morphologic and keratin protein levels, differentiation of HaCaT cells is still regulated by retinoic acid and Ca^{2+} concentrations. Morphologic organization into a regular squamous epithelial tissue architecture, however, has not yet been achieved in vitro, even when tested under conditions under which normal keratinocytes form a regular epidermis, i.e., in organotypic cocultures with mesenchymal cells (Smola et al. 1993; Boukamp et al. 1990a; Baur et al., in preparation; Ryle et al. 1989). Since rather normal morphogenesis of HaCaT cells is only achieved under more complex in vivo conditions, this failure indicates either defects in their endogenous regulatory programs or altered (decreased) sensitivity to external signals.

As known from other cell lines, the differentiation capacity of HaCaT cells is gradually reduced with continued passaging – the speed obviously depending on culture conditions – so that after more than 300 passages cells form dysplastic epithelia in surface transplants. Nevertheless, these cells, having lost many of their keratinization features, have not become tumorigenic nor acquired an invasive growth behaviour in vivo (Hülsen et al., in preparation). The loss of differentiation has been accelerated by forced proliferation at clonal densities with the consequence of increased proliferative activity in vitro and occasional benign tumor formation following subcutaneous injection in nude mice (Hülsen et al., in preparation). While this observation could indicate that loss of differentiation accompanies or even might favor tumor progression, this conclusion was not supported by other studies designed to interfere with the keratinocyte differentiation program. By transfection of the myogenic differentiation gene *myoD1* into HaCaT cells, their treatment by 5-aza-cytidine, and selection of an adhesion-deficient subclone, a cell population was isolated which had lost all of its biochemical and morphologic epidermal differentiation parameters. These cells were no longer able to form stratified epithelia (in vitro and in vivo) and had acquired typical fibroblast-like characteristics, but had not become tumorigenic, nor showed any other indication of tumor progression (Boukamp et al. 1992; Boukamp and Fusenig 1993). These studies did, however, substantiate earlier findings that in the process of "dedifferentiation" morphologic, i.e., histotypic, differentiation parameters are lost or reduced first, while cytodifferentiation markers (e.g., keratin expession) are largely unchanged or are altered much later. This correlates with the experience that morphologic alterations in tissue architecture (dysplasia) are the earliest indicators of preneoplastic changes. It also demonstrates that both phenomena are differentially regulated and that processes responsible for tissue architecture (e.g., cell–cell interactions) are more vulnerable by (obviously epigenetic) mechanisms under adverse environmental conditions.

Differentiation Changes with Tumorigenic Conversion

By different manipulations, early passage HaCaT cells were further transformed to tumorigenic cells forming benign or malignant epithelial tumors after subcutaneous injection into nude mice.

Transfection with the cellular Harvey-*ras* oncogene (c-Ha-*ras*) produced several cell clones which formed either slowly growing and eventually regressing, highly differentiated epithelial cysts (benign tumors) or progressively growing keratinized SCC (Boukamp et al. 1990b). Although the individual tumorigenic clones exhibited variations in the expression of differentiation parameters in vitro and in surface transplants in vivo, a classification into benign or malignant clones was not feasible on the basis of their differentiation potential (Ryle et al. 1989; Breitkreutz et al. 1991a,b, 1993a). In general, all tumorgenic clones maintained a high differentiation potential both at the biochemical level and according to histomorphologic criteria. This was particularly evident in surface transplants where both benign and malignant clones formed keratinizing epithelia, while only the malignant ones exhibited invasive growth behavior and elicited continued angiogenesis (Boukamp et al. 1990a; Tomakidi et al., in preparation). In this in vivo assay, however, a different regulation of keratinization parameters could be observed, distinguishing benign from malignant keratinocytes. Both expressed the keratins K1 and K10 in a fairly typical way, although with some variations. Interestingly, K1 and K10 were present even in the invasive parts of these malignant tumors, often in a fairly normal (suprabasal) tissue localization (Breitkreutz et al. 1991a, 1993a).

In addition, the basal-type keratins (K5 and K14), while being aberrantly expressed throughout the whole epithelium in early transplants (up to 2 weeks and comparable to early wound regeneration), were downregulated and in later transplants restricted to the expression in the basal layer(s). This was also seen in noninvasive (benign) and invasive (malignant) transplants. Moreover, also late differentiation markers such as involucrin component (the marker of cornified envelope) and filaggrin (the substrate of keratohyaline granules) were clearly identified using respective antibodies in differentiated areas of benign and malignant tissues, although filaggrin seemed to be more strongly expressed at a higher level (and broader tissue zone) in the benign transplants (Tomakidi et al., in preparation).

On the other hand, the expression of nonepidermal type keratins such as K4, K8, K13, K18, and K19 is usually seen in cultures of HaCaT cells and the derived benign and malignant clones and is differentially regulated by the mesenchymal environment in transplants. The simple epithelial keratins (K8, 18, and 19), being similarly expressed (at the RNA and protein levels) in 1-week-old transplants, are largely downregulated with time in the benign epithelia. This occurs, if at all, only to a minimal degree in malignant tissues, particularly visible with K18 and K19 (Lindberg and Rheinwald 1989). There was no particular localization of these aberrant cytoskeletal proteins at invasive tips of malignant transplants; they were usually distributed over large tumor areas. This focal expression at invasive parts, as described for human SCC (Markey et al. 1991), was sometimes but not always seen with vimentin, the cytoskeletal protein of mesenchymal cells (Tomakidi et al., in preparation).

Both benign and malignant transplants were clearly delineated towards the surrounding host mesenchyma by a continuous staining with antibodies against basement membrane components, such as collagen type IV and laminin. The reaction was of comparable intensity and thus a definite distinction between benign and malignant tissues could not be made on that basis. However, whether an uninterrupted and functionally normal basement membrane was formed cannot be substantiated at present.

In contrast, a differential regulation of integrins as major cell–cell and cell–matrix receptors was observed during the development of the transplants. Thus, integrin-$\alpha_6\beta_4$, usually localized at the basal pole of basal layer keratinocytes (Carter et al. 1990; Sonnenberg and Linders 1990; Sonnenberg et al. 1991), was initially expressed (at the RNA and protein level) throughout the whole epithelium. Within 2 weeks they became restricted to the basal zone in benign tissues with normalization of differentiation, but still spread over several epithelial layers in the malignant epithelium. This enlargement of the integrin expression zone was already observed in the thickened epithelium before invasion was obvious and similarly maintained in the invading tumor tissue. The significance of this finding – also as a potential diagnostic tool – is still not clear and needs further studies (Tennenbaum et al. 1992, 1993; Breitkreutz et al. 1993b).

Another receptor molecule which has been recently associated with invasion (E-cadherin; Mareel et al. 1993) was reduced in expression in HaCaT transplants, but still clearly positive in malignant clones, even in the invasive protrusions (Boukamp and Fusenig 1993). Thus, in this model system of highly differentiated cells, loss of E-cadherin is not a valid discriminator for invasive cells.

Conclusions

Although there is general consent that malignancy and differentiation are inversely correlated, clinical and experimental evidence clearly indicate that complete or substantial loss of the epithelial differentiation is not a prerequisite for malignant growth behavior. Major defects in differentiation are also not a prerequisite for premalignant stages, in particular for cellular immortalization, which is considered an essential and early step in the transformation process. Progressive dedifferentiation, on the other hand, often associated with advanced tumor stages, is also found in immortalized (i.e., by SV40 DNA), but not tumorigenic cell lines. Moreover, genetic manipulations causing epithelial dedifferentiation (e.g., *myoD* transfection in HaCaT cells) did not result in tumorigenic or malignant growth behavior (Boukamp et al. 1992; Boukamp and Fusenig 1993). Thus, substantial defects in differentiation, although usually linked to advanced malignancy, are obviously not obligatory or causal events in the carcinogenesis process. Nevertheless, the immortalized epithelial cell lines, i.e., the earliest stable transformation stages, even the highest differentiated ones (e.g., the HaCaT cell line) exhibit marked alterations in the differentiation program and its regulation. Whether these differentiation alterations are more a consequence of the severe genetic (chromosomal) aberrations common to all transformed cells (as a random process) or the result of selection processes for cells with reduced differentiation (and presumably faster proliferation) is still a matter of debate. A combination of both mechanisms seems probable in as far as cells with reduced terminal differentiation may adapt better to proliferation under adverse growth conditions. However, this remains to be demonstrated. This hypothesis would seem logic provided that the still rather hypothetical growth control which normal cells exert on tumor cells acts mostly (or only) in an indirect manner, namely by the induction of terminal differentiation. By enhancing this process – the theoretical basis of the concept of differentiation therapy – the proliferative compartment of a tumor tissue could be reduced, provided that the growth rate is not compensatorily stimulated to equal cell loss. In this respect the degree of differentiation achieved by therapeutic intervention would not be as important as the irreversible switch of proliferative cells into a (nonproliferative), terminally differentiating population. Thus, the delicate regulation of proliferation and differentiation is one of the basic questions to be addressed in order to evaluate the possibilities for differentiation therapy of tumors.

In epidermis or derived tumors one question has remained unanswered for a long time: are there differentiation stages identified by specific markers that obligatorily exclude or are incompatible with proliferation? In this regard the differentiation-specific keratins (K1 and K10) have been discussed as indicators (or even inducers) of postmitotic cells (Roop et al. 1988; van Neste et al. 1988). However, in our transplantation model the nontumorigenic HaCaT cells already express K1 in basal cells, and in epithelia formed by the tumorigenic clones proliferating cells can be observed in suprabasal areas positive for both keratins, at least in vitro. Furthermore, it is still not clear whether the usual compartmentalization of stratified epithelia is lost or seriously disturbed in tumors, at least in differentiating tumors, i.e., whether proliferation occurs in all cells in random distribution.

Our transplantation model is particularly well suited to help to answer these and related questions, since it allows at least for limited time periods the usual orientation and compartmentalization of a stratified epithelium with proliferative lower (mesenchyma-adjacent) and differentiating upper cell layers. This is even to some extent maintained in invasive tumor masses, allowing the discrimination of proliferative and differentiating compartments similar to the tissue of origin, the epidermis. Under these experimental conditions, interesting regulatory phenomena of growth and differentiation of keratinocytes in different transformation stages became apparent (Tomakidi et al., in preparation). From these and other studies it is evident that mesenchymal tissues (dermis, subcutis) exert growth control on cells in early stages of transformation, though in stage-related and model-dependent efficacy. Following subcutaneous injection, however, the cell lines immortalized in vitro are not only nontumorigenic but also growth restricted, irrespective of their differentiation potential. They form epithelial cysts in which cell proliferation stops completely and irreversibly within a few weeks.

As a consequence, these small and often regressing cysts no longer contain proliferating or even viable cells, but are composed of keratinized material, even when formed by those cell lines which did not exhibit much differentiation in vitro (Banks-Schlegel and Howley 1983; Boukamp et al. 1988). HaCaT cells of more advanced transformation stages formed cysts with continued proliferation in mesenchyma-adjacent areas, while keratinizing centripedally. These cells had obviously gained a certain degree of independence or insensitivity towards the growth constraint of the host mesenchyma. Since these cysts often regressed, but only after months, and their histomorphology was similar to keratoacanthomas, they represent experimental equivalents to benign epidermal tumor cells which partially and temporarily escaped the growth control of the mesenchymal environment.

From this we conclude that: (a) early tumor stages (immortal and benign cells) are still under the growth and differentiation control of the environment; (b) the sensitivity is lost or reduced in a stepwise manner with tumor progression; (c) the efficacy of control depends on tissue geometry, i.e., surface epithelia are less tightly controlled than epithelia surrounded by mesenchyma; (d) even malignant cells are initially (after transplantation) controlled in a similar way to benign cells but later more effectively escape this growth restraint; (e) this escape is not necessarily linked to a lower potential of epidermal differentiation, since invasive parts may show typical expression of many differentiation parameters.

Obviously proliferation, differentiation, and invasive growth are under different control mechanisms and not strictly interlinked. They must be regulated mostly by paracrine mechanisms, since the effects are observed in the absence of cell contact and thus are most probably mediated via diffusible factors. The identification of respective diffusible factors and the better understanding of their mode of action would greatly improve our situation in designing new therapeutic regimens. The major goal of this approach is to mimic and take advantage of the normal control mechanism of mesenchyma on growth and differentiation of ectopically positioned epithelium. Although it is not yet clear whether all tumor cells have maintained some responsiveness to regulators of growth and differentiation, the fact that differentiation can be enhanced in many model systems, strongly emphasizes the potential of such a therapeutic strategy to control cancer cells by more biological means.

References

Auersperg N, Krug PA, MacLaren JA, Watt FM, Myrdal SE (1989) Heterogeneous expression of keratin, involucrin, and extracellular matrix among subpopulations of a poorly differentiated human cervical carcinoma: possibly relationship to pattern of invasion. Cancer Res 49:3007–3014

Banks-Schlegel SP, Howley S (1983) Differentiation of human epidermal cells transformed by SV40. J Cell Biol 96:330–337

Bernard BA, Robinson SM, Semat A, Darmon M (1985) Reexpression of fetal characters in Simian virus 40-transformed human keratinocytes. Cancer Res 45: 1707–1716

Boukamp P, Fusenig NE (1993) "Trans-differentiation" from epidermal to mesenchymal/myogenic phenotype is associated with a drastic change in cell-cell and cell-matrix adhesion molecules. J Cell Biol 120:981–993

Boukamp P, Tilgen W, Dzarliewa-Petrusevska RT, Breitkreutz D, Haag D, Riehl RK, Bohnert A, Fusenig NE (1982) Phenotypic and genotypic characteristics of a cell line from squamous cell carcinoma of human skin. J Natl Cancer Inst 68:415–427

Boukamp P, Rupniak THR, Fusenig NE (1985) Environmental modulation of the expression of differentiation and malignancy in six human squamous cell carcinoma cell lines. Cancer Res 45:5582–5592

Boukamp P, Dzarliewa-Petrusevska RT, Breitkreutz D, Hornung J, Markham A, Fusenig NE (1988) Normal keratinization in a spontaneously immortalized aneuploid human keratinocyte cell line. J Cell Biol 106:761–771

Boukamp P, Breitkreutz D, Stark H-J, Fusenig NE (1990a) Mesenchyme-mediated and endogeneous regulation of growth and differentiation of human skin keratinoytes derived from different body sites. Differentiation 44:150–161

Boukamp P, Stanbridge EJ, Foo DY, Cerutti PA, Fusenig NE (1990b) C-Ha-ras oncogene expression in immortalized human keratinocytes (HaCaT) alters growth potential in vivo but lacks correlation with malignancy. Cancer Res 50:2840–2847

Boukamp P, Chen J, Gonzales F, Jones PA, Fusenig NE (1992) Progressive stages of "transdifferentiation" from epidermal to mesenchymal phenotype induced by MyoD1 transfection, 5-aza-2′-deoxycytidine treatment, and selection for reduced cell attachment in the human keratinocyte line HaCaT. J Cell Biol 116:1257–1271

Boukamp P, Breitkreutz D, Hülsen A, Altmeyer S, Tomakidi P, Fusenig NE (1993) In vitro transformation and tumor progression. In: Marks F, Hecker E, Jung EG, Tilgen W (eds) Skin carcinogenesis in man and in experimental models. Springer, Berlin Heidelberg New York (Recent results in cancer research, vol 128)

Bowden PE, Stark H-J, Breitkreutz D, Fusenig NE (1987) Expression and modification of keratins during terminal differentiation of mammalian epidermis. Curr Top Dev Biol 22:35–68

Breitkreutz D, Tilgen W, Boukamp P, Fusenig NE (1981) Correlation of prekeratin peptides and ultrastructure in epithelial cells of human skin tumours in vivo and in vitro. Anticancer Res 1:323–328

Breitkreutz D, Hornung J, Poehlmann J, Brown-Bierman L, Bohnert A, Bowden PE, Fusenig NE (1986) Environmental induction of differentiation-specific keratins in malignant mouse keratinocyte lines. Eur J Cell Biol 42:255–267

Breitkreutz D, Boukamp P, Stark H-J, Ryle C, Fusenig NE (1989) Response of established keratinocyte lines to modulators of epidermal differentiation. In: Reichert U, Shroot B (eds) Pharmacology and the skin, vol 3. Karger, Basel, pp 8–14

Breitkreutz D, Boukamp P, Ryle CM, Stark H-J, Roop DR, Fusenig NE (1991a) Epidermal morphogenesis and keratin expression in c-Ha-ras-transfected tumorigenic clones of the human HaCaT cell line. Cancer Res 51:4402–4409

Breitkreutz D, Boukamp P, Hülsen A, Ryle C, Stark H-J, Smola H, Thiekötter G, Fusenig NE (1991b) Human keratinocyte cell lines. In: Wilson G, Davis SS, Illum L (eds) Pharmaceutical applications of cell and tissue culture. Plenum, London, pp 283–296

Breitkreutz D, Stark H-J, Plein P, Baur M, Fusenig NE (1993a) Differential modulation of epidermal keratinization in immortalized (HaCaT) and tumorigenic human skin keratinocytes (HaCaT-ras) by retinoic acid and extracellular Ca^{2+}. Differentiation 54:201–217

Breitkreutz D, Stark H-J, Baur M, Thiekötter G, Smola H, Fusenig NE (1993b) Differenzielle Veränderungen epidermaler Integrinmuster in Modell-Epithelien transformierter benigner und maligner Keratinozyten (HaCaT-ras). In: Mahrle G, Krieg T (eds) Wundheilung und Wundverschluß. Springer, Berlin Heidelberg New York

Broders AC (1932) Practical points on the microscopic grading of carcinoma. NY State J Med 32:667–671

Carter WG, Kaur P, Gil SG, Gahr PG, Wayner EA (1990) Distinct functions for integrins $\alpha 3\beta 1$ in focal adhesions and $\alpha 6\beta 4$/bullous pemphigoid antigen in new stable anchoring contact (SAC) of keratinocytes: relation to hemidesmosomes. J Cell Biol 111:3141-3154

Chang SE (1986) In vitro transformation of human epithelial cells. Biochim Biophys Acta 823:161–194

Coulomb B, Lebreton C, Dubertret L (1989) Influence of human dermal fibroblasts on epidermalization. Invest Dermatol 92:122–125

Dürst M, Dzarliewa-Petrusevska RT, Boukamp P, Fusenig NE, Gissmann L (1987) Molecular and cytogenetic analysis of immortalized human primary keratinocytes obtained after transfection with human papillomavirus type 16 DNA. Oncogene 1:251–256

Easty DM, Easty GC, Baici A, Carter RL, Cederholm-Williams SA, Felix H, Gusterson B, Haemmerli G, Häuser-Urfer J, Heizmann CW, Marcel M, Stehrenberger B, Sträuli P (1986) Biological studies of ten human squamous carcinoma cell lines: an overview. Eur J Cancer 22:617–634

Eccles SA (1983) Differentiation and neoplasia. Invasion and metastasis; experimental systems. J Pathol 141:333–353

Fuchs E (1990) Epidermal differentiation: the bare essentials. J Cell Biol 111: 2807–2814

Fusenig NE (1994) Epithelial-mesenchymal interactions regulate keratinocyte growth and differentiation in vitro. In: Leigh I, Watt F, Lane B (eds) Keratinocyte handbook. Cambridge University Press, Cambridge (in press)

Fusenig NE, Breitkreutz D, Dzarlieva RT, Boukamp P, Bohnert A, Tilgen W (1983) Growth and differentiation characteristics of transformed keratinocytes from mouse and human skin in vitro and in vivo. J Invest Dermatol 81:168–175

Fusenig NE, Boukamp P, Breitkreutz D, Karjetta S, Petrusevska RT (1987) Oncogenes and malignant transformation of human keratinocytes. In: Cerutti PA,

Nyaard OF, Simic MG (eds) Anticarcinogenesis and radiation protection. Plenum, New York, pp 227–231
Fusenig NE, Boukamp P, Breitkreutz D, Hülsen A, Karjetta S, Stanbridge E (1989) Transformation of human skin epithelial cells in vitro: concepts of stages of transformation. Paper presented at workshop on cell transformation systems relevant to radiation-induced cancer in man, Dublin, Chap. 3
Fusenig NE, Breitkreutz D, Bohnert A et al. (1991a) Epithelial-mesenchymal interactions in tissue homeostasis and malignant transformation. In: Johnson NW (ed) Oral cancer. Cambridge University Press, Cambridge, pp 218–248
Fusenig NE, Breitkreutz D, Boukamp P (1991b) Differentiation potential of cancer cells. In: Masters JRW (ed) Human cancer in primary culture, a handbook. Kluwer Academic, New York, pp 55–80
Gabbert H, Wagner R, Moll R, Gerharz C-D (1985) Tumor dedifferentiation: an important step in tumor invasion. Clin Exp Metastasis 3:257–279
Harris CC (1987) Human tissues and cells in carcinogenesis research. Cancer Res 47:1–10
Heim S, Mandahl N, Mitelmann F (1988) Genetic convergence in tumour progression. Cancer Res 48:5911–5916
Hornung J, Bohnert A, Phan-Than L, Krieg T, Fusenig NE (1987) Basement membrane formation by malignant mouse keratinocyte cell lines in organotypic culture and transplants: correlation with degree of morphologic differentiation. J Cancer Res Clin Oncol 113:325–341
Kartasova T, Roop DR, Yuspa SH (1992) Relationship between the expression of differentiation-specific keratins 1 and 10 and cell proliferation in epidermal tumors. Mol Carcinog 6:18–25
Knight J, Gusterson BA, Cowley G, Monaghan P (1984) Differentiation of normal and malignant human squamous epithelium in vivo and in vitro: a morphologic study. Ultrastruct Pathol 7:133–141
Levitt ML, Gazdar AF, Oie HK, Schüller H, Thacher SM (1990) Cross-linked envelope-related markers for squamous differentiation in human lung cancer cell lines. Cancer Res 50:120–128
Lindberg K, Rheinwald JG (1989) Suprabasal 40 kd keratin (K19) expression as an immunohistologic marker of premalignancy in oral epithelium. Am J Pathol 134:98–98
Mackenzie I, Rittman G, Bohnert A, Breitkreutz D, Fusenig NE (1993) Influence of connective tissues on the in vitro growth and differentiation of murine epidermis. Epith Cell Biol 2:107–119
Mareel M, Bracke M, Van Roy F, Vakaet L (1993) Expression of E-cadherin in embryogenic ingression and cancer invasion. Int J Dev Biol 37:227–235
Markey AC, Lane BE, Churchill LJ, MacDonald DM, Leigh LM (1991) Expression of simple epithelial keratins 8 and 18 in epidermal neoplasia. J Invest Dermatol 97:763–770
McCance DJ, Kopan R, Fuchs E, Laimins LA (1988) Human papillomavirus type 16 alters human epithelial cell differentiation in vitro. Proc Natl Acad Sci USA 85:7169–7173
Moll R, Franke WW, Schiller DL, Geiger B, Krepler R (1982) The catalog of human cytokeratins: patterns of expression in normal epithelia, tumors and cultured cells. Cell 31:11–34
Moll R, Moll I, Franke WW (1984) Differences of expression of cytokeratin polypeptides in various epithelial skin tumours. Arch Dermatol Res 276:349–363
Moll R, Achtstätter T, Becht E, Balcarova-Ständer J, Ittensohn M, Franke WW (1988) Cytokeratins in normal and malignant transitional epithelium: maintenance of expression of urothelial differentiation features in transitional cell carcinomas and bladder carcinoma cell lines. Am J Pathol 132:123–144

Morgan PR, Shirlaw PJ, Johnson NW, Leigh IM, Lane EB (1987) Potential application of anti-keratin antibodies on oral diagnosis. J Oral Pathol 16:212–222
Nischt R, Roop DR, Mehrel T, Yuspa SH, Rentrop M, Winter H, Schweizer J (1988) Aberrant expression during two-stage mouse skin carcinogenesis of a type I 47-kDA keratin, K13, normally associated with terminal differentiation of internal stratified epithelia. Mol Carcinog 1:96–108
Osborn M, Weber K (1983) Tumor diagnosis by intermediate filament typing: a novel tool for surgical pathology. Lab Invest 48:372–394
Parkinson EK (1985) Defective responses of transformed keratinocytes to terminal differentiation stimuli. Their role in epidermal tumour promotion by phorbolesters and deep skin wounding. Br J Cancer 52:479–493
Rheinwald JG, Beckett M (1980) Defective terminal differentiation in culture as a consistent and selectable character of malignant human keratinocytes. Cell 22: 629–632
Rice RH, Green H (1979) Presence in human epidermal cells of a soluble protein precursor of the cross-linked envelope: activation of the cross-linking by calcium ions. Cell 18:681–694
Roop DR, Krieg TM, Mehrel T, Cheng CK, Yuspa SH (1988) Transcriptional control of high molecular weight keratin gene expression in multistage mouse skin carcinogenesis. Cancer Res 48:3245–3252
Ryle CM, Breitkreutz D, Stark H-J, Leigh IM, Steinert PM, Roop D, Fusenig NE (1989) Density-dependent modulation of synthesis of keratins 1 and 10 in the human keratinocyte line HaCaT and in ras-transfected tumorigenic clones. Differentiation 40:42–54
Schwartz RA (1988) Skin cancer: recognition and management. Springer, Berlin Heidelberg New York
Smola H, Thiekötter G, Fusenig NE (1993) Mutual induction of growth factor gene expression by epidermal-dermal cell interaction. J Cell Biol 122:417–429
Sonnenberg A, Linders CJT (1990) The $\alpha 6 \beta 1$ (VLA-6) and $\alpha 6 \beta 4$ protein complexes: tissue distribution and biochemical properties. J Cell Sci 96:207–217
Sonnenberg A, Calafat J, Janssen H, Daams H, Van der Raaij-Helmer LMH, Falcioni R, Kennel SJ, Aplin JD, Baker J, Loizidou M, Garrod D (1991) Integrin $\alpha 6 \beta 4$ complex is located in hemidesmosomes, suggesting a major role in epidermal cell-basement membrane adhesion. J Cell Biol 113:907–917
Steinert PM, Roop DR (1988) Molecular and cellular biology of intermediate filaments. Annu Rev Biochem 57:593–625
Stoler AB, Stenbäck F, Balmain A (1993) The conversion of mouse skin squamous cell carcinomas to spindle cell carcinomas is a recessive event. J Cell Biol 122: 1103–1117
Tennenbaum T, Yuspa SH, Grover A, Castronovo V, Sobel ME, Yamada Y, De Luca LM (1992) Extracellular matrix receptors and mouse skin carcinogenesis: altered expression linked to appearance of early markers of tumor progression. Cancer Res 52:2966–2976
Tennenbaum T, Weiner AK, Belanger AJ, Glick AB, Hennings H, Yuspa SH (1993) The suprabasal expression of $\alpha 6 \beta 4$ integrin is associated with a high risk for malignant progression in mouse skin carcinogenesis. Cancer Res 53:4803–4810
Tilgen W, Boukamp P, Breitkreutz D, Dzarliewa RT, Engstner M, Haag D, Fusenig NE (1983) Preservation of morphological, functional and karyotypic traits during long-term culture and in vivo passage of two human skin squamous cell carcinomas. Cancer Res 43:5995–6001
Van Neste DJJ, Staquet M-J, Leroy BP, DeCoster WJ (1988) Distribution pattern of psoriatic keratoblasts: computer-assisted image-analysis for combined evaluation of DNA synthesis and expression of 67 kD keratin polypeptides in the epidermis of stable plaques of psoriasis. J Invest Dermatol 90:382–386

Wille JJ, Maercklein PB, Scott RE (1982) Neoplastic transformation and defective control of cell proliferation and differentiation. Cancer Res 42:4620–4628

Woodworth CD, Bowden PE, Doninger J, Pirisi L, Barnes W, Lancaster WD, DiPaolo JA (1988) Characterization of normal human exocervical epithelial cells immortalized in vitro by papillomavirus types 16 and 18 DNA. Cancer Res 48:4620–4628

Wu YJ, Rheinwald JG (1981) A new small (40 kd) keratin filament protein made by some human squamous cell carcinomas. Cell 25:627

Yuspa SH, Kilkenny AE, Stanley J, Lichti U (1985) Keratinocytes blocked in phorbol ester-responsive early stage of terminal differentiation by sarcoma viruses. Nature 314:459–462

Action Spectrum for Photocarcinogenesis

F.R. de Gruijl

Dermatology/AZU, University of Utrecht, Netherlands

Abstract

The wavelength dependence of the carcinogenicity of ultraviolet (UV) radiation needs to be known in order to assess the carcinogenic risks of various UV sources, most notably the different solar UV spectra at ground level under depleting stratospheric ozone. This wavelength dependence cannot be extracted from human data (e.g., from epidemiology); it can, however, be directly obtained from animal experiments. Precise information on the wavelength dependence, the so-called action spectrum, was not available until recently: erythemal or mutagenic action spectra have been used as substitutes. However, experimental data on skin tumors induced in hairless mice (Skh:HR1) with various polychromatic sources have been building up. Our group has found that none of the substitute action spectra yield a statistically acceptable description of our data, and we have, therefore, derived a new action spectrum, dubbed the SCUP action spectrum (SCUP stands for Skin Cancer Utrecht-Philadelphia, because the action spectrum also fits experimental data from the former Skin and Cancer Hospital in Philadelphia). The SCUP action spectrum has a maximum at 293 nm, and in the UVA region above 340 nm the relative carcinogenicity per J/m^2 drops to about 10^{-4} of this maximum.

The effects of an ozone depletion on solar UV doses weighted with these different action spectra are compared: the erythemal and SCUP weighted dose come out as least sensitive with a 1.3% and 1.4% increase, respectively, for every 1% decrease in ozone.

Introduction

As early as the late nineteenth century, physicians reported on the increase in skin carcinoma in people working outdoors, and it was suggested that

Recent Results in Cancer Research, Vol. 139

sunlight might be the cause. It is clearly virtually impossible to prove this causal relationship directly for humans. Epidemiological data show an association between sunlight and skin cancer, but cannot prove a causal relationship. In fact, it is impossible to establish from epidemiological data alone which part of the solar spectrum is carcinogenic. One needs a priori knowledge to interpret the data in terms of ultraviolet (UV) radiation as causing skin cancer. This knowledge is most directly and completely obtained in animal experiments. There the process of UV carcinogenesis can be studied in depth.

Roffo (1939) reported that UV radiation, either from the sun or a mercury arc, caused skin cancer in rats and mice and that the carcinogenicity was lost when the radiation was filtered through window glass. From this observation it was concluded that short-wave UVB radiation (wavelengths <315 nm) is carcinogenic, because this radiation is mainly absorbed by window glass. The remaining UVA radiation appeared incapable of inducing skin cancers. This has been the state of knowledge on the wavelength dependency of UV carcinogenesis for decades.

How the carcinogenicity of UV radiation changes with wavelength became a topical question with the threat of increasing levels of solar UV radiation by a depletion of stratospheric ozone. The wavelength dependency is represented in a so-called action spectrum, and the one for sunburn (erythema) was used as a substitute for UV carcinogenesis, without much valid theoretical justification, according to Setlow (1974), who proposed to use an action spectrum based on DNA damage. In the experiments the animals have to be irradiated chronically in order to induce the skin cancers and to establish the wavelength depedence one would want to use monochromatic radiation of specific wavelengths. This is, however, unfeasible in actual practice, and hence polychromatic sources of different spectral compositions have been used to ascertain the carcinogenicity in different wavebands in UV radiation. The first animals experiments addressing this problem (Forbes et al. 1982) concentrated, of course, on UVB radiation (290–315 nm), the most effective wavelength region in the solar spectrum at the earth's surface. These data contained virtually no information outside the UVB range toward longer wavelengths in the UVA range (315–380 nm). The data proved to be insufficient to determine a proper action spectrum. Cole et al. (1986) found that the action spectrum for edema (MEE48) performed best on their data of UV tumorigenesis in albino hairless Skh:HR1 mice, but their data contained very little information on the carcinogenicity of UVA radiation.

Our group has been involved in a long-term program to determine the action spectrum for UV carcinogenesis in the Skh:HR1 mice. Sterenborg and Van der Leun (1987a) produced an action spectrum based on seven spectrally different UV sources, including a UVC source (254 nm) and a near-UVA source (main output > 340 nm). Slaper (1987) included one more UVA source, and modified the action spectrum. In addition, Kelfkens et al.

(1991a) completed an experiment with a custom-made fluorescent lamp (courtesy of Philips); the spectral output of this lamp is centered around 330 nm and fills a gap in the short-wave UVA range. These combined data provide an excellent testing set for any candidate action spectrum for UV carcinogenesis. Here will discuss the unsatisfactory performance of priorly available action spectra and the adequacy of the newly derived one.

Materials and Methods

When a group of albino hairless Skh:HR1 mice (which are immunocompetent) are daily exposed to UVB radiation, all of the mice will eventually develop skin tumors. The rate at which the tumors occur depends on the daily dose: a daily dose of 1.5 kJ/m^2 UV from a Westinghouse FS40 sunlamp will produce tumors of at least 1 mm in diameter in 50% of the animals in about 75 days; with 0.75 kJ/m^2 per day it takes about 100 days. A lower daily dose delays the tumor incidence by a certain factor. Thus, various UVB sources can be compared in their carcinogenicity. More specifically, one can express the carcinogenicity of a daily exposure from a certain UVB lamp in terms of an equivalent daily exposure from an FS40 sunlamp. The data obtained with the FS40 sunlamp (De Gruijl et al. 1983) form a frame of reference. These FS40 data provide a relationship between the daily UV dose, D, and the time until 50% of the mice have 1-mm tumors (t_{50}). D varied by a factor of 33, and t_{50} ranged from 74 to 503 days. Now we can compare the carcinogenic effects of various lamps by their t_{50}s and express the t_{50}s in equivalent daily FS40 doses. If we normalize such an equivalent daily dose, E, to 1.0 for t_{50} = 300 days (i.e., 115.4 J/m^2 per day <400 nm, from a FS40) we find

$$E = (283/(t_{50} - 17))^{1.61} \tag{1}$$

Thus, we have defined a dimensionless equivalent daily dose, which we can calculate from the t_{50} of a certain chronic exposre regimen.

In contrast to UVB radiation, UVA radiation induces an early predominance of benign papillomas, which results in a slower build-up of tumors. Hence, UVA and UVB tumor responses are not directly comparable, but when we reject the obvious papillomas from the UVA data we again see tumor incidences that parallel those under UVB sources (Kelfkens et al. 1991a). The induction kinetics of carcinomas under either UVB or UVA radiations appear, therefore, to be identical.

We have used the data acquired with eight different UVA UVB sources, which are summarized in Table 1 with their wavelength ranges and wavelengths of maximum output. The mice were dorsally exposed daily in all of the experiments. For each of the lamps the average daily UV doses (in J/m^2) on the backs of the mice are given in Table 1. The equivalent daily doses

Table 1. Summary of lamps used as UV sources: spectral range set at 1% cutoff

Lamp	Spectral range (nm)	Peak(s) (nm)	Daily dose (J/m^2)	Equivalent dose (*E*)	Relative error (*e*)
TLX	270–305	280	72	0.93	0.10
TL12	275–375	313	555	5.61	0.10
FS40	275–390	313	269	2.33	0.04
TL01	305–367	312	1 040	2.47	0.09
TL01*	306–368	312	1 375	1.68	0.16
EFL330	317–>400	345/365	70 000	0.45	0.06
TL09*	328–>400	358/365	238 000	0.81	0.08
HPA*	332–>400	365/373/385	220 000	0.83	0.10

corresponding to the average physical daily doses of the lamps are also given in Table 1.

The TLX, EFL330, and TL01* lamps are not commercially available and were custom made by Philips. All the lamps are fluorescent tubes, with the exception of the HPA, a high pressure lamp. The TLO9 and EFL330 lamps were filtered with ordinary window glass. The TL01* lamp had a glass envelope which differed from that of the commercially available TL01. The TLX and the HPA lamps were filtered with liquid filters in quartz (TLX) or glass (HPA) containers.

The daily exposure times were shorter than 2 h, except for the EFL330 and TL09* lamps, which took 12 h daily to deliver the required doses. According to Kelfkens et al. (1991b), the 12-h daily dose is equivalent to a 25% higher 1.25-h daily dose, i.e., spreading the same dose over a longer daily exposure period increases the tumorigenicity. We have corrected the EFL330* and TL09* daily doses for this effect.

To see whether an action spectrum properly describes our data set, we matched the spectrally weighted effective daily dose, *W*, to the equivalent carcinogenic daily dose, *E*. To this end, *W* had to be multiplied with a matching factor, *f*, which minimizes

$$\chi^2 = \Sigma_i \frac{(\ln(<E_i>/E_i))^2}{e_i^2} \qquad (2)$$

where i = 1 . . . 8 for the different lamps, E_i the measured value of *E* for lamp i, and e_i is the relative error in E_i, $<E_i> = f.\ W_i$ is the expected value of E_i according to the action spectrum. An optimum *f* value was computed for each tested action spectrum.

As an action spectrum is usually dimensionless, *W* has the dimension of a daily dose (J/m^2 per day). This means that *f* has the inverse dimension. If the action spectrum is normalized to 1.0 in its maximum at wavelength λ_m, then $1/f$ is the estimated daily dose of λ_m radiation for t_{50} = 300 days.

Multiplying the action spectrum with f yields spectral weights which directly estimate E.

The action spectra included in this study are:

1. The erythemal (24 h) action spectrum published by Parrish et al. (1982)
2. Its synthetic version by McKinlay and Diffey (1987)
3. The edemal action spectrum for mice, MEE48 (Cole et al. 1986), extended at the 10^{-4} level above 330 nm
4. The action spectrum for tumorigenesis in mice, SteSla, derived by Sterenborg and modified by Slaper (1987)
5. The most recent update of the action spectrum for tumorigenesis in hairless mice, SCUP (De Gruijl et al. 1993)
6. An action spectrum for mutagenesis (Peak et at. 1984) corrected for transmission through mouse epidermis (Sterenborg and Van der Leun 1987b)

Results

The overall performances of the action spectra are summarized by χ^2 in Table 2. The $1/f$ daily doses (for t_{50} = 300 days) are also given with the wavelengths, λ_m, to which they apply.

Mutagenic action spectra corrected for epidermal transmission have served as synthetic carcinogenic action spectra. We could not obtain a

Table 2. Results of matching the action spectra to the Utrecht data set

Action spectrum	χ^2 (*df*)	$1/f$ dose (J/m^2 per day)	λ_{max} (nm)
Mutagenic +transmission	328 (7)	18.1	295
McKinlay-Diffey	843 (7)	53.3	<298
Parrish et al. (24 h)	804 (7)	50.6	296
Sterenborg-Slaper	200 (7[a])	29.5	302
MEE48 (extended)	53.2 (7)	23.7	297
SCUP	3.4 (3)	23.8	293

SCUP, Skin Cancer Utrecht-Philadelphia.
[a] The seven degrees of freedom is not really correct: this action spectrum was derived earlier from a part of the present data set.

satisfactory fit with such an action spectrum ($\chi^2 = 328$ with $df = 7$). From Table 2 it becomes evident that the erythema action spectra also perform poorly. The most recently added data, that of the EFL330 were not included in the Sterenborg-Slaper action spectrum, which tends to overestimate the effectiveness of the EFL330 lamp. The EFL330 data contribute 70 to a total of 200 for the χ^2 of the Sterenborg-Slaper action spectrum. Of the available action spectra, the extended version of the MEE48 performs best. However, the χ^2 values are too large for a good fit to the data.

We have recently published in detail how a new action spectrum can be derived from data gathered with polychromatic sources (De Gruijl et al. 1993); the resulting SCUP action spectrum was based on the present data set and the experimental data from the former Skin and Cancer Hospital in Philadelphia. The actual fit of this new action spectrum is satisfactory, as can be seen in Table 2; $\chi^2 = 3.4$ with $df = 3$. The degrees of freedom have been lowered because this action spectrum required five parameters to be determined from the experimental data. The success of this fit can be ascertained by comparing Fig. 1a and b: in Fig. 1a we see t_{50} versus the unweighted daily UV dose for various experiments, and in Fig. 1b these same data are shown with the SCUP-weighted daily UV dose. In Fig. 1a, the points are scattered in accordance with the effectiveness of the UV source used, and in Fig. 1b all the points are focused on a common dose–time relationship.

A comparison of this SCUP action spectrum with the human erythemal action spectrum is shown in Fig. 2. The presently tested action spectral all bear a crude resemblance to one another, and most of them have been used in some form or other to assess carcinogenic UV doses. The appropriate

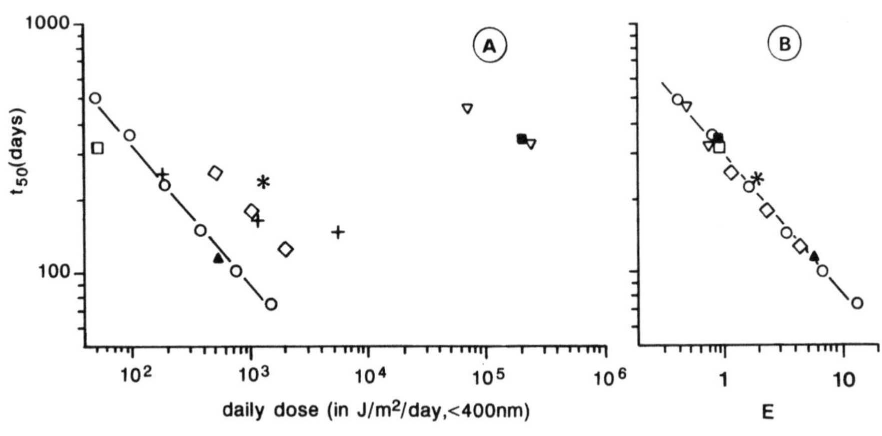

Fig. 1.A,B. The median tumor induction times (t_{50}) versus daily ultraviolet (UV) dose for various lamps. **A** Unweighted UV doses. **B** Skin Cancer Utrecht-Philadelphia (SCUP)-weighted UV doses (multiplied by f to estimate the equivalent dose E, see Table 2). □, TLX; ○, FS40; ▲, TL12; ◇, TL01; *, TL01*; ▼, EFL330; ▽, TL09*; ■, HPA*

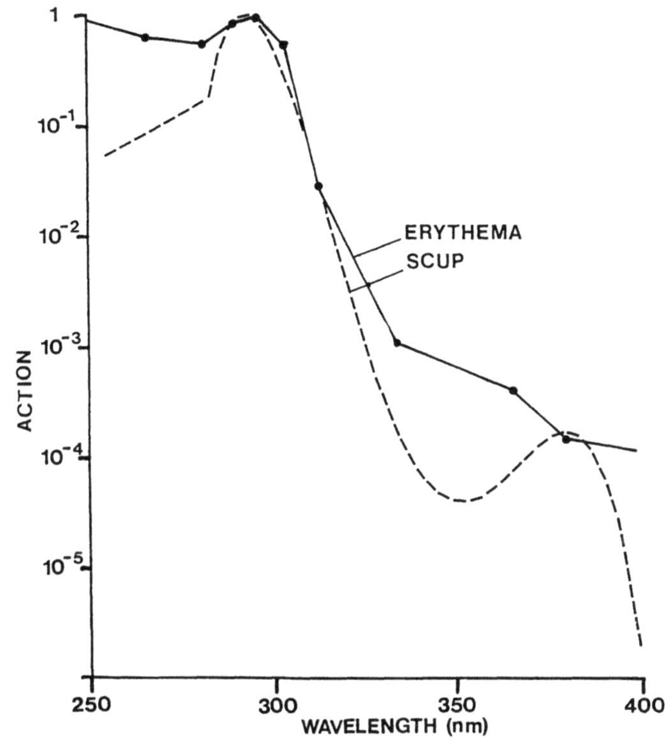

Fig. 2. Comparison of the erythemal action spectrum (*solid line*) and the Skin Cancer Utrecht-Philadelphia (SCUP) action spectrum (*dashed line*)

carcinogenic dose is especially important in assessments of increases in skin cancer as a consequence of a stratospheric ozone depletion. The so-called radiation amplification factor, RAF, is a number which concisely represents how strong the (annual ambient) UV dose reacts to a change in ozone: for a 1% decrease in ozone, the carcinogenic UV dose will increase by the RAF. Table 3 gives the RAF for the present action spectra.

Discussion

A fundamental premise in the present approach is that exposures of different wavelengths can be weighted and added up to a total effective dose. This is the so-called concept of photoaddivity. There is no a priori certainty that a UVA exposure would add to a UVB exposure. However, our group has recently found that this is indeed the case for UV carcinogenesis in the hairless mouse (Berg et al. 1993). Moreover, the simple fact that one can derive an operationally valid action spectrum from this first principle of photoadditivity indicates the validity of the premise.

Table 3. Radiation amplification factors (RAF)

UV dose weighted by:	RAF	
	30° N. Lat.	0°–65° N. Lat.
Mutations through epidermis[a]	1.56	1.54–1.60
Sterenborg-Slaper[a]	1.59	1.58–1.59
MEE48[a]	1.54	1.50–1.56
SCUP	1.40	1.39–1.41
Erythema (Parrish et al. 1982[a])	1.31	1.25–1.33
Erythema (McKinlay and Diffey 1987[a]; Kelfkens et al. 1990)[a]	1.15	1.08–1.18

SCUP, Skin Cancer Utrecht-Philadelphia; N. Lat., northern latitude.
[a] From Kelfkens et al. 1990.

Because of the widely varying effectiveness of UV sources, the experimental data span a large range of daily doses (in J/m^2) and tumor induction times (see Fig. 1a). A good action spectrum should introduce an optimum coherency between spectrally weighted doses and induction times (Fig. 1b). This provides a good basis to ascertain the suitability of an action spectrum. The χ^2 obtained from the match of an action spectrum to the data is a measure for the coherency introduced into the data, i.e., the smaller the χ^2, the larger the coherency. Moreover, the χ^2 allowed us to make a statistical assessment of the coherency. The mutagenic action spectra corrected for epidermal thickness appeared to be inadequate, as were the erythemal action spectra. The earlier action spectra for skin cancer in hairless mice, the extended MEE48 action spectrum and the Sterenborg-Slaper action spectrum, did not perform well enough either. The recently derived SCUP action spectrum (De Gruijl et al. 1993) was presented with $\chi^2 = 3.4$ with $df = 3$. As the SCUP action spectrum has been (partially) derived from the present data, the match to the data should, of course, be quite good, albeit at the expense of losing a few degrees of freedom. It should be stressed here that the SCUP action spectrum has large margins of uncertainty in the UVA region (>340 nm), and it is not well defined below 280 nm.

The RAF for the different action spectra are presented in relation to ozone decreases and UV increases (Table 3). The value of 1.4 for the SCUP-weighted UV doses comes close to the erythema-weighted one of 1.3. It could be argued that the murine SCUP action spectrum needs to be corrected for humans because of the thicker human epidermis. Such corrections can be made (de Gruijl and van der Leun, 1994), and they lower the RAF somewhat, bringing it in the range of RAF for erythema (this correction in SCUP results in a relative increase in the carcinogenicity of UVA versus UVB). As erythemal doses have frequently been substituted for carcinogenic doses in risk assessments for ozone depletion, it is not to be expected that using a SCUP-weighted dose will change these assessments to any appreciable extent (De Gruijl and van der Leun 1993).

Acknowledgements. The author wishes to thank the Dutch Cancer Foundation and the Dutch Ministery of Housing, Physical Planning, and Environment for their financial support to our research program. The Dutch Academy of Sciences awarded a fellowship to the author. The cooperation with Philips has been, and still is, vital to our program. The work of other present and former members of our group is gratefully acknowledged.

References

Berg RJW, de Gruijl FR, van der Leun JC (1993) Interaction between ultraviolet A and ultraviolet B radiations in skin cancer induction in hairless mice. Cancer Res 53:4212–4217
Cole CA, Forbes PD, Davies RE (1986) An action spectrum for photocarcinogenesis. Photochem Photobiol 43:275–284
de Gruijl FR, van der Leun JC (1993) Influence of ozone depletion on the incidence of skin cancer, quantitative prediction. In: Young AR, Björn LO, Moan J, Nultsch W (eds) Environmental UV photobiology. Plenum, New York, pp 89–112
de Gruijl FR, van der Meer JB, van der Leun JC (1983) Dose-time dependency of tumor formation by chronic UV exposure. Photochem Photobiol 37:53–62
de Gruijl FR, Sterenborg HJCM, Forbes PD, Davies RE, Cole C, Kelfkens G, Van Weelden H, Slaper H, van der Leun JC (1993) Wavelength dependence of skin cancer induction by ultraviolet irradiation of albino hairless mice. Cancer Res 53:53–60
de Gruijl FR, van der Leun JC (1994) Estimate of the wavelength dependency of ultraviolet carcinogenesis in humans and its relevance to the risk assessment of a stratospheric ozone depletion. Health Phys 67:317–323
Forbes PD, Davies RE, Urbach F, Berger DS, Cole CA (1982) Simulated stratospheric ozone depletion and increased ultraviolet radiation: effects on photocarcinogenesis in hairless mice. Cancer Res 42:2796–2803
Kelfkens G, De Gruijl FR, van der Leun JC (1990) Ozone depletion and increase in annual carcinogenic ultraviolet dose. Photochem Photobiol 52:819–823
Kelfkens G, de Gruijl FR, van der Leun JC (1991a) Tumourigenesis by short-wave ultraviolet-A: papillomas versus squamous cell carcinomas. Carcinogenesis 12:1377–1382
Kelfkens G, van Weelden H, de Gruijl FR, van der Leun JC (1991b) The influence of dose rate on ultaviolet tumorigenesis. J Photochem Photobiol B 10:41–50
McKinlay AF, Diffey BL (1987) A reference action spectrum for ultraviolet induced erythema in human skin. In: Passchier WF, Bosnjakovic BFM (eds) Human exposure to ultraviolet radiation: risks and regulations. Elsevier Science, Amsterdam, pp 83–87
Parrish JA, Jaenicke KF, Anderson RR (1982) Erythema and melanogenesis action spectra of normal human skin. Photochem Photobiol 36:187–191
Peak MJ, Peak JG, Moehring MP, Webb RB (1984) Ultraviolet action spectra for DNA dimer induction, lethality and mutagenesis in E. coli with emphasis on the UVB region. Photochem Photobiol 40:613–620
Roffo AH (1939) Über die physikalische Aetiologie der Krebskrankheit. Strahlentherapie 78:328–350

Setlow RB (1974) The wavelengths in sunlight effective in producing cancer: a theoretical analysis. Proc Natl Acad Sci USA 71:3363–3366
Slaper H (1987) Skin cancer and UV exposure: investigations on the estimation of risks. PhD thesis, University of Utrecht
Sterenborg HJCM, van der Leun JC (1987a) Action spectra for tumorigenesis by ultraviolet radiation. In: Passchier WF, Bosnjakovic BFM (eds) Human exposure to ultraviolet radiation: risks and regulations. Elsevier Science, Amsterdam, pp 173–190
Sterenborg HJCM, van der Leun JC (1987b) Change in epidermal transmission due to UV-induced hyperplasia in hairless mice: a first approximation of the action spectrum. Photodermatology 5:71–82

Processing of Directly and Indirectly Ultraviolet-Induced DNA Damage in Human Cells

T.M. Rünger[1], B. Epe[2], and K. Möller[1]

[1] Department of Dermatology, University of Würzburg, Josef-Schneider Strasse 2, 97080 Würzburg, Germany
[2] Department of Toxicology, University of Würzburg, Versbacher Strasse 9, 97080 Würzburg, Germany

Abstract

Mutations caused by ultraviolet (UV)-induced DNA damage represent the initial genetic changes in the tumorigenesis of UV-induced skin cancer. Different wavelengths of UV radiation cause different kinds of DNA damage and mutations. UVB (290–320 nm) generates pyrimidine dimers by direct excitation of the DNA molecule. UVA (320–400 nm) can damage the DNA only indirectly through a photosensitized reaction. This indirect action is mediated mainly by singlet oxygen, which generates purine base modifications, and has been implicated in the carcinogenic effects of UVA. In order to study the processing of directly and indirectly UV-induced DNA damage in human cells, we first treated the replicating plasmid pRSVcat with up to 10 kJ/m^2 UVB or with the photosensitizer methylene blue plus visible light (which generates singlet oxygen) in vitro. Then, the damaged plasmid was transfected into normal or repair deficient xeroderma pigmentosum complementation group A (XP-A) cells. DNA repair was assessed by measuring activity of reactivated chloramphenicol acetyltransferase (CAT) enzyme, encoded by the plasmid's cat gene, in cell extracts after 3 days. While XP-A cells exhibited a significantly reduced repair of UVB-induced DNA damage, they showed a normal repair of singlet oxygen-induced DNA damage. This indicates a differential DNA repair pathway for directly and indirectly UV-induced DNA damage in human cells. Irradiation of the plasmid with UVA alone did not result in a genotoxic effect. Only in conjunction with a cell extract, which provides all candidate cellular photosensitizers, did we find a reduced CAT activity after transfection. This indicates that the genotoxicity of UVA is mediated by a cellular photosensitizer.

Recent Results in Cancer Research, Vol. 139

Introduction

Exposure of the skin to ultraviolet (UV) irradiation is the most important risk factor for skin cancer (NIH Consensus Conference 1989). Mutations caused by UV-induced DNA damage can represent the initial genetic changes in skin carcinogenesis if they activate oncogenes or inactivate tumor suppressor genes.

Both short-wave UVB (290–320 nm) and longer-wave UVA (320–400 nm) have been shown to induce nonmelanoma skin cancer in animal models, mainly mice (van Welden et al. 1988; Staberg 1983). Experiments with melanoma-prone mongrels of the platy fish Xiphophorus showed that both UVB and UVA were able to induce malignant melanoma, but that UVA was especially effective (Setlow et al. 1993). The authors suggest that 90%–95% of human malignant melanoma might be induced by UVA.

Different wavelengths of UV irradiation cause different kinds of damage to the DNA molecule and consequently also different kinds of mutations. While the absorption maximum of the DNA molecule is at 260 nm, UVB (290–320 nm) is still capable of exciting the DNA molecule directly and subsequently damaging it directly. Here, the most important DNA photoproducts are the pyrimidine dimers (Brash 1988; Mitchell and Nairn 1988). In skin tumors, mutations in oncogenes or tumor suppressor genes were found in loci with two adjacent pyrimidines, candidate sites for the formation of such pyrimidine dimers (Sarasin 1989; Ananthaswamy and Pierceall 1990; Ziegler et al. 1993). Due to absorption of shorter wavelengths in the stratum corneum of an intact epidermis, 300 nm has been shown to be the most effective wavelength to induce the formation of pyrimidine dimers in the biologically important basal layer of the epidermis (Freeman et al. 1989).

If the UV radiation is first absorbed by another cellular molecule, the DNA molecule can be damaged indirectly after energy or electron transfer. Such a photosensitized reaction can be mediated by endogenous (e.g., porphyrines, flavines) or exogenous (e.g., psoralenes, tetracycline) photosensitizers. Modifications of the DNA molecule by excited photosensitizers (Foote 1991) can be direct reactions (type I photosensitized reaction) or, more importantly, can be mediated through reactive oxygen species, mainly singlet oxygen (type II photosensitized reaction). Singlet oxygen does not generate pyrimidine dimers, but purine base modifications. The most important and mutagenic lesion is the 8-hydroxy-guanine (7,8-dihydro-8-oxoguanosine), which tends to produce G:C to T:A transversions by pairing with adenine instead of cytosine during replication (Epe 1991; Cheng et al. 1992). These indirect reactions are likely to be the mechanisms of the mutagenic, genotoxic, and cytotoxic effects of UVA (320–400 nm), since UVA is not capable of exciting and damaging the DNA molecule directly (Tyrrell and Keyse 1990; Tyrell and Pidoux 1989; Lundgren and Wulf 1988;

Churchill et al. 1991; Gange and Rosen 1986). The nature of the endogenous photosensitizer that mediates these effects remains to be established. The generation of oxidative DNA damage (8-hydroxy-guanine) by visible light (Pflaum et al. 1994) or by UVB (Beehler et al. 1992) has recently been reported.

Genetic stability is an important prerequisite for the maintenance of the integrity and function of each cell. That is why even prokaryotic, and even more so eukaryotic, cells possess complex systems of DNA repair enzymes for the repair of all kinds of DNA damage, including the above-mentioned types of UV-induced DNA damage.

Xeroderma pigmentosum (XP) is an autosomal recessive disorder, in which an increased risk of developing UV-induced skin cancer is due to a defect in the repair of UV-induced DNA damage (Kraemer et al. 1987a; Cleaver 1968; Hoeijmakers 1993). Eight different complementation groups reflect a heterogeneity with probably eight different genetic defects. Recently, the identification and characterization of some XP genes (Tanaka et al. 1990; Hoeijmakers 1993) has increased our knowledge of the so far barely understood human DNA repair system. The biological relevance of oxidative DNA damage is underlined by the identification of a repair endocuclease specific for such lesions, the FPG protein (formamidopyrimidine-DNA glycosylase) (Tchou et al. 1991).

XP is a valuable model system for the pivotal role of DNA repair in prevention of UV-induced skin cancer. The fact that UV-induced skin cancer also occurs in individuals with normal DNA repair capacities indicates that the repair of UV-induced DNA damage can be incomplete in normal cells. Differences in individual DNA repair capacities have been shown to affect individual cancer and skin cancer risk (Alcalay et al. 1990; Pero et al. 1989; Wei et al. 1993; Kovacs and Langemann 1991).

We have been using transient plasmid vectors to study the processing of different kinds of UV-induced DNA damage within human cells. The plasmids were either damaged by irradiation with UVB, which causes directly UV-induced DNA damage (pyrimidine dimers), or with singlet oxygen, which is probably the agent responsible for indirectly UV-induced DNA damage. These damaged plasmids were then introduced into repair-proficient or repair-deficient human host lymphoblast cells. Expression of the plasmid-encoded chloramphenicol acetyltransferase (CAT), which depends on successful repair of the DNA damage in that plasmid gene by host cell enzymes, was then assayed by CAT activity in cell extracts 3 days after transfection. The better the host cells were able to repair the DNA damage on the plasmid, the higher the resulting CAT activity was. While DNA repair-deficient XP cells exhibited a significantly lower CAT activity than normal cells after transfection of UVB-irradiated plasmids, their capacity to repair oxidative DNA damage was not impaired. UVA did not exhibit genotoxic effects unless it was used in conjunction with a cell extract.

This indicates that the genotoxicity of UVA is mediated by a cellular photosensitizer.

Methods

Cells

Epstein-Barr virus-transformed lymphoblast cell lines were either established in our laboratory following the protocol described by Neitzel (1986) (KM, BD, TR) or purchased from the Human Genetic Mutant Cell Repository (Camden, New Jersey, USA) (GM3715, GM3657, GM0621, GM0130, GM1805, GM2250, and GM2248). The cells were grown in RPMI 1640 medium supplemented with 17% fetal calf serum in 5% CO_2 and used during exponential growth.

Plasmid Treatment

One of the following four treatments were used to damage the plasmid pRSVcat:

1. Plasmids at a concentration of 30 μg/ml were irradiated with 1 kJ/m^2, 5 kJ/m^2, and 10 kJ/m^2 UVB (Philips TL21 lamps; emission maximum, 315 nm; spectrum, 275–365 nm) at 0°C.
2. Plasmids were treated with singlet oxygen, generated by methylene blue (10 μg/ml) and light (1, 5, and 10 min illumination with visible light, 1000 W Osram halogen lamp, 47 W/m^2 between 400 and 800 nm). Plasmid concentration was 75 μg/120 μl. The DNA damage profile induced by this treatment has been described earlier by Müller et al. (1990) using DNA repair endonucleases. It comprises mainly FPG protein-sensitive sites and hardly any single strand breaks, pyrimidine dimers, or AP sites. It is identical to the DNA damage profile produced by $NDPO_2$, a chemically clean source of singlet oxygen.
3. Plasmids were irradiated with 500 kJ/m^2, 1000 kJ/m^2, or 2500 kJ/m^2 UVA (Mutzhaas, UVASUN 2000; emission maximum, 365 nm; spectrum, 320–440 nm at 0°C in water (without any photosensitizers).
4. Plasmids were irradiated with 500 kJ/m^2, 1000 kJ/m^2, or 2500 kJ/m^2 UVA (Mutzhaas, UVASUM 2000; emission maximum, 365 nm; spectrum, 320–440 nm). Here a 20% crude, ultrasonically produced cell extract, which provided all candidate intracellular photosensitizers, was present during irradiation. Irradiation was performed at 0°C in order to prevent plasmid modification by enzymes of the cell extract. Prior to further usage, the treated plasmids were purified by cesium chloride gradient, in order to eliminate relaxed or linear plasmid DNA, possibly still produced by endonucleases.

Plasmid Assay

The plasmid pRSVcat contains the *cat* gene in a configuration that allows expression of the CAT protein in human cells. Five micrograms of pRSVcat were used to transfect 15 × 10^6 cells, using the electroporation procedure (Gene Pulser, BioRAD: 250 v, 960 μFD capacitor, 400 μl serum-free medium, time constant between 20 and 30 ms). The cells were then transferred to 25 ml prewarmed complete medium and allowed to grow. After 3 days a cell extract was produced by three freeze–thaw cycles with ethanol in dry ice and subsequent rewarming to 37°C. CAT activity in that cell extract was determined with the one-vial procedure described by Neumann et al. (1987) and Eastmann (1987). Calibration was done with different concentrations of CAT (Boehringer Mannheim) and a linear relationship was found between 0.5 and 0.001 units CAT. In addition, total protein was determined in each extract (Coomassie-blue, BioRAD). The mean specific activity was 0.6 units CAT/mg protein.

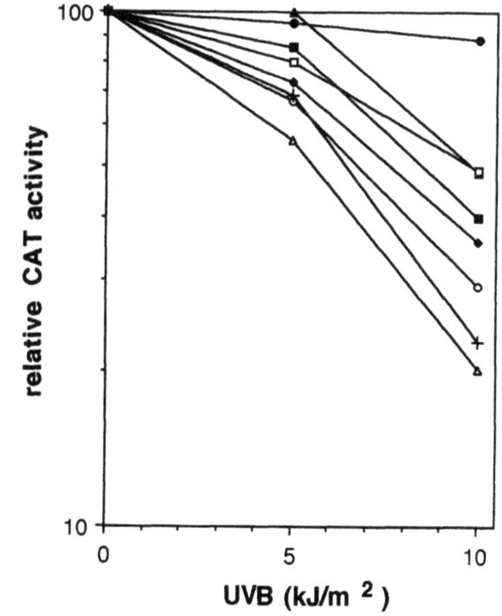

Fig. 1. Relative chloramphenicol acetyltransferase (CAT) activity (as percentage of untreated control) in cell extracts of eight normal lymphoblast lines after transfection of ultraviolet (UV) B-irradiated plasmid pRSVcat, reflecting repair of UVB-induced DNA damage within these eight normal cell lines. Values are means of at least two independent samples. □, GM3657; ▲, GM3715; ○, GM0621; ■, GM1308; ◆, GM1805; Δ, KM; +, BD; ●, TR

Results

Repair of Directly Ultraviolet-Induced DNA Damage

Figure 1 shows the capacity of eight normal lymphoblast cell lines to repair UVB-induced DNA damage. The decline of relative CAT activity with increasing doses of UVB indicates that even normal cells cannot repair all damage completely, e.g., with 5 kJ/cm^2, a dose often reached during sun exposure or in a therapeutic setting, the mean host cell reactivation rate (reflecting DNA repair performance) is only 77%. This figure also shows a considerable variation between the normal cell lines. However, our data cannot answer the question of whether these differences have any clinical relevance, e.g., reflect individually different cancer risks. Cells from a patient with xeroderma pigmentosum complementation group A showed a significantly reduced ($p < 0.01$) repair of UVB-induced DNA damage (Fig. 2), thus confirming the already well-known DNA repair deficiency with our assay.

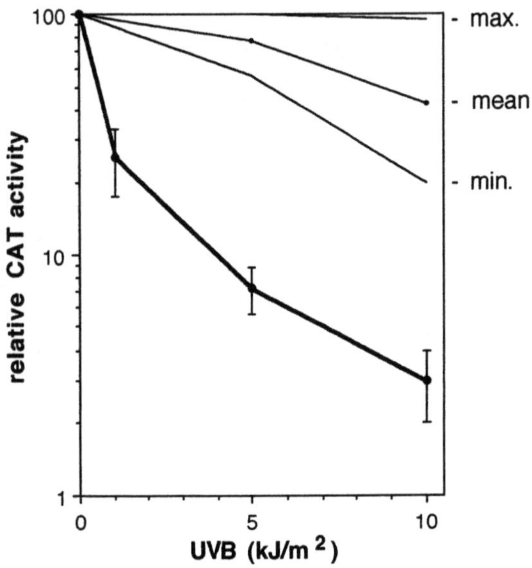

Fig. 2. Relative chloramphenicol acetyltransferase (CAT) activity (as percentage of untreated control) in cell extracts of the xeroderma pigmentosum (complementation group A) lymphoblast line GM2250 after transfection of ultraviolet (UV) B-irradiated plasmid pRSVcat, reflecting significantly reduced repair of UVB-induced DNA damage within that DNA repair-deficient cell line. Values are means of three independent samples. The mean, minimum, and maximum values from the results with eight normal cell lines (see Fig. 1) are shown as the normal range

Repair of Indirectly Ultraviolet-Induced DNA Damage

Figure 3 shows the capacity of seven normal lymphoblast cell lines to repair DNA damage induced by singlet oxygen. The capacity of normal cells to repair this kind of DNA damage is also limited and also shows considerable individual variation. In contrast to UVB-induced DNA damage, cells from the same XP patient were able to repair this oxidative DNA damage as well as the normal cells (Fig. 4).

In order to prove that genotoxic effects of UVA are indeed mediated by an indirect, photosensitized reaction with the DNA molecule, we performed the same experiments with UVA irradiation of the plasmid with and without presence of cellular photosensitizerss, supplied by a diluted cell extract. While no effects were seen when the plasmids were irradiated in an aqueous solution without any photosensitizers, plasmids irradiated in the presence of a cell extract exhibited a reduced CAT activity (Fig. 5), clearly indicating that genotoxicity of UVA is mediated by cellular photosensitizers and that such DNA damage is not completely repaired by normal, repair-proficient cells. Figure 6 shows that a cell line from a patient with XP complementation group C did not show a further reduced repair of such lesions, as compared to the two normal lines in Fig. 5.

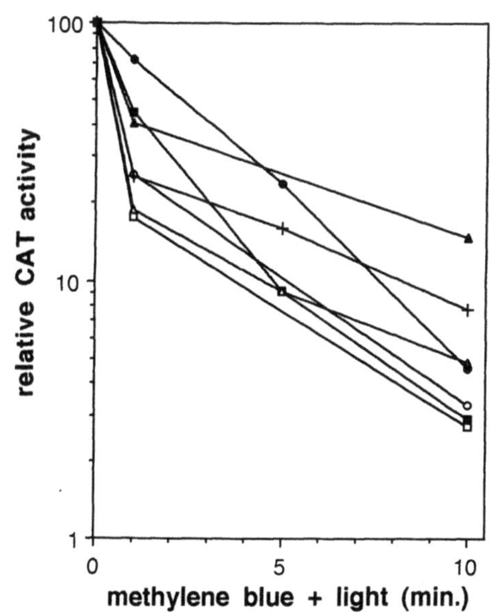

Fig. 3. Relative chloramphenicol acetyltransferase (CAT) activity (as percentage of unirradiated control) in cell extracts of seven normal lymphoblast lines after transfection of the plasmid pRSVcat treated with singlet oxygen, reflecting repair of oxidative DNA damage within these eight normal cell lines. Singlet oxygen was generated by photoexcitation with visible light of the photosensitizer methylene blue. Values are means of at least two independent samples. □, GM3657; ▲, GM3715; ○, GM0621; ■, GM1308; △, KM; +, BD; ●, TR

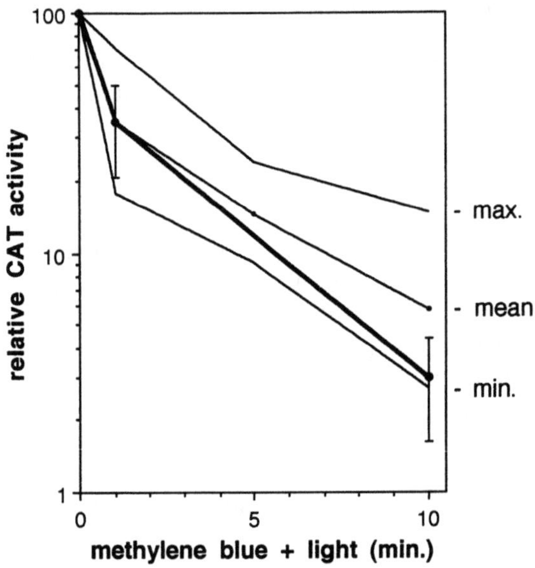

Fig. 4. Relative chloramphenicol acetyltransferase (CAT) activity (as percentage of unirradiated control) in cell extracts of the xeroderma pigmentosum (complementation group A) lymphoblast line GM2250 after transfection of the plasmid pRSVcat treated with singlet oxygen, reflecting a normal repair of oxidative DNA damage within that otherwise DNA repair-deficient cell line. Singlet oxygen was generated by photoexcitation with visible light of the photosensitizer methylene blue. Values are means of three independent samples. The mean, minimum, and maximum values from the results with seven normal cell lines (see Fig. 3) are shown as the normal range

Discussion

In our work we have taken advantage of the versatility of host cell reactivation assays with transfected plasmids to study the processing and genotoxicity of several different kinds of DNA damage.

With directly UV-induced damage on plasmid DNA we were able to demonstrate the known DNA repair defect in XP complementation group A cells. Athas et al. (1991), Kraemer et al. (1987), and Protiç-Sabliç and Kraemer (1985, 1986) have used similar plasmid assays for the same purpose with very similar results.

In contrast, XP-A cells were indistinguishable from normal cells in their ability to repair singlet oxygen-induced (probably representing indirectly UV-induced) DNA damage. This finding is in accordance with the results of Nocentini (1992), who did not find a reduced repair of singlet oxygen-induced DNA damage during host cell reactivation of Herpes simplex virus or SV40 virus in XP-A cells. This indicates that directly and indirectly UV-induced DNA damage is processed differently within human cells.

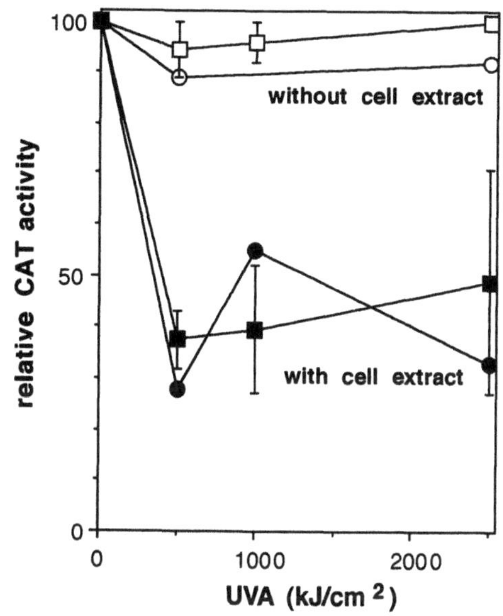

Fig. 5. Relative chlorampheuicol acetyltransferase (CAT) activity (as percentage of unirradiated control) in cell extracts of the the two normal lymphoblast cell lines GM0130 (○, ●) and TR (□, ■) after transfection of ultraviolet (UV) A-irradiated plasmid pRSVcat, irradiated either in an aqueous solution without photosensitizers (*open symbols*) or in the presence of a cell extract, providing all candidate cellular photosensitizers (*black symbols*)

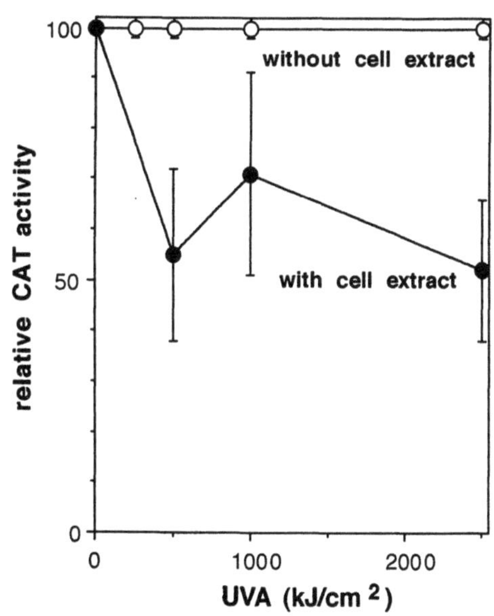

Fig. 6. Relative chloramphenicol acetyltransferase (CAT) activity (as percentage of unirradiated control) in cell extracts of the the xeroderma pigmentosum (complementation group C) lymphoblast cell lines GM2248 (○, ●) after transfection of ultraviolet (UV) A-irradiated plasmid pRSVcat, irradiated either in an aqueous solution without photosensitizers (*open symbols*) or in the presence of a cell extract, providing all candidate cellular photosensitizers (*black symbols*)

Although UVA is not able to damage the DNA molecule directly, it still is carcinogenic in animal models and might even play a pivotal role in tumorigenesis of malignant melanoma (Setlow et al. 1993; Swerdlow et al. 1988). Van Weelden et al. (1988) have found that the carcinogenic risks of tanning by UVA and of tanning by UVB are in the same order of magnitude in hairless mice.

Indirectly UV-induced DNA damage is believed to be responsible for the carcinogenic potential of UVA. We were able to show that genotoxicity of UVA is indeed caused by an indirect effect on DNA, mediated by photosensitizers (and singlet oxygen). The biologic relevance of indirectly UV-induced DNA damage is also supported by the finding that the antioxidative vitamins C and E have photoprotective effects (Mathews-Roth et al. 1987; Record et al. 1991; Darr et al. 1992). Our findings strongly support the notion that UVA, including UVA1, cannot be regarded harmless to the skin, either when used for cosmetic purposes or for therapy.

Acknowledgements. This work was supported by a grant from the Deutsche Forschungsgemeinschaft within the Sonderforschungsbereich 172 "Molecular Mechanisms of Carcinogenic Primary Lesions."

References

Alcalay J, Freeman SE, Goldberg LH, Wolf JE (1990) Excision repair of pyrimidine dimers induced by simulated solar irradiation in the skin of patients with basal cell carcinoma. J Invest Dermatol 95:506–509

Ananthaswamy HN, Pierceall WE (1990) Molecular mechanisms of ultraviolet radiation carcinogenesis. Photochem Photobiol 52:1119–1136

Athas WF, Hedayati MA, Matanoski GM, Farmer ER, Grossman L (1991) Development and field-test validation of an assay for DNA repair in circulating human lymphoblasts. Cancer Res 51:5786–5793

Beehler BC, Przybyszeski J, Box HB, Kulesz-Martin MF (1992) Formation of 8-hydroxyguanosine with DNA of mouse keratinocytes exposed in culture to UVB and H_2O_2. Carcinogenesis 13:2003–2007

Brash DE (1988) UV mutagenic photoproducts in Escherichia coli and human cells: a molecular genetics perspective on human skin cancer. Photochem Photobiol 48:59–66

Cheng KC, Cahill DS, Kasai H, Sishimura S, Loeb LA (1992) 8-Hydroxy-guanine, an abundant form of oxidative DNA damage, causes G to T and A to C substitutions. J Biol Chem 267:166–172

Churchill ME, Peak JG, Peak MJ (1991) Repair of near-visible- and blue-light-induced DNA single-strand breaks by CHO cell lines AA8 and EM9. Photochem Photobiol 54:639–644

Cleaver JE (1968) Defective repair replication of DNA in xeroderma pigmentosum. Nature 218:652–656

Darr D, Combs S, Dunston S, Manning T, Pinnel S (1992) Topical vitamin C protects porcine skin from ultraviolet radiation-induced damage. Br J Dermatol 12:247–253

Eastman A (1987) An improvement to the novel rapid assay for chloramphenicol acetyltransferase gene expression. Biotechniques 5:730–732
Epe B (1991) Genotoxicity of singlet oxygen. Chem Biol Interact 80:239–260
Foote CS (1991) Definition of type I and type II photosensitized oxidation. Photochem Photobiol 54:659–663
Freeman SE, Hacham H, Gange RW, Maytum DJ, Sutherland JC, Sutherland BM (1989) Wavelength dependence of pyrimidine dimer formation in DNA of human skin irradiated in situ with ultraviolet light. Proc Natl Acad Sci USA 86:5605–5609
Gange RW, Rosen CF (1986) UVA effects on mammalian skin and cells. Photochem Photobiol 43:701–705
Hoeijmakers JHJ (1993) Nucleotide exision repair II: from yeast to mammals. Trends Genet 9:211–217
Kovacs E, Langemann H (1991) Differences in the kinetics of DNA repair in cancer patients and healthy controls. Oncology 48:312–316
Kraemer KH, Lee MM, Scotto J (1987a) Xeroderma pigmentosum. Cutaneous, ocular, and neurologic abnormalities in 830 published cases (review article). Arch Dermatol 123:241–250
Kraemer KH, Protiç-Sabliç M, Bredberg A, Seidman M (1987b) Plasmid vectors for the study of DNA repair and mutagenesis. In: Hönigsmann H (ed) Current problems in dermatology. Karger, Basel, pp 166–181
Lundgren K, Wulf HC (1988) Cytotoxicity and genotoxicity of UVA irradiation in chinese hamster ovary cells measured by specific locus mutations, sister chromatid exchanges and chromosome aberrations. Photochem Photobiol 47: 559–563
Mathews-Roth MM, Krinsky NI (1987) Carotenoids affect development of UV-B induced skin cancer. Photochem Photobiol 46:507–509
Mitchell D, Nairn RS (1988) The (6-4) photoproduct and human skin cancer. Photodermatol 5:61–66
Müller E, Boiteux RP, Cunningham RP, Epe B (1990) Enzymatic recognition of DNA modifications induced by singlet oxygen and photosensitizers. Nucleic Acids Res 18:5969–5973
National Institutes of Health Consensus Development Conference Statement (1989) Sunlight, ultraviolet radiation, and the skin, vol 7, no 8
Neitzel H (1986) A routine method for the establishment of permanent growing lymphoblastoid cell lines. Hum Genet 73:320–326
Neumann JR, Morency CA, Russian KO (1987) A novel rapid assay for chloramphenicol acetyltransferase gene expression. Biotechniques 5:444–447
Nocentini S (1992) Cellular responses to hematoporphyrin-induced photo-oxidative damage in Fanconi anemia, xeroderma pigmentosum and normal human fibroblasts. Mutat Res 284:275–285
Pero RW, Johnson DB, Markowitz M, Doyle G, Lund-Pero M, Seidegard J, Halper M, Miller DG (1989) DNA repair synthesis in individuals with and without a family history of cancer. Carcinogenesis 10:693–697
Pflaum M, Boiteux S, Epe B (1994) Visible light generates oxidative DNA base modifications in high excess of strand breaks in mammalian cells. Carcinogenesis (in press)
Protiç-Sabliç M, Kraemer KH (1985) One pyrimidine dimer inactivates expression of a transfected gene in xeroderma pigmentosum cells. Proc Natl Acad Sci USA 82:6622–6626
Protiç-Sabliç M, Kraemer KH (1986) Host cell reactivation by human cells of DNA expression vectors damaged by utraviolet radiation or by acid-heat treatment. Carcinogenesis 7:1776–1770

Record IR, Dreosti IE, Konstantinopoulos M, Buckley RA (1991) The influence of topical and systemic vitamin E on ultraviolet light-induced skin damage in hairless mice. Nutr Cancer 16:219–225

Sarasin A (1989) Molecular mechanisms of mutagenesis in mammalian cells: present and future. Mutat Res 220:51–53

Setlow RB, Grist E, Thompson K, Woodhead AD (1993) Wavelengths effective in induction of malignant melanoma. Proc Natl Acad Sci USA 90:6666–6670

Staberg B (1983) The carcinogenic effect of UV-A irradiation. J Invest Dermatol 81:517–519

Swerdlow AJ, English JS, MacKie RM, O'Doherty CJ, Hunter JA, Clark J, Hole DJ (1988) Fluorescence light, ultraviolet lamps and risk of cutaneous melanoma. Br Med J 297:647–650

Tanaka K, Miura N, Satokata I, Miyamoto I, Yoshida MC, Satoh Y, Kondo S, Yasui A, Okayama H, Okada Y (1990) Analysis of a human DNA excision repair gene involved in group A xeroderma pigmentosum and containing a zinc-finger domain. Nature 348:73–76

Tchou J, Kasai H, Shibutani S, Chung MH, Laval J, Grollman AP, Nishimura J. (1991) 8-Oxoguanine (8-hydroxyguanine)-DNA glysosylase and its substrate specificity. Proc Natl Acad Sci USA 88:4690–4694

Tyrrell RM, Keyse SM (1990) New trends in photobiology. The interaction of UVA radiation with cultured cells. J Photochem Photobiol B 4:349–361

Tyrrell RM, Pidoux M (1989) Singlet oxygen involvement in the inactivation of cultured human fibroblasts by UV A (334 nm, 365 nm) and near-visible (405 nm) radiations. Photochem Photobiol 49:407–412

Van Weelden H, de Gruijl FR, van der Putter SCJ, Toonstra J, van der Leun JC (1988) The carcinogenic risks of modern tanning equipment: is UV-A safer than UV-B? Arch Dermatol Res 280:300–307

Wei Q, Matanoski GM, Farmer ER, Hedayati MA, Grossman L (1993) DNA repair and aging in basal cell carcinoma: a molecular epidemiology study. Proc Natl Acad Sci USA 90:1614–1618

Ziegler A, Leffell DJ, Kunala S, Sharma HW, Gailani M, Simon JA, Halperin AJ, Baden HP, Shapiro PE, Bale AE, Brash DE (1993) Mutation hotspots due to sunlight in the p53 gene of nonmelanoma skin cancers. Proc Natl Acad Sci USA 90:4216–4220

Photodynamic Action of Ultraviolet A: Induction of Cellular Hydroperoxides

S. Schmitz[1], C. Garbe[1], K. Jimbow[2], A. Wulff[1], H. Daniels[1], J. Eberle[1], and C.E. Orfanos[1]

[1] Department of Dermatology, The Free University of Berlin, University Medical Center Steglitz, Hindenburgdamm 30, 12200 Berlin, Germany
[2] Division of Dermatology and Cutaneous Sciences, University of Alberta, Canada

Abstract

Long-wavelength ultraviolet radiation (UVA) can cause cancer. A carcinogenic mechanism involved may be the induction of harmful reactive oxygen species resulting from photodynamic effects. UVA is generally assumed to induce photodynamic effects, but evidence from experiments with viable biological materials has been indirect until present. Here we measured the induction of (lipid) hydroperoxides as direct indicators of photodynamic reactions. Cultured human fibroblasts were irradiated with 10 J UVA/cm^2. The induced hydroperoxides were measured by an enzymatic method using glutathione peroxidase and glutathione reductase (GR). Additionally, reduced glutathione (GSH) was determined as parameter for the constitutive antioxidant defense. UVA was found to increase lipid hydroperoxides in fibroblasts by 116% ($p<0.001$), when compared to nonirradiated controls. Conversely GSH was decreased in the irradiated cells by 51% ($p<0.001$). Because of the induced hydroperoxides, it is concluded that the UVA effects were mediated by a photodynamic mechanism. The photodynamic mechanism resulted in the formation of reactive oxygen species and the consumption of constitutive antioxidants. This suggests a role for antioxidants during the photodynamic mechanism. Photodynamic mechanisms may play a crucial role in carcinogenic events, especially after UVA.

Introduction

Ultraviolet radiation (UVR) is classified into long-wavelength UVA (380–315 nm), short-wavelength UVB (315–280 nm), and UVC (280–200 nm). The need for different mechanisms of UV effects became evident when UVA was shown to damage DNA despite not being absorbed by DNA.

Recent Results in Cancer Research, Vol. 139

Thus an "indirect" mechanism was required to explain DNA damage after UVA. In contrast, UVB and UVC may be absorbed by DNA and lead to "direct" damage. The clarification of the mechanisms involved in biological UV action is oncologically important, because recent studies have attributed carcinogenic risks to UVA (Schmitz et al. 1994).

Only radiation which is absorbed can result in photobiological effects. The absorbing molecules are called chromophores. Chromophores, which become excited and reactive after radiation, are referred to as sensitizers. In a sensitization process, a sensitizer (S) initially absorbs a photon and is elevated from its singlet ground state to a singlet excited state (S^1). The short-lived excited singlet state sensitizer (S^1) converts to longer-lived, triplet excited state sensitizer (S^3), which may interact with other cellular target molecules (Dall' Acqua and Martelli 1991). In this article we restrict the use of the term "sensitizer mediated" to oxygen-independent reactions. In sensitizer-mediated reactions the sensitizer itself reacts with a functional target molecule. An example for a sensitizer-mediated mechanism is psoralens and ultraviolet A (PUVA) therapy. The irradiated psoralen molecules become excited and cross-link with pyrimidine bases of DNA (Dall' Acqua and Martelli 1991).

The sensitizer-mediated mechanism is very distinct from oxygen-dependent, "photodynamic" (PD) mechanisms, which result in the formation of reactive oxygen species (ROS). ROS are reactive molecules and may mediate damage to other cell molecules. The oxygen dependence as defining criterion for "photodynamic" mechanisms dates back to the beginning of this century (Spikes 1991). Though all PD reactions are oxygen dependent by definition, the immediateness of O_2 involvement has led to distinguish two different types of PD reaction pathways (Girotti 1990; see Fig. 1): (1) In the type I PD reaction pathway the excited triplet state sensitizer (S^3) reacts with a secondary molecule without initial participation of oxygen; the activated secondary molecule then reacts with oxygen; (2) in the type II PD reaction pathway, the S^3 reacts directly with oxygen. Later products, e.g., (lipid) hydroperoxides (ROOH), may be the same for both type I and II PD reaction pathways. ROOH are suitable markers for PD reactions, because they result from both PD pathways.

Here we irradiated cultured human fibroblasts with UVA and investigated the formation of ROOH, since direct evidence for a PD mechanism in biologically viable experimental models was not yet available. To measure ROOH we adapted a previously described method (Allen et al. 1990). The principle of analysis was: (a) reduction of ROOH by glutathione peroxidase (G-Px), an enzyme which reacts with both hydrogen peroxide and organic hydroperoxides, resulting in the formation of stoichiometric amounts of GSSG; (b) elimination of the remaining GSH through derivatization with *N*-ethylmaleimide (NEM); (c) conversion of the GSSG to GSH with glutathione reductase (GR). The resulting GSH was measured in a reaction with the

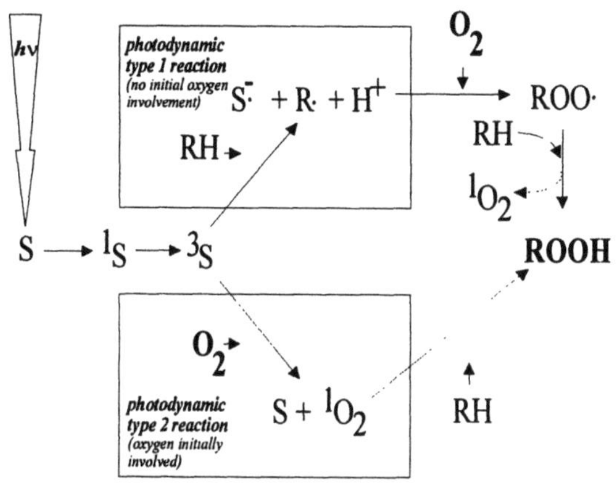

Fig. 1. Nonstoichiometric scheme illustrating the mechanism of the photodynamic (PD) induction of hydroperoxides (*ROOH*) by both PD reaction types (see also the introduction to the text). *S*, sensitizer (uppercase 1 indicating the singlet-excited state, uppercase 3 indicating the triplet-excited state of the sensitizer); *RH*, secondary molecule; *ROO*·, peroxyl radical; O_2, molecular oxygen; $^1O_2$, singlet oxygen. + and − indicate positive and negative charges;· signifies unpaired electrons of "free radicals"; *hν* stands for electromagnetic radiation, such as ultraviolent (UV) light

chromogen dithiobisnitrobenzoic acid (DTNB) and indicated the amount of ROOH.

As a modification to the original method we introduced an initial washing step to eliminate constitutive cellular GSSG. An additional enzymatic step using phosholipase A_2 (PLA_2; O'Gara et al. 1989) was used in half of the samples to improve the measurability of lipid hydroperoxides and to achieve higher yields of ROOH. As additional parameter to ROOH we measured the influence of UVA on levels of the constitutive antioxidant GSH, which has been shown to protect against UVA-induced DNA damage (Applegate et al. 1993). The influence of constitutive GSH on ROOH was studied by depleting constitutive GSH in the fibroblasts with the γ-glutamyl-cysteine synthetase inhibitor buthionine sulfoximine (BSO).

With the described techniques we were able demonstrate the induction of hydroperoxides in human cultured fibroblasts by UVA and its effect on GSH as part of the constitutive antioxidant defense. The induction of lipid hydroperoxides in human fibroblasts provides experimental evidence for the existence of a PD mechanism in viable cells after UVA irradiation.

Materials and Methods

Chemicals. All chemicals were purchased from Sigma Chemical Company (St. Louis, MO, USA) and were of the highest available purity. Butylated hydroxytoluene (1 μM) and desferrioxamine (20 μM) were supplements in all media and liquids used in the processing of irradiated samples and controls.

Cell Culture. Human skin fibroblasts were grown in primary culture from human foreskins as described by Freshney (1987). The cells were grown under standard culture conditions using RPMI 1640 (Gibco-Life-Technologies, Gaithersburg, MD, USA) supplemented with 10% fetal bovine serum as medium. After the fourth passage the cells were grown to confluence in 75-cm^2 tissue culture flasks (Costar, Cambridge, MD, USA). Fresh medium was supplemented before each irradiation.

Irradiation. For UVA irradiations an illumination table with peak irradiance at 360 nm (UV/PUVA 180, Waldmann, Schwenningen, Germany) was used. The flasks with the cells were irradiated from the bottom with 10 J cm^{-1}, which was measured as effective dose of penetrating UVA at the cell monolayer level. During the irradiation all irradiated culture flasks were constantly rotated to adjust for dose inhomogenities of the irradiation field. Some culture flasks with cells were wrapped in aluminum foil and served as sham-irradiated controls. The temperatures of the irradiated media was measured before and after irradiations; temperatures remained above 35°C during UVA exposures of 30 min. The pH of the media did not change, as was checked before and after irradiations. Immediately after the irradiation, media were decanted and substituted with ice-cold phosphate-buffered saline (PBS). From then on the flasks were kept at 4°C and were processed expeditiously. The irradiation technique from the bottom of the flasks served to exclude any potentially contaminating UVB remnants, which were filtered out. In contrast to UVB, the plastic-penetrating UVA was able to reach the cells. A second advantage of the irradiation from the bottom of the flasks was that the irradiant UV did not pass through growth media, which might contain noncellular photosensitizers and result in nonspecific PD effects.

Sample Preparation. Cells were scraped off the bottom of their flasks at 4°C, counted in a hemocytometer, and washed twice with PBS. All processing of the samples was done at 4°C. For cell fractionation the cells were transferred to microfuge tubes. After centrifugation (192 g, 10 min; Sorvall RC-5C, DuPont de Nemours, Bad Homburg v.d.H., Germany), the supernatants were decanted and the pellets resuspended in 200 μl 20-μM ethylene diamine tetraacetate (EDTA; 4°C). After 10 min all cells were swollen and partially ruptured. The tubes were shock frozen in liquid nitrogen, slowly warmed to 4°C, and centrifuged (13 000 rpm, 20 min; Minifuge, Eppendorff, Hamburg, Germany). The pellets were resuspended in 20-μM EDTA. Another cycle of freezing–thawing resulted in the fractionation of all cells, as was evaluated microscopically. The samples were then aliquoted and frozen in liquid nitrogen.

Measurement of Lipid Hydroperoxides. A previously described enzymatic two-step method based on the reaction of lipid hydroperoxides with G-Px was used (Allen et al. 1990). The freeze-ruptured cells were washed twice with 20-μM EDTA (13000 rpm, 20 min, 4°C; Minifuge) to remove cytosolic oxidized glutathione (GSSG). Here an enzymatic step using phospholipase A_2 (PLA_2; Boehringer/M., Mannheim, Germany) was added to the original assay. The enzyme served to breakdown phosphatidylcholine in cell membranes, which contained lipid hydroperoxides that would theoretically become better substrates for G-Px after digestion with PLA_2 (Thomas and Girotti 1988). The previous sample preparations were thawed, divided, and half of them supplemented with 10 U porcine PLA_2. All samples, with and without PLA_2, were supplemented with Na-phosphate buffer (73 mM) and 1 mM $CaCl_2$ to a total volume of 200 μl and incubated at 37°C for 2 h.

Following the original procedure (Allen et al. 1990), 50 μl 1-μM GSH (Boehringer/M., Mannheim, Germany) and 20 μl with 0.2 U G-Px were added, and Na-phosphate buffer was added to total volume of 0.5 ml each sample as described. After a 10-min incubation period, 50 μl 125-mM *N*-ethylmaleimide (NEM) was added. After thorough mixing the unreacted GSH was derivatized for 15 min at room temperature. Excess NEM was then hydrolytically removed by titration to pH 11 with 8 M KOH. After leaving the samples for 5 min at room temperature, the samples were readjusted to pH 7.4 with 1 M HCl.

Measurement of Reduced Glutathione. GSH was measured by the GR DTNB (dithiobisnitrobenzoic acid)-recycling assay as described (Allen et al. 1990). In addition to the derivatized GSH, which indicated lipid hydroperoxides, we determined constitutive GSH levels from separate aliquots.

For the measurement of lipid hydroperoxides, 1-ml spectrophotometer cuvettes (path, 1 cm) were filled with 100 μl pH-adjusted sample suspension from the preceding PLA_2 and G-Px incubations; then 700 μl 0.3-mM NADPH (reduced nicotine adenine dinucleotide phosphate; Boehringer/M., Mannheim, Germany) and 100 μl 10-mM DTNB were added. When the contents of the cuvettes had equilibrated to room temperature, 1 U GR (Boehringer/M., Mannheim, Germany) was added, and the change in the absorbance at 412 nm was measured using a recording spectrophotometer (Beckman, Fullerton, CA, USA). Peroxide concentrations were calculated from butyl hydroperoxide (Bt-OOH) standards, which had been processed in parallel to the samples.

For the measurement of cellular GSH, the aliquoted supernatants from centrifuged freeze-ruptured cells were used. One hundred microliters of supernatant from each of the freshly thawed samples was added to 1-ml cuvettes and measured by the GR-DTNB recycling assay, as described for the lipid hydroperoxide measurements. Cellular GSH quantities were then calculated by comparison with known GSH standards. To some fibroblasts, BSO in a final concentration of 10 μM (Lautier et al. 1992) had been supplemented 18 h prior to irradiation to study the effect of glutathione depletion on UV-inducible peroxides.

Statistical Evaluation. The significance of the disparities between the observed means of the parameters measured was evaluated by analysis of variance (ANOVA), as calculated using standard computer software (Excel 4.0, Microsoft Corp., Redmont, WA, USA).

Results

For better comparability between the parameters, all data displayed (Figs. 2–5) relate to independent irradiation experiments made with the same cell line on the same day and processed in parallel at the same time. Results became more variable when fibroblasts from different donors were irradiated, but remained always repeatable in principle (not shown).

Because of the complexity resulting from three enzymatic conversions, we used butyl hydroperoxide (Bt-OOH) as standard, which was processed in parallel to the samples through all analytical steps. Theoretically, the quantification of ROOH required only GSH standards, since ROOH should

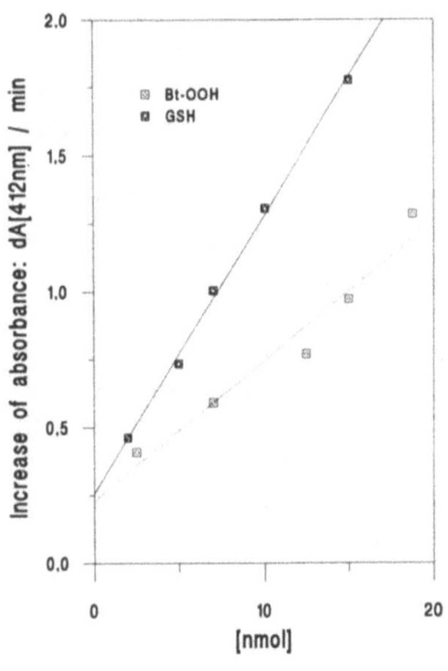

Fig. 2. Butyl hydroperoxide (*Bt-OOH*) and reduced glutathione (*GSH*) standards and molar to change of absorbance. Dilutions of Bt-OOH were processed in parallel to samples after freeze-rupturing of the cells. GSH standards were fresh dilutions added directly to the glutathione–reductase reaction. The shown graphs refer to the data presented in Figs. 3–5

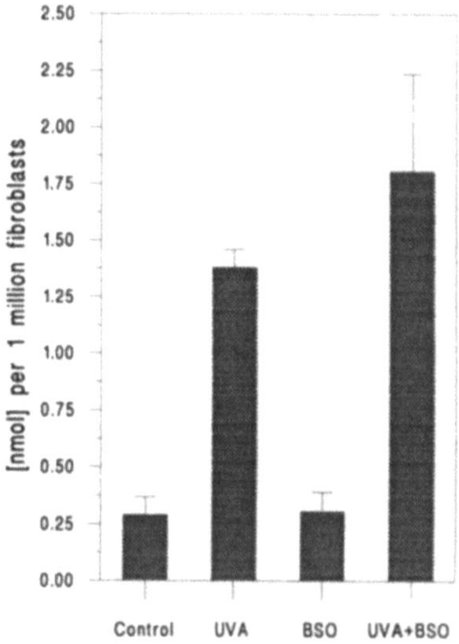

Fig. 3. The effect of 10 J ultraviolet A (*UVA*)/cm^2 and buthionine sulfoximine (*BSO*) on cellular hydroperoxides as measured without phospholipase A_2 (PLA_2) treatment of the samples. Mean values from three independent experiments with standard deviations

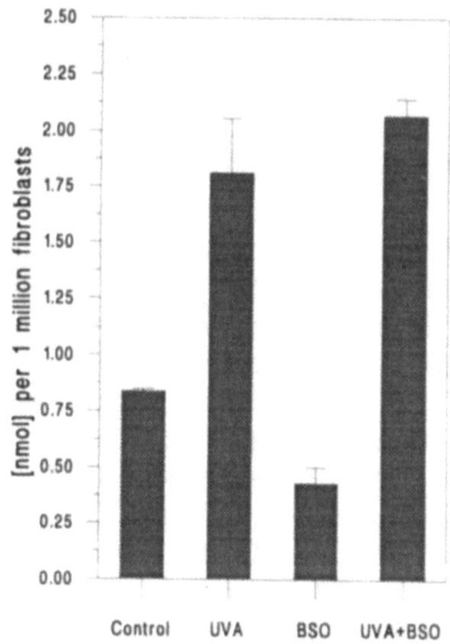

Fig. 4. The effect of 10 J ultraviolet A (*UVA*)/cm^2 and buthionine sulfoximine (**BSO**) on cellular lipid hydroperoxides as measured with phospholipase A_2 (PLA_2) treatment of the samples. Mean values from three independent experiments with standard deviations

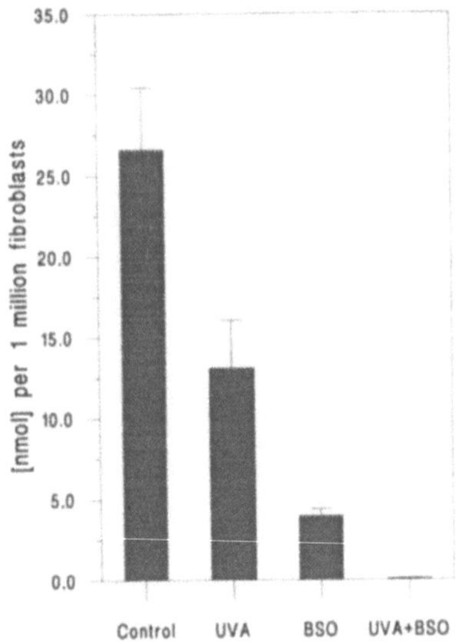

Fig. 5. The effect of 10 J ultraviolet A (*UVA*)/cm^2 and buthionine sulfoximine (*BSO*) on cellular reduced glutathione (GSH). Mean values from three independent experiments with standard deviations

convert to GSH on an equimolar basis. As demonstrated (Fig. 2), the analytical yields of the processed Bt-OOH standards were less than for plain GSH standards, which had been dissolved from the pure chemical. The slope for Bt-OOH was slightly reduced in its increment, but remained linear in the analytical range (2–20 mmol standard).

Irradiation of the fibroblasts with 10 J UVA/cm^2 resulted in measurable increases of ROOH, even when the samples were later processed without PLA_2. The effect of UVA alone was a 374% ($p < 0.001$) increase of ROOH when compared to sham-irradiated controls. The effect was even more pronounced in BSO-pretreated cells, where UVA induced a 520% ($p < 0.001$) increase, which was not significantly different when compared to the effect of UVA alone, however.

Processing of the samples with PLA_2 (Fig. 4) resulted in overall higher yields of measurable ROOH. Compared to the non-PLA_2-treated controls, UVA increased ROOH by 523% ($p < 0.001$) or in combination with GSH pretreatment by 611% ($p < 0.001$). Since PLA_2 treatment also increased preexisting ROOH in sham-irradiated controls (188%, $p < 0.001$, compared to non-PLA_2-treated sham-irradiated controls), the relative effects of UVA in PLA_2-treated samples were less then in non-PLA_2-treated cells (+116%, $p < 0.001$ for UVA; +146%, $p < 0.001$ for UVA after BSO pretreatment).

When studying the influence of UVA on constitutive cellular GSH (Fig. 5), a GSH-consuming effect (−51%, $p < 0.01$, compared to sham-irradiated controls) was detected. BSO alone depleted GSH by 85% ($p < 0.001$); the combination of UVA and BSO treatment resulted in 97% decrease of GSH ($p < 0.001$).

Discussion

At present a PD mechanism is assumed to be the principal mechanism of UVA-induced biological damage (Peak and Peak 1986). However, there exists little direct evidence for this mechanism for viable biological materials. It is known that many UVA effects, e.g., DNA damage and induction of erythema in vivo, are dependent on the presence of molecular oxygen, but this is rather indirect evidence. The determination of specific sensitizers would be helpful, but would be no proof for their role in PD reaction.

Direct evidence for a PD mechanism can be derived only from the measurement of specific products of PD reactions. Parameters of oxidative stress after UVA irradiations have been determined before (Morlière et al. 1991; Moysan et al. 1993). However, the measured thiobarbituric acid reactive substances (TBARS) were late-stage breakdown products of lipid peroxides with limited specificity of PD reactions. Such TBARS may result from increased cellular prostaglandin turnover as well, which was substantiated by studies by Cohen and DeLeo (1993), who found that UVA induced phospholipase A_2 activation in mammalian cell membrane preparations. Additionally, the same group demonstrated a stimulating effect of UVA on arachidonic acid release and cyclooxygenase activity in mammalian cells (Hanson and DeLeo VA 1989).

Thus hydroperoxides would be better indicators for PD reactions, since hydroperoxides may arise as direct products from PD reactions (Fig. 1). Problematically, the measurement of ROOH in cultured cells after UVR would require a highly sensitive method. Several methods have been reported for the measurement of hydroperoxides. A standard procedure is determination by iodometry (Buege and Aust 1978). Problems arise when high analytical sensitivities are required, such as in cell culture material. The sensitivity problem has been overcome partially by a specially designed apparatus (Thomas et al. 1989). Other modern spectrophotometric methods exist, but they lack the sensitivity required for the measurement of lipid hydroperoxides in cell culture (Thomas and Poznansky 1990). The cyclooxygenase assay might provide sufficient sensitivity (Miller et al. 1991), but the need for prostaglandin H synthase has limited the utility of this assay. The luminol chemiluminescence assay (Yamamoto et al. 1990) and ^{13}C nuclear magnetic resonance spectroscopy (Frankel et al. 1990) of hydrogen peroxide are highly sensitive, but require specialized equipment.

Our method is based on a recently reported highly sensitive method (Allen et al. 1990). The method is similar to a previously reported method for high-performance liquid chromatography (HPLC; O'Gara et al. 1989), but utilizes standard laboratory equipment. The assay depends on the enzymatic conversion of ROOH, yielding stoichiometric amounts of GSSG. By decreasing the amounts of constitutive GSSH in cells, this method became applicable to cell culture material. The elimination of GSSG was necessary, since physiological concentrations of constitutive GSSG are present in the micromolar range and might mask ROOH-indicating GSSG. A washing step was sufficient to decrease the constitutive GSSG to non-interfering levels.

The difference in molar absorbance between Bt-OOH and GSH standards (Fig. 2) was probably caused by the technical complexity of the procedure. For this reason the use as a quantitative assay was only possible when ROOH concentrations were calculated from peroxide standards. The latter had always been processed in parallel to the samples.

The incubation of samples with PLA_2 was found to be less important. PLA_2 treatment was introduced because it resulted in a theoretically higher specificity for lipid hydroperoxides and a higher yield in measurable ROOH (Fig. 4). Interestingly, a UVA effect was evident in both the PLA_2-treated (Fig. 4) and -untreated sample preparations (Fig. 3). There may be two explanations for the similar effectiveness: (1) Substrate molecules for G-Px other than PLA_2-releasable fatty acid hydroperoxides might result from UVA or (2) constitutive PLA_2 might become active during UVA irradiation.

Both explanations would support a PD mechanism of UVA, the first explanation because all hydroperoxides induced by UVA may be PD (Fig. 1) and G-Px reacts only with hydroperoxides. Not displayed is the fact that hydrogen peroxide may result from a type I PD reaction in which superoxide anion is formed and consecutively dismutates in the presence of superoxide dismutase (Girotti 1990). The second explanation would support such a mechanism because PLA_2 may facilitate the G-Px reaction only when the peroxides "trapped" in the fatty acids of phosphatidylcholine are hydroperoxides.

The GSH-depleting effect of UVA (Fig. 5) is consistent with previous reports which found UVA to decrease cellular levels of GSH in fibroblasts (Moysan et al. 1993) and may indicate the involvement of constitutive antioxidants as a protection mechanism against the PD effects of UVA. The decrease of GSH may be explained by its functioning as a cofactor to other enzymes, e.g., G-Px, or by acting as a consumable free radical scavenger. UVA has previously been demonstrated to affect the antioxidant systems and to increase oxidative stress in cultured human fibroblasts (Moysan et al. 1993). It is interesting to note that GSH levels were demonstrated to determine the frequency of both spontaneous and UVA-inducible mutations in cultured human cells (Applegate et al. 1992).

The goal of this study was to determine specific products of PD reactions after UVA irradiation. A PD mechanism had been assumed previously, but products specific for PD reaction have not been measured, at least not in biological materials. Our confirmatory data may be the first to provide direct evidence for the PD nature of UVA. Defining the PD mechanism in contrast

Table 1. Classification of mechanisms involved in the mediation of cellular ultraviolet (UV) effects

Class	Mechanism of UV action	Oxygen dependence	Primary chromophores	Cellular targets	Possible UV spectra involved	Occurrence of mechanism (examples)
A	Photo-dynamic[a] induction of ROS	Yes	Cellular	Random (e.g., DNA, proteins, membranes)	UVA, UVB	Cosmetic tanning, PUVA therapy, therapeutic UVB
B	Sensitizer–target interaction[b]	No	Cellular	Specific (DNA, (functional molecules?)	UVA, (other UV?)	PUVA therapy, (other UV-applications?)
C	Direct DNA interaction	No	DNA	DNA	UVB, UVC	Therapeutic UVB, germicidal lamp

ROS, reactive oxygen species; PUVA, psoralens and ultraviolet A.
[a] The two photodynamic reaction pathways were not used for classification, since biological effects are difficult to distinguish.
[b] For example, psoralen DNA cross-links.

to the other mechanism of UVR results in three distinct biologically relevant mechanisms (Table 1): (1) class A, the PD mechanism, which is dependent on the presence of oxygen; (2) class B, a sensitizer-mediated mechanism, resulting in oxygen-independent sensitizer target interactions, such as the specific interaction of UV-exited psoralens with DNA; and (3) class C, the direct interaction of UVR with cellular DNA.

Though most biological effects of UVA would be class A mediated, UVA therapy with psoralens (PUVA) is sensitizer mediated. Though experimental evidence for the class B mechanism is derived from the study of PUVA therapy, the possibility of other wavelengths having similar effects as the existence of unidentified class B sensitizers cannot be dismissed. It should be mentioned that even PUVA may result in PD effects (Potapenko 1991) and should therefore be attributed to both class A and B mechanisms. In contrast to UVA, the shorter-wavelength UVB and UVC spectra may be absorbed by DNA and result in direct DNA damage (class C mechanism). UVB, which is less easily absorbed by DNA than UVC, may theoretically induce PD effects if sensitizer and oxygen requirements are met.

The above classification was deduced from oxygen and sensitizer requirements for specific UV spectra. The utility of these classes of UV mechanisms lies in the identification of functionally distinct UV effects and in their prevention. It is evident that a class A mechanism resulting in ROS at multiple cellular sites should have different effects than a class C mechanism where a specific cellular targets is affected. The classification may be also useful in matching specific physiological and possibly therapeutic defense mechanisms.

We conclude that the measurement of hydroperoxides provides direct evidence for the PD effects of UVA, which result in the formation of potentially harmful ROS. The involvement of ROS clearly distinguish UVA effects from other spectra of UVR. The identification of specific classes of UV effect mechanisms may improve our understanding of the pathogenesis of skin cancer and may be necessary for understanding physiological and possible therapeutical defense mechanisms against UVR.

References

Allen KD, Kuang C-J, Morin CL (1990) Determination of picomole quantities of hydroperoxides by a coupled glutathione peroxidase and glutathione disulfide specific glutathione reductase assay. Anal Biochem 186:108–111

Applegate LA, Lautier D, Frenk E, Tyrrell RM (1992) Endogeneous glutathione levels modulate the frequency of both spontaneous and long wavelength ultraviolet induced mutations in human cells. Carcinogenesis 13:1557–1560

Buege JA, Aust SD (1978) Microsomal lipid peroxidation. Methods Enzymol 52: 302–310

Cohen D, DeLeo VA (1993) Ultraviolet radiation-induced phospholipase A_2 activation occurs in mammalian cell membrane preparations. Photochem Photobiol 57:383–390

Dall' Acqua F, Martelli P (1991) Photosensitizing action of furocoumarins on membrane components and consequent intracellular events. J Photochem Photobiol B 8:235–254
Frankel EN, Neff WE, Weisleder D (1990) Determination of methyl linoleate hydroperoxides by ^{13}C nuclear magnetic resonance spectroscopy. Methods Enzymol 186:380–387
Freshney RI (1987) Culture of animal cells, 2nd edn. Liss, New York
Girotti AW (1990) Lipid peroxidation in photodynamic systems. In: Vigo-Pelfrey C (ed) Membrane lipid peroxidation. CRC Press, Boca Raton, pp 203–218
Hanson DL, DeLeo VA (1989) Long wave ultraviolet radiation stimulates arachidonic acid release and cyclooxygenase activity in mammalian cells in culture. Photochem Photobiol 49:423–430
Lautier D, Luscher P, Tyrrell RM (1992) Endogeneous glutathione levels modulate both constitutive and UVA radiation/hydrogen peroxide inducible expression of the human heme oxygenease gene. Carcinogenesis 13:227–232
Miller JF Jr, Kulmacz RJ, Lands WEM (1991) Use of a voltage-responsive timer to quantitiate hydroperoxides by the cyclooxygenase assay. Anal Biochem 193:55–66
Morlière P, Moysan A, Santus R, Huppe G, Maziere JC, Dubertret L (1991) UVA-induced lipid peroxidation in cultured human fibroblasts. Biochim Biophys Acta 1084:261–268
Moysan A, Marquis I, Gaboriau F, Santus R, Dubertret L, Morlière P (1993) Ultraviolet A-induced lipid peroxidation and antioxidant defense systems in cultured human fibroblasts. J Invest Dermatol 100:692–698
O'Gara CY, Maddipati KR, Marnett LJ (1989) A sensitive electrochemical method for quantitative hydroperoxide determination. Chem Res Toxicol 2:295–300
Peak MJ, Peak JG (1986) Molecular photobiology of UVA. In: Urbach F, Gange RW (eds) The biological effects of UVA radiation. Praeger, New York, pp 42–52
Potapenko A (1991) Mechanisms of photodynamic effects of furocoumarins. J Photochem Photobiol B 9:1–33
Schmitz S, Garbe C, Tebbe B, Orfanos CE (1994) Langwellige ultraviolette Strahlung (UVA) und Hautkrebs. Hautarzt 45:517–525
Spikes JD (1991) The origin and meaning of the term "photodynamic" (as used in "photodynamic therapy", for example). J Photochem Photobiol B 9:369–374
Thomas JP, Girotti AW (1988) Photooxidation of cell membranes in the presence of hematoporphyrin derivative: reactivity of phospholipid and cholesterol hydroperoxides with glutathione peroxidase. Biochim Biophys Acta 962:297–307
Thomas PD, Poznansky MJ (1990) A modifid tetramethylbenzidine method for measuring lipid hydroperoxides. Anal Biochem 188:228–232
Thomas SM, Jessup W, Gebicki JM, Dean RT (1989) A continuous-flow automated assay for iodometric estimation of hydroperoxides. Anal Biochem 176:353–359
Yamamoto Y, Frei B, Ames BN (1990) Assay of lipid hydroperoxides using high-performance liquid chromatography with isoluminal chemiluminescence detection. Methods Enzymol 186:371–380

Dall'Acqua F, Martelli P (1991) Photosensitizing action of furocoumarins on membrane components and consequent intracellular events. J Photochem Photobiol B 8:235–254

Frankel EN, Neff WE, Weisleder D (1990) Determination of methyl linoleate hydroperoxides by ^{13}C nuclear magnetic resonance spectroscopy. Methods Enzymol 186:380–387

Frimer AA (1985) Singlet O₂. CRC Press, Boca Raton

Girotti AW (1990) Lipid peroxidation in photodynamic systems. In: Vigo-Pelfrey C (ed) Membrane lipid peroxidation. CRC Press, Boca Raton, pp 203–218

[illegible]

[illegible]

*Analysis of N-*ras *Mutations in Human Cutaneous Melanoma: Tumor Heterogeneity Detected by Polymerase Chain Reaction/Single-Stranded Conformation Polymorphism Analysis*

A. van Elsas[1], S. Zerp[1], S. van der Flier[1], M. Krüse-Wolters[1], A. Vacca[2], D.J. Ruiter[3], and P. Schrier[1]

[1] Department of Clinical Oncology, University Hospital, P.O. Box 9600, 2300 RC Leiden, The Netherlands
[2] Department of Biomedical Sciences and Human Oncology, School of Medicine, Bari, Italy
[3] Department of Pathology, University Hospital, Nijmegen, The Netherlands

Abstract

Determination of the activation state of oncogenes as well as tumor suppressor genes is a main subject of interest in the analysis of the mechanism of tumor initiation. In human melanoma, the c-*myc* and N-*ras* oncogenes have been found to be activated in approximately 50% and 15% of the analyzed material, respectively. These studies have mostly been done on fresh tumor material or cell lines. Only in a few cases has an attempt been made to look at tumor heterogeneity or clonality with respect to the activation of oncogenes. We have adjusted the polymerase chain reaction (PCR)/single-stranded conformation polymorphism analysis (SSCP) technique to screen paraffin-embedded melanoma material for the presence of N-*ras* mutations and found genetic defects at particular progression stages. In one melanoma of the skin, we were able to sublocalize an N-*ras* mutation in the intraepidermal tumor part, that was absent in the part deeply invading the dermal layer. We conclude that a thorough investigation of N-*ras* activation in human melanoma should include analysis of histologically different parts of the tumor.

Introduction

Genetic analysis of many forms of human cancer has led to the concept that aberrant expression of oncogenes and inactivation of tumor suppressor genes are causally involved in tumor initiation and progression (Bishop 1991; Weinberg 1991; Fearon and Vogelstein 1990). Oncogenes exert crucial tasks in the regulation of growth and differentiation of normal cells at diverse levels, such as signal transduction and transcription regulation. Deregulation of oncogene function ("activation") may occur through point mutation or overexpression, thereby potentially leading to uncontrolled cell

Recent Results in Cancer Research, Vol. 139

growth. Tumor suppressor genes in normal cells are equally important in the modulation of proliferation, for instance by providing for negative regulatory signals in the cell cycle. In this case, inactivation of the gene product may contribute to tumor development.

Several oncogenes have been implicated in the induction and progression of human melanoma. Overexpression of c-*myc* has been reported to occur in half of the melanoma cell lines analyzed (Alitalo et al. 1987; Versteeg et al. 1988), whereas the N-*ras* oncogene was also found to be activated by a point mutation in 6%–19% of the analyzed material (primary, metastatic, and cell lines; Van't Veer et al. 1989; Bos 1989). We have shown that a primary tumor can be divided into at least two different cell populations on the basis of the occurrence of two different point mutations in the N-*ras* gene which have metastasized to different locations (Van't Veer et al. 1989). This observation suggested that N-*ras* activation in this tumor was a relatively late event in the oncogenic transformation of the melanocytic cell, preceding the formation of a macroscopic tumor mass and leading to two different mutations in distinct daughter cells.

In an attempt to further characterize the importance of N-*ras* activations in human melanoma development, we analyzed a number of melanoma materials, both fresh and paraffin-embedded biopsies. The combination of a crude DNA extraction of pathologically subdivided tumor parts and polymerase chain reaction (PCR)/single-stranded conformation polymorphism (SSCP) analysis (Orita et al. 1989a; Murakami et al. 1991; Pelletier et al. 1991) resulted in the identification of a superficial spreading melanoma with an N-*ras* mutation in the intraepidermal population that was absent in the deeply invading tumor cells. These data suggest that the adapted PCR-SSCP technique in parallel with histological analysis allows for sensitive detection of point mutations in distinct regions of melanoma tumors.

Materials and Methods

Collection of Tumor Material

Paraffin slides of melanoma material were collected through a collaborative study on N-*ras* mutations in human melanoma in the EORTC melanoma group. Tumor samples had been routinely fixed and paraffin embedded. Slides of 5- to 10-μm thickness were cut, H-E stained, and examined for diagnosis, proportion of tumor cells, and sublocalization of different progression stages, wherever possible.

DNA Extraction and Polymerase Chain Reaction/Single-Stranded Conformation Polymorphism Analysis

Tissue pooled from two or three slides was deparaffinized using xylene extraction. Xylene was removed by alcohol washes and the tissue pellet dehydrated with acetone. Protein was digested in 100 μl PK2 buffer (10 m*M* Tris pH 8.3, 1 m*M* EDTA, 0.5% Tween-20) containing 50 μg proteinase K/ml (Boehringer, Mannheim, Germany) overnight at 56°C. The resulting mixture was heated to 95°C for 5 min, stored on ice for 15 min, and cleared by centrifugation. Soluble material was further purified according to Boom et al. (1990). Briefly, DNA was adsorbed to silica preparations (Janssen Chimica, Beersse, Belgium) in guanidiumthiocyanate-containing buffer, washed, and eluted in 10 m*M* Tris pH 8, 1 m*M* EDTA at 56°C. This material was stored at 4°C. The DNA extract (0.5–3 μl) was used for amplification of N-*ras*-specific exon 1 and 2 sequences using the following primers: for exon 1 5′-GACTGAGTACAAACTGGTGG-3′ and 5′-GGGCCTCAC CTCTAGGTG-3′ were used yielding a fragment of 118 bp; for exon 2 a 103-bp fragment was generated using 5′-GGTGAAACCTGTTTGTTGGA-3′ and 5′-ATACACAGAGGAAGCCTTCG-3′ (Suzuki et al. 1990). The 20 μl amplification mixture further consisted of 250 μ*M* dATP, dTTP, dGTP, 50 μ*M* dCTP (Pharmacia, Woerden, the Netherlands), 500 n*M* of each primer, 0.04 units of Tth polymerase, 2 μl 10X buffer (Sphaero Q, Leiden the Netherlands), and 0.4 μCi dCTP (Amersham, Little Chalfont, England; 3000 Ci/mmol). Cycling was performed using the following program: 4 min 95°C, 36 cycles (30 s 95°C, 60 s 50°C, 30 s 72°C), 5 min 72°C. Four microliters of the amplified mixture was mixed with gel-loading buffer without NaOH. Half of this solution was denatured at 95°C for 4 min and loaded next to the nondenatured sample onto an 8% polyacrylamide gel, containing either 10% glycerol and 1 × TBE or 5% glycerol and 0.5 × TBE. Gels were run for 4–6 h at 30 W and room temperature. Vacuum-dried gels were exposed to Fuji RX X-ray film for 6–72 h.

Sequence Analysis and Spot Blot Hybridization

The DNA extract was reamplified for sequence analysis as described above using 250 μ*M* of each dNTP. The PCR fragment was gel purified using the Mermaid procedure (Stratagene, La Jolla, USA). Ten to 50 ng of this fragment was sequenced using γ-^{32}P-labeled primers and the T7 system (Pharmacia).

For quantification purposes, 1 μl DNA extract was spotted onto GeneScreen filter (Dupont NEN, Boston, USA) and dried. Hybridization with a probe specific for human *alu* repeat sequences (pBLUR8) (Jelinek et al. 1980) was done overnight at 65°C. After three consecutive washes in 6 ×

SSC, 2 × SSC, 0.1 × SSC/0.1% sodium dodecyl sulfate (SDS) at 65°C, the filter was exposed to Fuji RX X-ray film.

Results

*Optimization of DNA Extraction and Polymerase Chain Reaction Conditions for Single-Stranded Conformation Polymorphism Analysis of N-***ras**

The quality and amount of genomic DNA extracted from paraffin slides is crucial for a successful PCR result. Several DNA isolation procedures were tested for their yield in amplifiable material (Goelz et al. 1985; Shibata et al. 1988; von Weizsacker et al. 1991). First, it was found that through phenol/chloroform extractions of crude DNA solutions most DNA was lost. Second, the crude isolate may contain pollutants that interfere with efficient amplification. For melanotic melanoma samples, we found that in the presence of melanin, the N-*ras* fragments could only be generated if the DNA extract was strongly diluted. To overcome this problem, we purified the DNA extract employing silica preparations that specifically bind nucleic acids. Contaminations were removed by several washes of the silica-bound DNA (Boom et al. 1990), which highly improved PCR efficiency (not shown).

As opposed to the use of end-labeled PCR primers (Orita et al. 1989b), radiolabeled deoxycytidine triphosphate (dCTP) was incorporated during amplification to detect PCR fragments on SSCP gels. At a fivefold decreased amount of unlabeled dCTP (50 μM; Fig. 1a, every third lane) as compared to the other nucleotides (250 μM), a maximal incorporation of α-^{32}P-dCTP was found, whereas with further dilutions of the unlabeled dCTP, an increasing amount of aberrant fragments was generated (Fig. 1a, right lanes). Since it is difficult to standardize the DNA yield from paraffin slides, we next tested whether the amount of genomic DNA extracted was predictive of PCR efficiency for the N-*ras* exon 1 and 2 fragments. A series of isolates from paraffin-embedded material was spotted onto a nylon membrane and hybridized with a radiolabeled probe specific for human *alu* repeat sequences (Jelinek et al. 1980). A DNA extract from melanoma cell line IGR39D (Schrier et al. 1991) with known concentration was applied as a reference. One microliter of the extract was used for a PCR-SSCP analysis of N-*ras* exon 1 fragment (118 bp). As shown in Fig. 1b, PCR yield was not obviously related to the DNA concentration, since some samples showed excellent amplification with a DNA content less than 1 ng per μl (e.g., 164, 203, 204), whereas two other samples containing 10 ng/μl or more did not (157, 165). Contaminants probably determine PCR yield in general. Finally, we found that the length of the PCR product was reciprocally related to PCR efficiency, reflecting the degree of degradation in this paraffin-embedded material (not shown).

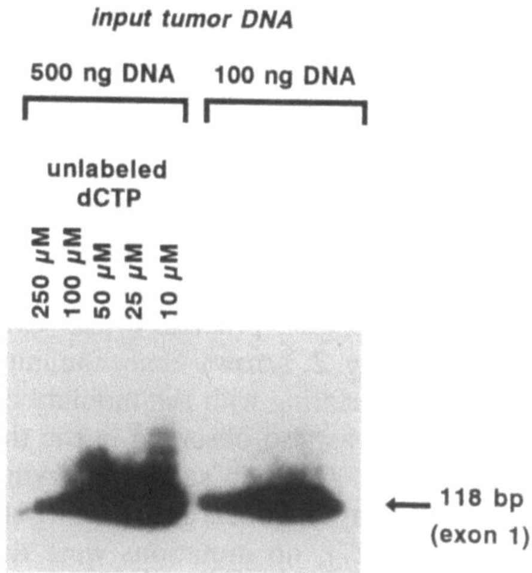

a

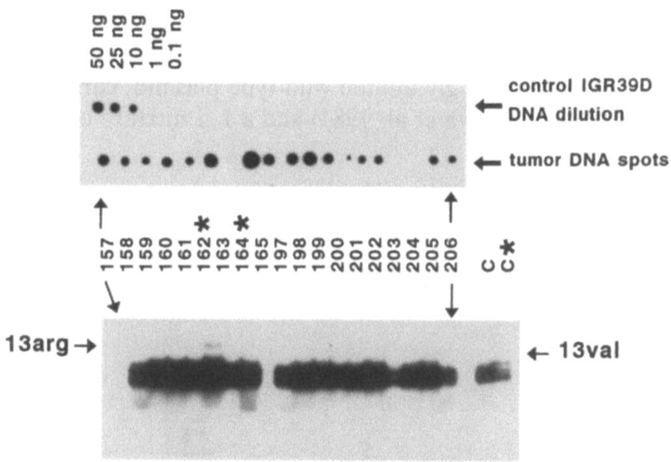

b

Fig. 1a,b. Detection of polymerase chain reaction (PRC)-amplified N-*ras* sequences in paraffin-embedded melanoma materials. **a** PCR reactions were performed at different concentrations of deoxycytidine triphosphate (dCTP) as indicated. The amount of α-^{32}P-dCTP was kept constant. **b** DNA was purified from 19 different paraffin-embedded tumors. One microliter was quantified by hybridization to the human *alu* sequence-specific probe pBLUR8 and comparison to a series of dilutions with known DNA concentration. Another microliter was used for PCR/single-stranded conformation polymorphism (SSCP) analysis of N-*ras* exon 1. Samples are indicated by *numbers*, mutations by an *asterisk*, and shifting bands by *arrows*

Single-Stranded Conformation Polymorphism Analysis of Mutations

To investigate the reliability of our technique, we next tested a series of melanoma samples with known N-*ras* status (Van't Veer et al. 1989). From one patient several metastasized tumors were analyzed (86047-1 to -5) together with normal liver DNA. All metastases were previously shown to carry a C to A mutation in codon 61 of the N-*ras* gene. As compared to the control amplification of two plasmids containing the wild-type N-*ras* exon 2 sequences (pNras, pNras13V), an extra single-stranded conformation was observed (Fig. 2, arrow). Since the mutation was present in both strands and possibly interfering with the mobility of all formed tertiary conformations, a slight shift was also observed in the three other single-stranded bands (Fig. 2, asterisk). Another sample carrying the same base transition (Fig. 2, 88010) displays identical gel mobility shifts. In two remaining tumor samples (84007, 85027), no mutations were detected in exon 2. Similar tests were carried out using samples containing exon 1 aberrations. All previously established mutations were detected in our PCR-SSCP system (not shown).

The SSCP gel shown in Fig. 1b is representative for the sensitivity of the analysis. The two right lanes (C and C*) were loaded with amplification product from strongly diluted wild-type plasmid, carrying the genomic N-*ras* gene (pNras; Brown et al. 1984) and a 1:1 mixture of wild-type and 13gly →

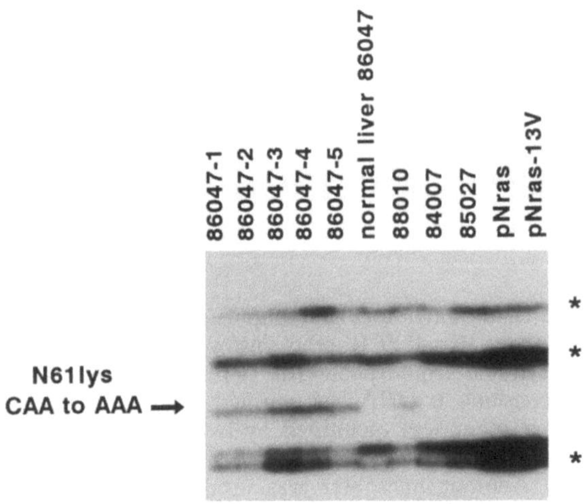

Fig. 2. Polymerase chain reaction (PCR)/single-stranded conformation polymorphism (SSCP) analysis of N-*ras* mutations in human melanoma material. PCR-SSCP analysis of exon 2 N-*ras* was performed as described in "Methods". From patient 86047, five different metastases were included (*lanes 1–5*), as well as normal liver biopsy material (*lane 6*). Samples 88010, 84007, and 85027 (*lanes 7–9*) were derived from different patients. Plasmids pNras (*C, lane 10*: wild-type human genomic N-*ras*) and pNras13V (*C**, *lane 11*: 13-Gly → Val N-*ras*) were amplified as controls

val mutant plasmid (pNras13V). One strand of the point-mutated fragment (position 2, G → T) clearly shifted up (13val). Two samples (162, 164) from the series of isolates applied showed another mutation in codon 13 (position 1 G → C), which leads to a different shift (13arg). A possible pitfall of the SSCP analysis is exemplified by the observation that a second gel run under different conditions (twice as much glycerol and TBE) did not show these mutation-specific shifts (not shown). Wild-type alleles were almost always strongly present, since separation of tumor cells from normal skin or stroma cells is not feasible.

*Differential N-*ras* Mutation Analysis*

We analyzed a primary melanoma section from a superficial spreading melanoma (left side of the back), 2-mm Breslow thickness and Clark level IV. This primary tumor was removed and the sections allowed for the separation of intraepidermal (microinvasive) tumor cells and cells progressively invading the dermal layer. A mutation in exon 2 of N-*ras* was detected by SSCP (Fig. 3a) and sequenced. A CAA to CTA transition was found in codon 61, whereas the normal allele was also present (Fig. 3b). This may either indicate a heterozygous mutation, biclonality with respect to the N-*ras* mutation status, or contamination with normal cells. Surprisingly, the mutation was only present in the intraepidermal tumor part. This may argue for biclonality of the tumor with respect to N-*ras* mutation, resulting in cell populations with and without an N-*ras* mutation. Another explanation

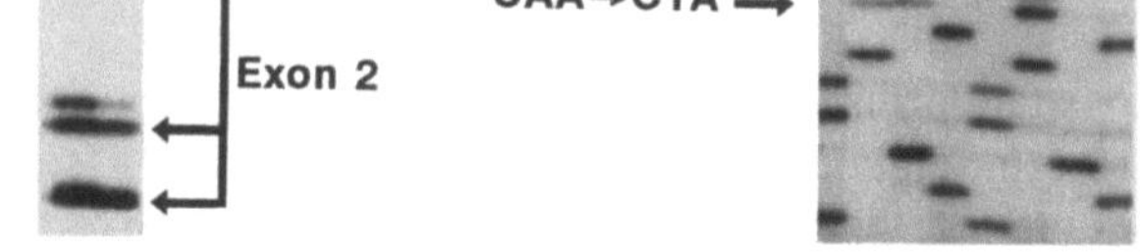

Fig. 3. Sublocalization of mutant N-*ras* to a noninvasive part of a melanoma tumor. Tumor 60 was histologically subdivided as melanoma in situ (60A; noninvasive part), and a progressive region (60B; invasive part). By histological criteria, 60A consisted of the shoulder region of a superficial spreading melanoma Clark II (approximately 10% tumor cells in the isolated sample), whereas 60B was Clark III-IV (±80% tumor cells). *Left*, polymerase chain reaction (PCR)/single-stranded conformation polymorphism analysis of exon 2 sequences. *Right*, sequence analysis of 60A and 60B. Normal N-*ras* encodes CAA (Gln) in codon 61

would be that the mutation is present in the normal surrounding skin tissue, since this particular region of the slide contained only approximately 10% tumor cells, whereas the invasive region consisted of 80% tumor cells. This possibility, though, is considered to be highly unlikely, since normal cells have never been found to carry a mutant *ras* allele.

Discussion

*Sensitivity of Single-Stranded Conformation Polymorphism Analysis of N-***ras** *Mutations*

Analysis of *ras* oncogene mutations in tumor material can be performed using several techniques, such as direct sequencing (Tada et al. 1990), restriction enzyme polymorphism analysis (Mitsudomi et al. 1991), RNAse protection (Forrester et al. 1987), denaturing gradient gel electrophoresis (DGGE; Myers et al. 1987), and oligonucleotide hybridization (Verlaan-de Vries et al. 1986). These procedures share a disadvantage with the SSCP analysis, as they are dependent upon PCR efficiency and therefore upon DNA quality. It has been reported that RNAse protection analysis does not detect all possible point mutations (Myers et al. 1985), and restriction enzyme polymorphism analysis and oligonucleotide hybridization are elaborate and time consuming. The use of DGGE requires extended PCR primer pairs and specialized material to create exact gradients, but otherwise renders very accurate results. We chose PCR-SSCP analysis for the detection of N-*ras* gene mutations for its simplicity and efficiency (O'Rahilly et al. 1991).

Making use of a DNA purification method based upon the binding of DNA to silica preparations, we were able to generate a very sensitive PCR-SSCP system. Accuracy of SSCP was checked in a series of melanoma materials with known mutations. All lesions previously identified by oligonucleotide hybridization (Van't Veer et al. 1989) were readily detectable.

*Heterogeneity with Respect to N-***ras**

A standardized protocol was developed to analyze N-*ras* mutations in paraffin-embedded archival material. First, a section was microscopically examined, and when heterogeneity was observed the tumor was divided in distinct parts. In one such case (invasive superficial spreading melanoma), discrepancy of N-*ras* mutation status between two different tumor stages was detected: a mutant allele (N61-leu) present in the shoulder region of the tumor, whereas it was absent from the deeply invading tumor cells. This implies that the N-*ras* mutation occurred relatively early in development of this particular lesion, because at least two primary tumor cell populations with distinct N-*ras* mutation status were likely present and had grown out.

Since it is generally assumed that *ras* mutations at position 61 activate the protein and lead to transformation (Land et al. 1983) or progression (Fearon and Vogelstein 1990), our finding on the presence of the mutation in the intraepidermal tumor part only is surprising. It argues against a role of N-*ras* in the invasive progression of this particular tumor. Apparently, cells in the heterogeneous primary tumor without the *ras* mutation have acquired properties to deeply invade the dermal layer independent of the *ras* status (Waghorne et al. 1988). The N-*ras* mutation that was found in the microinvasive part of the primary tumor could have been induced through ultraviolet irradiation (UVR; Van der Lubbe et al. 1988; Pierceall and Ananthaswamy 1991; Pierceall et al. 1992), since the DNA sequence in the opposite strand of the mutation in N-*ras* contains tentative pyrimidine dimerization sites (Dobetsky et al. 1987). The fact that the mutation was detected in a sample consisting of 10% tumor cells only stresses the high sensitivity of the PCR-SSCP method. Using this technique we are currently extending our previous observation that N-*ras* activation in cutaneous malignant melanoma may have occurred through UVR (Van't Veer et al. 1989).

References

Alitalo K, Koskinen P, Makela TP, Saksela K, Sistonen L, Winqvist R (1987) myc oncogenes: activation and amplification. Biochim Biophys Acta 907:1–32

Bishop JM (1991) Molecular themes in oncogenesis. Cell 64:235–248

Boom R, Sol CJ, Salimans MM, Jansen CL, Wertheim van Dillen PM, van der Noordaa J (1990) Rapid and simple method for purification of nucleic acids. J Clin Microbiol 28:495–503

Bos JL (1989) ras oncogenes in human cancer: a review. Cancer Res 49:4682–4689

Brown R, Marshall CJ, Pennie SG, Hall A (1984) Mechanism of activation of an N-ras gene in the human fibrosarcoma cell line HT1080. EMBO J 3:1321–1326

Dobetsky EA, Grosovsky AJ, Glickman BW (1987) The specificity of UV-induced mutations at an endogenous locus in mammalian cells. Proc Natl Acad Sci USA 84:9103–9107

Fearon ER, Vogelstein B (1990) A genetic model for colorectal tumorigenesis. Cell 61:759–767

Forrester K, Almoguera C, Han K, Grizzle WE, Perucho M (1987) Detection of high incidence of K-ras oncogenes during human colon tumorigenesis. Nature 327:298–303

Goelz SE, Hamilton SR, Vogelstein B (1985) Purification of DNA from formaldehyde fixed and paraffin embedded human tissue. Biochem Biophys Res Commun 130:118–126

Jelinek WR, Toomey TP, Leinwand L, Duncan CH, Biro PA, Choudary PV, Weissman SM, Rubin CM, Houck CM, Deininger PL, Schmid CW (1980) Ubiquitous, interspersed repeated sequences in mammalian genomes. Proc Natl Acad Sci USA 77:1398–1402

Land H, Parada LF, Weinberg RA (1983) Tumorigenic conversion of primary embryo fibroblasts requires at least two cooperating oncogenes. Nature 304: 596–602

Mitsudomi T, Viallet J, Mulshine JL, Linnoila RI, Minna JD, Gazdar AF (1991) Mutations of ras genes distinguish a subset of non-small-cell lung cancer cell lines from small-cell lung cancer cell lines. Oncogene 6:1353–1362

Murakami Y, Hayashi K, Sekiya T (1991) Detection of aberrations of the p53 alleles and the gene transcript in human tumor cell lines by single-strand conformation polymorphism analysis. Cancer Res 51:3356–3361

Myers RM, Lumelsky N, Lerman LS, Maniatis T (1985) Detection of single base substitutions in total genomic DNA. Nature 313:495–498

Myers RM, Maniatis T, Lerman LS (1987) Detection and localization of single base changes by denaturing gradient gel electrophoresis. Methods Enzymol 155: 501–527

O'Rahilly S, Choi WH, Patel P, Turner RC, Flier JS, Moller DE (1991) Detection of mutations in insulin-receptor gene in NIDDM patients by analysis of single-stranded conformation polymorphisms. Diabetes 40:777–782

Orita M, Iwahana H, Kanazawa H, Hayashi K, Sekiya T (1989a) Detection of polymorphisms of human DNA by gel electrophoresis as single-strand conformation polymorphisms. Proc Natl Acad Sci USA 86:2766–2770

Orita M, Suzuki Y, Sekiya T, Hayashi K (1989b) Rapid and sensitive detection of point mutations and DNA polymorphisms using the polymerase chain reaction. Genomics 5:874–879

Pelletier J, Bruening W, Kashtan CE, Mauer SM, Manivel JC, Striegel JE, Houghton DC, Junien C, Habib R, Fouser L, Fine RN, Silverman BL, Haber DA, Housman D (1991) Germline mutations in the Wilms' tumor suppressor gene are associated with abnormal urogenital development in Denys-Drash syndrome. Cell 67:437–447

Pierceall WE, Ananthaswamy HN (1991) Transformation of NIH3T3 cells by transfection with UV-irradiated human c-Ha-ras-1 proto-oncogene DNA. Oncogene 6:2085–2091

Pierceall WE, Kripke ML, Ananthaswamy HN (1992) N-ras mutation in ultraviolet radiation-induced murine skin cancers. Cancer Res 52:3946–3951

Schrier PI, Versteeg R, Peltenburg LTC, Plomp AC, Van't Veer LJ, Krüse-Wolters KM (1991) Sensitivity of melanoma cell lines to natural killer cells: a role for oncogene-modulated HLA expression? Semin Cancer Biol 2:73–83

Shibata DK, Arnheim N, Martin WJ (1988) Detection of human papilloma virus in paraffin-embedded tissue using the polymerase chain reaction. J Exp Med 167: 225–230

Suzuki Y, Orita M, Shiraishi M, Hayashi K, Sekiya T (1990) Detection of ras gene mutations in human lung cancers by single-strand conformation polymorphism analysis of polymerase chain reaction products. Oncogene 5:1037–1043

Tada M, Omata M, Ohto M (1990) Analysis of ras gene mutations in human hepatic malignant tumors by polymerase chain reaction and direct sequencing. Cancer Res 50:1121–1124

Van der Lubbe JL, Rosdorff HJ, Bos JL, Van der Eb AJ (1988) Activation of N-ras induced by ultraviolet irradiation in vitro. Oncogene Res 3:9–20

Van't Veer LJ, Burgering BMTh, Versteeg R, Boot AJM, Ruiter DJ, Osanto S, Schrier PI, Bos JL (1989) N-ras mutations in human cutaneous melanoma on sun-exposed body sites. Mol Cell Biol 9:3114–3116

Verlaan-de Vries M, Bogaard ME, Van den Elst H, Van Boom JH, Van der Eb AJ, Bos JL (1986) A dot-blot screening procedure for mutated ras oncogenes using synthetic oligodeoxynucleotides. Gene 50:313–320

Versteeg R, Noordermeer IA, Krüse-Wolters KM, Ruiter DJ, Schrier PI (1988) c-myc downregulates class I HLA expression in human melanomas. EMBO J 7:1023–1029 von Weizsacker F, Labeit S, Koch HK, Oehlert W, Gerok W, Blum HE (1991) A simple and rapid method for the detection of RNA in formalin-fixed, paraffin-embedded tissues by PCR amplification. Biochem Biophys Res Commun 174: 176–180

Waghorne C, Thomas M, Lagarde A, Kerbel RS, Breitman ML (1988) Genetic evidence for positive selection and overgrowth of primary tumors by metastatic cell subpopulations. Cancer Res 48:6109–6114

Weinberg RA (1991) Tumor suppressor genes. Science 254:1138–1146

Skin Cancer and Warts in Immunosuppressed Renal Transplant Recipients

I.M. Leigh[1,2] and M.T. Glover[1,2]

[1] Department of Dermatology, Royal London Hospital Trust, London E1 1BB, UK
[2] ICRF Skin Tumour Laboratory, London Hospital Medical College, 56 Ashfield Street, London E1 2BL, UK

Abstract

Non-melanoma skin cancer (NMSC) is increasingly recognised as a complication of long-term immunosuppression and has been particularly studied in renal transplant recipients (RTR). A population study of renal transplant recipients has been performed with analysis of those features contributing to a high rate of detection of NMSC, such that 40% patients with fair skin have NMSC 5 years after transplantation. 90% of the total patient population have warts 5 years after transplantation, many being atypical and in sun-exposed sites. Therefore, contributory factors in these patients include not only the global immunosuppression, ultraviolet radiation (UVR)-induced mutagenesis and photoimmunosuppression, but also the widespread presence of human papillomavirus (HPV) infection, including the unusual epidermodysplasia verruciformis (EV)-associated cutaneous oncogenic HPV.

Introduction

Basal cell carcinomas (BCC) and squamous cell carcinomas (SCC) of the skin are an enormous clinical problem in fair-skinned populations, and in the United States alone more than 500 000 new cases are diagnosed annually. The mortality from non-melanoma skin cancers (NMSC) is low compared to other malignancies, but both mortality and incidence are rising and affecting younger people. Major risk factors include the total amount of cumulative ultraviolet (UV) irradiation, particularly in patients working out of doors; this risk is increased by fair skin which burns easily and reduced by increased pigmentation, such that patients of colour have a much lower risk of NMSC.

Ultraviolet (UV) B radiation (280–320 nm) appears to be the wavelength most responsible for induction of most skin cancers. UVA can cause skin

Recent Results in Cancer Research, Vol. 139

cancer in animals, when given in high doses (Strickland 1986), but UVC is usually filtered out by the ozone layer in the stratosphere. UV radiation produces a particular type of DNA damage when photoadduction produces pyrimidine dimers (cyclobutane type) and pyrimidine (6-4) pyrimidone lesions (Brash 1988). These UV-induced photoproducts are normally preferentially excised from transcriptionally active chromatin by DNA repair mechanisms. The mutation and transformation of the cells following UV-induced damage depends on the efficiency of DNA repair (Friedberg 1985). When individuals are deficient in the ability to repair pyrimidine dimers, as in xeroderma pigmentosum, then transformation and tumour development is more likely to occur (Cleaver and Bootsma 1975).

Human papillomaviruses (HPV) are small, double-stranded DNA viruses with more than 60 subtypes (de Villiers 1989). The high-risk genital HPV16 and HPV18 are implicated in cervical carcinoma (Zur Hausen 1991) and significantly associated with skin cancer in the anogenital region, but seldom in non-genital skin (Piercall et al. 1991). The major association of HPV with NMSC occurs in the uncommon hereditary skin condition epidermodysplasia verruciformis (EV), when patients develop atypical warts and subsequently skin cancer in sun-exposed sites (Lutzner et al. 1984). This structurally distinct subset of HPV is therefore known as EV-HPV (Pfister 1984; Fuchs and Pfister 1990). These viruses have also been found occasionally in the skin and mucosal malignancies, which have been reported in immunosuppressed individuals to be occurring at a much higher rate than in the normal population. The number of epidermal tumours appears to rise with increasing time from transplantation (Table 1). We therefore undertook a population study of all individuals attending the Royal London Hospital renal transplant service to determine the presence of cutaneous warts and skin cancer.

Table 1. Percentage of renal transplant recipients with epidermal tumours

Reference	Time since transplantation (years)	Percentage
Hardie et al. (1980)	>1	3
Hardie et al. (1980)	>9	44
Bencini (1983)	<5	12.5
Bencini (1983)	>5	24
Boyle et al. (1984)	2–5	4
Boyle et al. (1984)	9	36
Barr et al. (1989)	<5	1.5
Barr et al. (1989)	>5	12

Clinical Survey

All patients who had surviving renal allografts attending the regional transplant service at the Royal London Hospital were given an appointment to attend the skin clinic, but poor attendance resulted in patients being examined in the renal transplant clinic. All patients were examined by a dermatologist and the site and distribution of skin lesions documented. All lesions thought to be potentially malignant, and any indurated or inflamed warts were removed and examined histologically by a pathologist. Tissue was also taken for immunocytochemistry, for viral typing and for tissue culture. Findings from these studies will be reported separately. Our initial findings indicated the need for regular dermatological review and frequent surgery, so an extra weekly clinic was set up in the skin department, running concurrently with the transplant clinic, to encourage regular attendence by the patients.

Patient Characteristics

A total of 291 patients were examined (Table 2). The mean age of patients at the time of transplantation was 36.9 year (range, 3.7–65.5 years). Mean duration of transplantation at the time of examination was 57.4 months (range, 3–260 months) and mean duration of dialysis preceding transplantation was 47.5 months (range, 0–263 months). The 94 (33%) patients transplanted before 1985 received immunosuppression with 1.5 mg azathioprine/kg and 10 mg prednisolone daily. The 197 (67%) patients transplanted since 1985 also receive cyclosporin A at a dose producing a blood level of 100–200 μg/l. These patients had not received systematic advice on sun avoidance.

Presence of Warts

A total of 59% of the patients had warts (Fig. 1). There was an increased prevalence of warts with increasing time from transplantation such that by 5

Table 2. Patient characteristics

Characteristics	
Total population (n)	291
Mean age at transplantation	37 years
Median duration of transplantation	42 months
Number with viral warts	172 (59%)
Number of patients with NMSC	62

NMSC, non-melanomatous skin cancer.

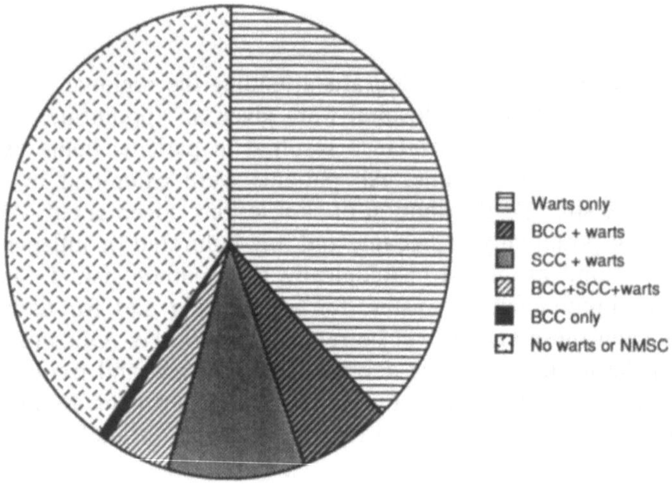

Fig. 1. Warts and non-melanoma skin cancer in 291 renal transplant recipients. *BCC*, basal cell carcinoma; *SCC*, squamous cell carcinoma

years after transplantation 90% of the patients had warts. The prevalence of warts was not related to skin type (unlike NMSC). In patients who had undergone transplantation less than 5 years before, the warts were most commonly palmoplantar and generally few in number. In older patients and those who had undergone transplantation more than 5 years before, there was a tendency to develop flat warts on sun-exposed skin, particularly over the backs of the hands (Fig. 2a). In patients with fair skin and a history of moderate or high sun exposure, these warts were confluent in places. In enthusiastic sunbathers, sheeted warts could be seen over the trunk, the limbs, and the dorsa of the feet. Male patients tended to develop sheets of warts in the beard area (Fig. 2b). The sheeted and flat warts were often not recognised by the patients, who regarded them as merely "dry skin".

Illustrative Case History

A 49-year-old telephone engineer developed end-stage renal failure as a result of chronic glomerulonephritis in 1978. After 3 years' haemodialysis, at the age of 35, he had a cadaveric renal transplant. He received maintenance immunosuppression with 125 mg azathioprine/day and 10 mg prednisolone/day. He continued to work out of doors full-time and sunbathed whenever possible. He was first seen in the dermatology department in 1991, 10 years post-transplant. He had type II skin. There were very numerous flat warts over his trunk, arms, backs of the hands, legs and dorsa of the feet. The warts were particularly striking in the V of the neck (Fig. 2c). Histology of a

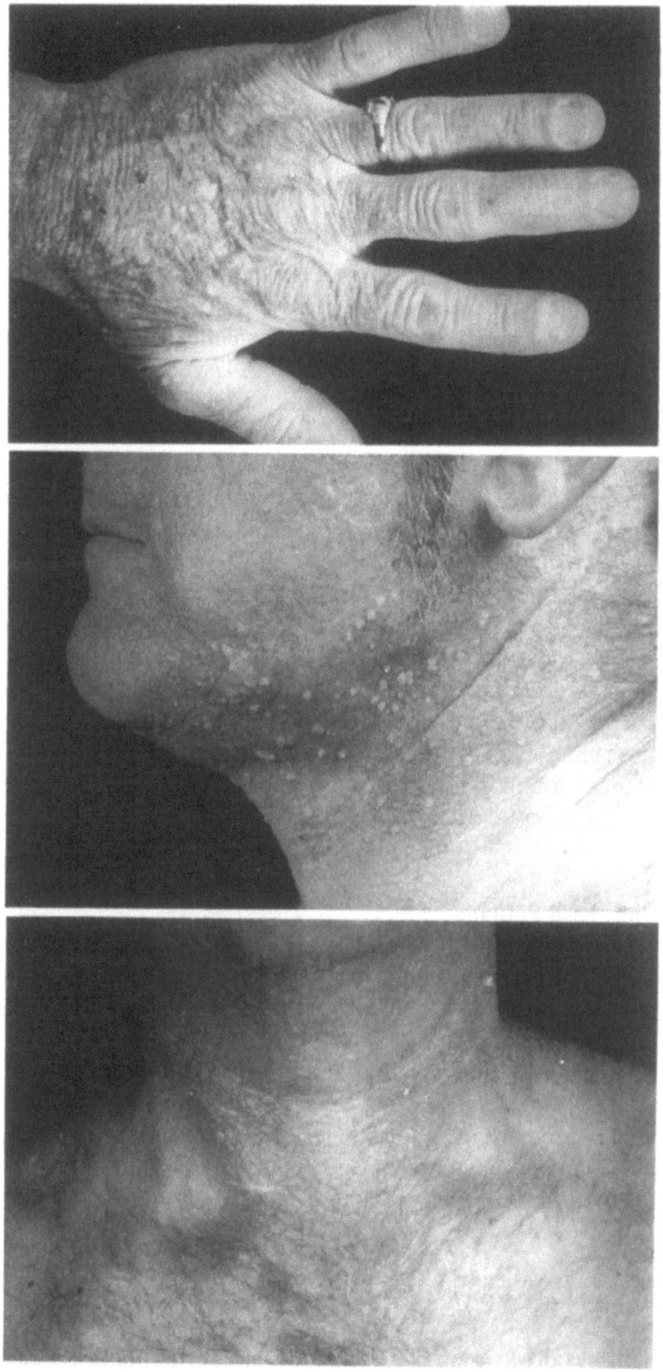

a

b

c

Fig. 2a–c. Warty lesions in renal transplant recipients. **a** Dorsal hand showing a mixture of flat warts and warty keratoses. **b** Widespread warts spread around beard area by shaving. **c** Confluent warts in V of neck of frequent sunbather lesion on the back of the hand showed SCC. Biopsies from the thigh and the V of neck showed basal dysplasia. Over the past year the warts have increased in number and those on sun-exposed sites have become thicker.

Non-melanoma Skin Cancer

One or more NMSC was diagnosed in 62 patients (Fig. 1). The presence of lesions was dependent on skin type, as only 30% of all patients who had undergone transplantation 5 years before had NMSC, but selecting patients with types I and II skin gave a prevalence of 40% NMSC at 5 years. The mean age of onset of skin cancer was 47 years (range, 30–67 years). During the course of this study we removed BCC or SCC from 41 patients which had not been previously noted by the patient or by their own physicians.

A total of 43 patients had a total of 75 invasive SCC and 57 in situ SCC. In some patients new tumours would appear over a period of 2–3 weeks. The SCC generally presented as inflamed or indurated keratotic lesions, often arising within warty areas, most frequently on the back of the hand (Fig. 3a). SCC were sometimes clinically similar to warts (Fig. 3b,c), though usually with an indurated base. Kerato-acanthoma-like lesions were removed from five patients. Like the SCC, these usually arose from warty areas, and they were difficult to distinguish from SCC histologically.

A total of 35 patients developed a total of 65 BCC. Only two patients had more than five BCC each. The BCC were clinically and histologically similar to those found in non-immunosuppressed patients, predominantly appearing, on sun-exposed areas; 12 of the BCC patients also had SCC.

High-Risk Patients

Eight patients had extensive areas of epidermal dysplasia, particularly over the backs of the hands, the forearms and the forehead, with multiple invasive and in situ SCC and rapidly growing and recurring lesions (Fig. 3d). Four have needed excision and grafting of the dorsa of both hands (Glover et al. 1994b). Eight patients are taking long-term etretinate to limit the rate of development of dysplastic lesions. A total of 15 patients present particular problems in management and require examination at 4- to 8-week intervals for identification and treatment of new tumours.

Typical Case History

A 44-year-old man with chronic glomerulonephritis received a cadaveric renal transplant at the age of 22, after 3 months of haemodialysis. Nine years later, because of chronic rejection, he returned to dialysis for 5 years

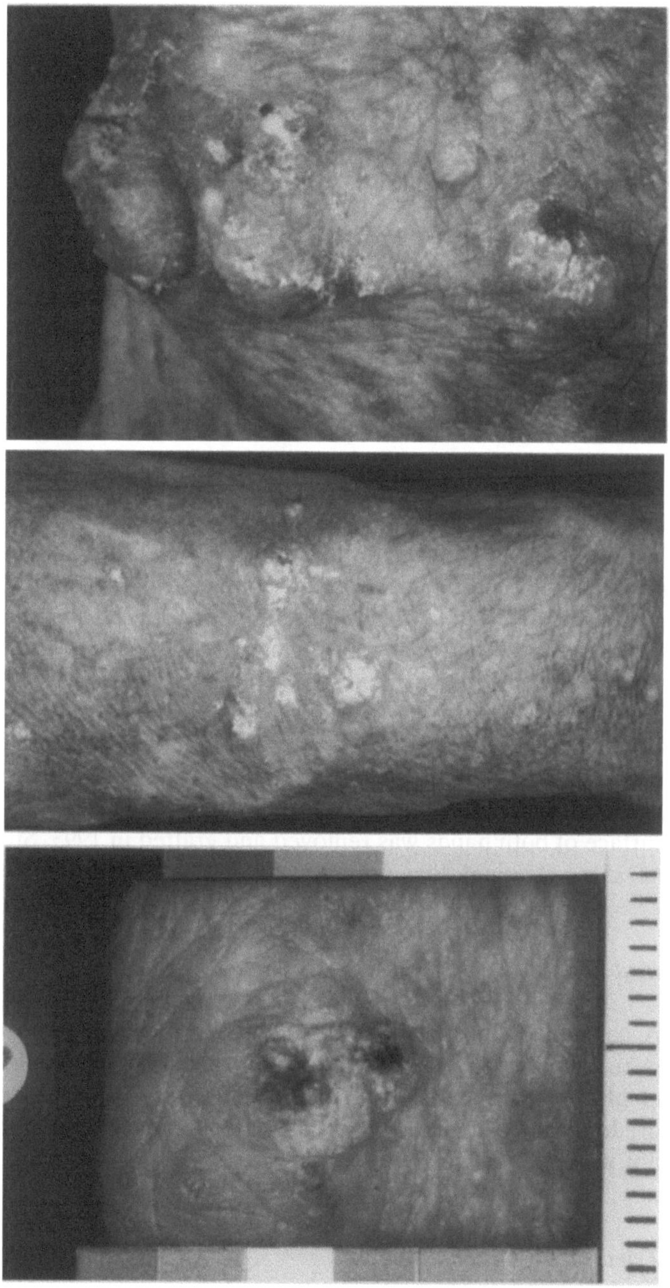

a

b

c

Fig. 3a–d. Non-melanoma skin cancer in renal transplant recipients. **a** Multiple keratotic lesions in area of field change. **b** Multiple squamous cell carcinomas on sun-exposed forearm. **c** Typical warty squamous cell carcinoma, looking rather indolent but with an indurated base. **d** Rapidly growing and recurring squamous cellcarcinoma in a high-risk patient

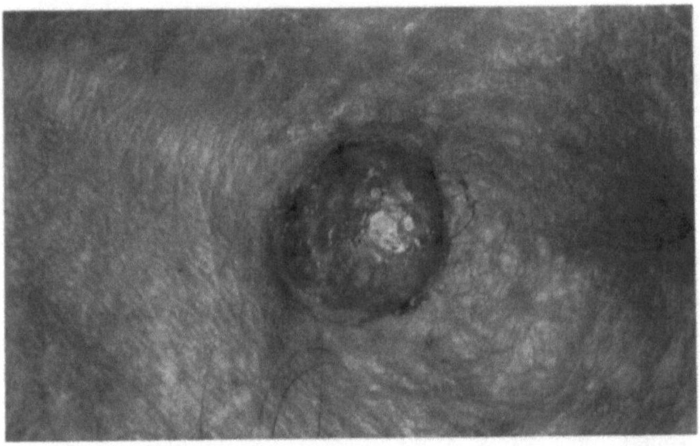

Fig. 3d

before receiving a second renal allograft. After 5 years this also failed, leading to a third transplant in 1989. He received maintenance immunosuppression with 360 mg cyclosporin A/day, 150 mg azathioprine/day and 10 mg prednisolone/day. His work was all indoors, but he spent much of his leisure time involved in outdoor sporting activity. He has type III skin. He was first seen in the skin department in 1991, 22 years after his first transplant. He had numerous warts on the backs of the hands and forearms, with several very indurated lesions. SCC were removed from several areas on the backs of the hands, and Bowenoid keratoses were removed from the forearms, face and upper trunk. Because of the widespread dysplasia the entire dorsal surface of both hands was removed and grafted in 1993. Since he was started on 25 mg etretinate/day 6 months ago he has no further malignancies.

Oral Lesions

A controlled study of lip and intraoral lesions was performed and patients were found to have a high rate of lip cancer and leukoplakia (14.4%; King et al. 1994), again in sun-exposed sites (Fig. 4a). Intraoral lesions were predominantly oral hairy leukoplakia and gingival hyperplasia (Fig. 4b) and not warts or oral cancer.

Typical Case History

A 38-year-old taxi driver developed end-stage renal failure as a result of chronic glomerulonephritis. After 6 months of haemodialysis, he had a cadaveric renal transplant at the age of 35. Maintenance immunosuppression consisted of 125 mg azathioprine/day, 10 mg prednisolone/day and 300 mg

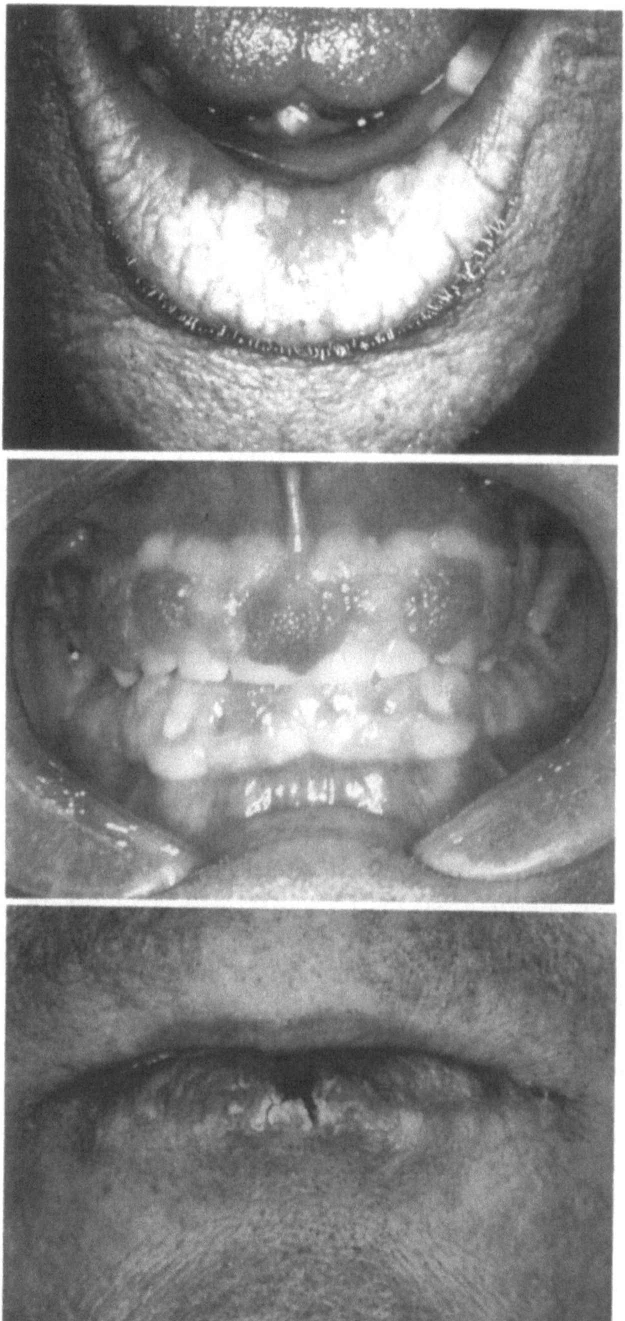

a

b

c

Fig. 4a–c. Oral lesions in renal transplant recipients. **a** Warty leukoplakia of sun-exposed lips. **b** Gingival hyperplasia. **c** Squamous cell carcinoma of lower lip cyclosporin A/day. He had lived in Australia between the ages of 12 and 17 years and had burnt to the point of blistering on a number of occasions. He had spent 3 years as a taxi driver, but had previously had indoor jobs. He had skin type II. He began to develop warts within a year of transplantation. When we first saw him 3 years post-transplant, he had an SCC on his nose and on the lower lip (Fig. 4c) and Bowenoid keratoses on the cheek and lower leg. Since then he has had several further Bowenoid keratoses removed from the cheeks.

Genital Disease

Renal transplant recipients (RTR) also have a higher risk of carcinoma of the cervix, vulva and perineum, which is poorly documented apart from in the American registries (Penn 1988) and reports from the Edinburgh studies (Alloub et al. 1989). There were 190 males and 101 females in our study (i.e. 35% females) and cervical smears were traced from GP and hospital records. Ten women (10%) were found to have known cervical disease: two had cervical intraepithelial neoplasia (CIN) 1, two had CIN-3, two had invasive carcinoma of the cervix and four had dysplasia on smear. The patients were reluctant to attend for colposcopy and examination and this is likely to be an underestimate of the true numbers.

Case History

A 33-year-old woman with Alport's syndrome received a cadevaric renal transplant 10 years ago after 2 years of peritoneal dialysis. Immunosuppression consisted of 125 mg azathioprine/day and 10 mg prednisolone/day. Cervical biopsy in 1983 showed dysplasia, which was treated with cryocautery. Dysplasia was detected on smear again in 1987, with micro-invasive SCC evident on subsequent cone biopsy of the cervix. Following total abdominal hysterectomy, dysplastic cells were found in a smear of the vaginal vault, and histology of the upper, anterior vaginal wall showed appearances consistent with HPV infection. She failed to return for treatment. When we first saw her in 1992, she had very few cutaneous warts but had extensive vulval, peri-anal and vaginal warts. Histology of biopsies from all these sites showed evidence of HPV infection and full-thickness dysplasia.

Epidemiology

A standard questionnaire concerning life-time sun exposure through work and leisure activities was completed for each patient. Patients who had lived in a tropical or sub-tropical climate for 6 months or more or who had had an outdoor occupation in the UK for 5 years or more were classified as high sun exposure. Patients who sunbathed for more than 14 days per year or who had outdoor activities for more than 10 h a week were classified as having high recreational sun exposure. Patients were asked a standard question about tanning ability and tendency to burn in order to establish skin type.

A total of 50% of the 291 patients had skin types I or III, 35% skin type III and 15% had skin types IV–VI. Risk factors for the development of tumours were found to be: gender (men predominating); dosage of prednisolone; age at transplantation; skin type and cumulative UV exposure; and time on dialysis prior to transplantation (Glover et al., in preparation).

Histopathology

Previous studies have suggested that SCC in RTR show certain features which were thought to be suggestive of wart virus infection, including:

- Multinucleate giant cells
- Koilocytes
- Warty architecture
- Parakeratotic peaks
- Keratohyaline granules
- Inflammatory infiltrate
- Benign surface
- Clonal nests
- Papillomatosis of edge
- Acanthosis of edge
- Basal dysplasia of edge

Price et al. (1988) compared tumours from a small number of immunosuppressed and non-immunosuppressed patients and found characteristic multinucleate cells/monster cells in the immunosuppressed individuals. There were also a number of atypical mitoses, a generally warty architecture and a vesicular chromatin pattern with prominent nucleoli. Blessing et al. (1989) also found evidence of a verrucous architecture with symmetry of lesions, central pointing of epidermal ridges, parakeratotic peaks surmounting papillae, hypergranulosis and koilocytes. In an open study we found additional features that we considered characteristic of pleomorphism, a benign surface to squamous carcinomas (basal dysplasia) and reduced inflammation (Fig. 5a,b). However, a masked controlled study comparing 40 tumours from immunosuppressed with 40 tumours from a control non-immunosuppressed population showed no statistically significant differences when scored for the supposedly discriminating features (Glover, in preparation). This suggests that unbiased observers could not distinguish tumours from immunosuppressed patients as having distinct viral features.

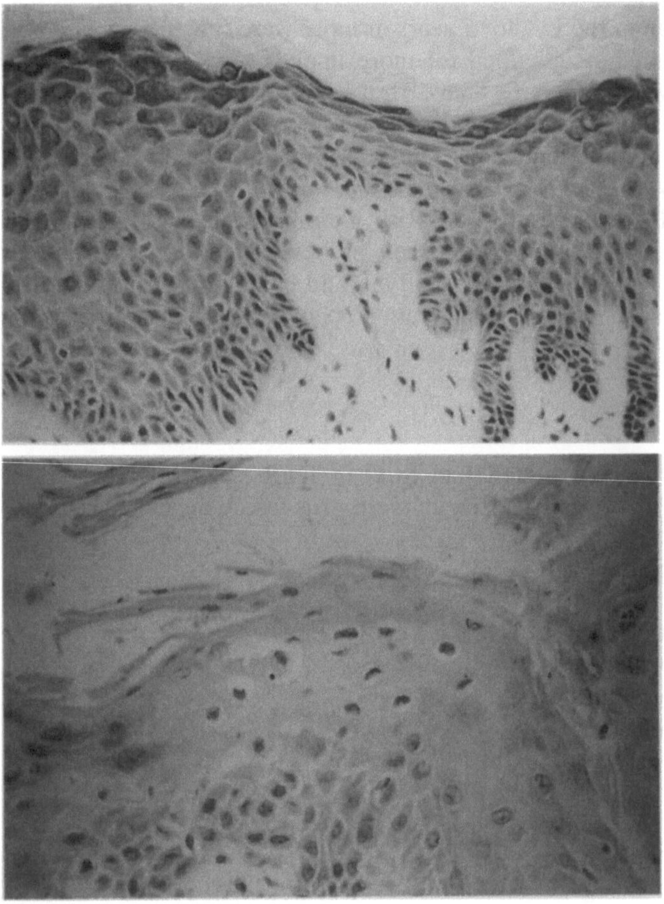

a

b

Fig. 5a,b. Histopathology of warty dysplastic keratosis showing basal dysplasia (**a**) and relative maturation to surface with crenated pyknotic nuclei and suggestion of koilocytosis (**b**)

Characteristics of Epidermal Tumours: Keratin

Previous studies have shown that epidermal SCC are associated with a loss of epidermal differentation keratins K1 and K10, a conservation of keratinocyte keratins K5 and K14 and a progressive induction of simple epithelial keratins K8 and K18 (Leigh et al. 1993). A notable early feature of microinvasive tumour was found to be the basal expression of keratin 17 (Proby et al. 1994). No difference was found between lesions from immunosuppressed and immunocompetent individuals.

Presence of Virus

We have established primary cultures of keratinocytes from 24 lesions of varying degrees of squamous atypia from nine of the above patients. Using a mixed probe for cutaneous HPV on Hirt extracts, ten of 14 cultures screened for the presence of episomal HPV DNA were positive and three cultures were positive when screened with a probe for cutaneous oncogenic HPV DNA 5 or 8. Episomal copy was universally lost with continued passage (Purdie et al. 1993), as is found in cultures of normal anogenital warts (Williams et al. 1994). Cultures of malignant origin exhibited extended life-span and developed immortalised lines which have been briefly characterised by morphology and growth requirements. The results of virus typing of tissue samples are currently in progress, but are complicated by the large number of viruses found.

Discussion

Our study indicates a very high rate of NMSC in RTR in the UK, which is not noted for high sun exposure, reaching 45% of patients who underwent transplantation more than 15 years before. Additionally, a sub-group of these patients are identified as being at special risk, requiring identification and close monitoring. Most of this high-risk group have fair skin and have had outdoor occupations with relatively high sun exposure. They show widespread epidermal dysplasia and have multiple NMSC from as early as 35 years of age. Because the tumours may be aggressive, these patients require extensive excision and grafting of dysplastic skin, plus long-term etretinate to control the development of new malignant lesions.

Immune Function

Long-term immunosuppression clearly disturbs the process of immune surveillance that normally controls malignant progression (Klein and Klein 1977). Objective means of assessing degrees of immunosuppression are lacking and at present it is impossible to determine which patients are over-immunosuppressed or when immunosuppression may be reduced without jeopardising graft function. Non-specific tests of immunity in RTR show generally depressed spontaneous cell-mediated cytotoxicity and antibody-dependent cell-mediated cytotoxicity. RTR with skin cancer show responses similar to those without skin cancer apart from decreased responses to allogenic lymphocytes and recall antigens (Kelly et al. 1984).

There is some evidence that immunogenetic factors may play a part in susceptibility to NMSC, with the demonstration of a possible protective effect of HLA-A11 against NMSC in RTR (Bouwes-Bavink et al. 1991), perhaps reflecting efficient presentation of antigens induced by SCC and possibly also by HPV, through A11 to cytotoxic T lymphocytes. This protective effect of A-11 has not been confirmed in our study (Glover et al. 1993), probably because other factors implicated in tumorigenesis such as the effects of UV radiation and length of immunosuppression override the immunogenetic factors.

Immunosuppressive Therapy

The drugs used to achieve immunosuppression may have effects beyond simple immunosuppression. The active metabolite of azathioprine, 6-thioguanine, is a known tumour promotor and initiator amd the concentration of 6-thioguanine has been found to be higher in RTR with dysplastic lesions than in matched subjects without dysplastic lesions. Taylor et al. found a lag phase of 3.5 years following transplantation before dysplastic keratoses were detected, but that subsequently appearance of new lesions increases linearly (Taylor and Shuster 1992). Tumour initiation by azathioprine was proposed to occur during this lag phase. Since 1985 a proportion of patients have received cyclosporin A rather than azathioprine. Whether this regime is associated with lower levels of malignancy is difficult to establish at this stage, since the time span of observation of cyclosporin A is so much shorter than that of azathioprine. Evidence to date is contradictory, some studies reporting a greater cumulative prevalence of dysplastic skin lesions in RTR receiving cyclosporin A than in those receiving azathioprine for a similar period (Shuttleworth et al. 1988), others finding fewer skin cancers in patients treated with cyclosporin A (Sheil 1977) and some finding no difference (Bunney et al. 1990) Ultimately, it seems likely that reduction in the overall levels of immunosuppression to a minimum will be of greater importance than the nature of the individual agents used.

Ultraviolet Radiation

UV radiation is of overwhelming importance in the aetiology of skin cancer in RTR. Cumulative sun exposure is strongly associated with the development of SCC (Hardie et al. 1980; Boyle et al. 1984; Barr et al. 1989; Bouwes-Bavink et al. 1991). In our study the SCC occurred predominantly on sun-exposed sites such as the dorsa of the hands and forearms and the forehead and were most frequent and troublesome in fair-skinned individuals (skin types I and II) who had either had outdoor occupations or had spent at least 3 months in the tropics or sub-tropics.

UV irradiation equivalent to recreational sun exposure can cause selective systemic immunosuppression (Parrish 1983). In mice UVB induces a subset of T suppressor lymphocytes, which can transfer the ability to prevent rejection of UVB-induced tumours (Kripke 1981). Epicutaneous delivery of

DNA repair endonuclease can abolish this UV-induced immunosuppression in mice (Kripke et al. 1992). In humans UVB can suppress allergic contact dermatitis to a potent sensitiser such as dinitrochlorobenzene in 40% of normal volunteers. However, 92% of patients with a history of NMSC showed suppression of allergic contact dermatitis following UVB (Yoshikawa et al. 1990), indicating that susceptibility to UVB immunosuppression may be a risk factor for the development of NMSC. This response needs to be tested in RTR.

Human Papillomaviruses

Clinically all but one of our patients developing SCC had large numbers of warts, and the SCC commonly arose within wart-covered sun-exposed skin. Parallels can be drawn with the rare genetic skin disease EV, which provides a convincing cutaneous model for HPV-induced tumorigenesis. EV patients are presumed to have an immune defect, as yet poorly defined, that leads to infection with multiple unusual HPV types, especially HPV 5 and 8. These EV HPV have been reported from the warts and tumours of small numbers of RTR (Lutzner et al. 1983; Gassenmaier et al. 1986; Obalek et al. 1992). The transforming genes of HPV 16 and 18 (E6 and E7) are strongly implicated in cervical cancer, when E6 proteins complex with the tumour suppressor p53 (Wernesset et al. 1990), leading to its degradation via a ubiquitin-dependent pathway (Scheffner et al. 1990). Since p53 arrests the cell cycle for DNA repair following damage, accelerated p53 degradation will tend to permit replication of abnormal DNA. The E7 protein of HPV 16 and 18 bind similarly to the retinoblastoma protein (Scheffner et al. 1991). However, the transforming gene (E6) of HPV8 does not bind to p53 and therefore the mechanism of cellular transformation from EV HPV is not yet understood (Iftner et al. 1988). Although EV HPV have been found in RTR, most studies show no HPV DNA in the tumour cells (Dyall-Smith et al. 1991; Rudlinger and Grob 1989). It is possible that both warts and skin cancers are favoured by the combination of drug-induced immunosuppression and photo-immunosuppression and simply "co-habit", so HPV is an innocent bystander. Our pathological and virological data also suggests that virus is not commonly found in the tumours, but a hit and run mechanism has some attractions. Also the close proximity of viral lesions to cancers may have indirect effects of tumour growth via local upregulation of cytokines (such as interleukin-6 IL-6) or interference with other cellular proteins (such as p53/Rb) required to limit DNA damage from UV radiation.

Conclusions

It seems likely that in most renal transplant recipients UV, the agents used to achieve long-term immunosuppression and possibly HPV act synergistically to produce the high rates of SCC. The relative importance of the different factors is likely to vary from patient to patient, depending on their degree of sun exposure, skin type, degree of immunosuppression and genetic factors such as HLA type. For most RTR warts and epidermal dysplasia do not represent more than an inconvenience and are seen as a small price to pay for the benefits of a well-functioning renal allograft. However, there is a proportion of patients, generally those with fair skin who have had high levels of sun exposure, who have severe and widespread cutaneous dysplasia requiring very close supervision and extensive surgery.

References

Alloub MI, Barr BB, McLaren KM, Smith IW, Bunney MH, Smart EE (1989) HPV infection and CIN in women with renal allografts. Br Med J 298:153–156

Barr B, Benton E, McLaren K et al (1989) Human papillomavirus infection and skin cancer in renal allograft recipients. Lancet 1:124–129

Bencini PL, Montagnino G, De-Vecchi A et al (1983) Cutaneous manifestations in renal transplant recipients. Nephron 34:79–83

Blessing K, McLaren K, Benton E et al (1989) Histopathology of skin lesions in renal allograft recipients: an assessment of viral features and dysplasia. Histopathology 14:129–139

Bouwes-Bavinck J, Vermeer B, van der Woude F et al (1991) Relation between skin cancer and HLA antigens in renal transplant recipients. N Engl J Med. 325:843–847

Boyle J, Briggs JD, Mackie RM, Junor BJR, Aitchison TC (1984) Cancer, warts and sunshine in renal transplant patients: a case control study. Lancet 1:702–705

Brash DE (1988) UV mutagenic photoproducts in Escherichia coli and human cells: a molecular genetics perspective on human skin cancer. Photochem Photobiol 48:59–66

Bunney M, Benton E, Barr B et al (1990) The prevalence of skin disorders in renal allograft recipients receiving cyclosporin A compared with those receiving azathioprine. Nephrol Dial Transplant 5:379–382

Cleaver, JE, Bootsma, D (1975) Xeroderma pigmentosum: biochemical and genetic characteristics. Annu Rev Genet 9:19–38

de Villers EM (1989) Heterogeneity of the human papillomavirus group. J Virol 63:4898–4903

Dyall-Smith D, Trowell H, Mark A, Dyall-Smith M (1991) Cutaneous squamous cell carcinomas and papillomaviruses in renal transplant recipients: a clinical and molecular biological study. J Dermatol Sci 2:139–146

Friedberg EC (1985) DNA damage and human disease. In: Friedberg EC (ed) DNA repair. Freeman, New York, pp 505–574

Fuchs PG, Pfister H (1990) Papillomaviruses in epidermodysplasia verruciformis. Papillomavirus Rep 1(4):1–4

Gassenmaier A, Fuchs P, Schell H, Pfister H (1986) Papillomavirus DNA in warts of immunosuppressed renal allograft recipients. Arch Dermatol Res 278:219–223

Glover MT, Bodmer J, Bodmer W, Kennedy LJ, Brown J, Navarette C, Kwan JTC, Leigh IM (1993) HLA antigen frequencies in renal transplant recipients and non-immunosuppressed patients with non-melanoma skin cancer. Eur J Cancer 29:520–524

Glover MT, Hanby AM, Gerio R, Leigh IM (1994a) Squamoproliferative lesions in renal transplant recipients: do the histopathological features differ from those in immunocompetent patients? (in press)
Glover MT, Proby CM, Naranjan N, Deakes J, Kwan JTC, Leigh IM (1994b) Skin cancer in renal transplant recipients: the extent of the problem and a strategy for management. Br J Plastic Surg 47:86–89
Glover MT, Deekes J, Kwan JTR, Proby CM, Leigh IM. The major risk factor for skin cancer in renal transplant patients (in preparation)
Hardie I, Strong R, Hartley L et al (1980) Skin cancer in Caucasian renal allograft recipients living in a sub-tropical climate. Surgery 87:177–183
Iftner T, Bierfelder S, Csapo Z, Pfister H (1988) Involvement of human papillomavirus type 8 genes E6 and E7 in transformation and replication. J Virol 62:3655–3661
Kelly G, Shiel A, Taylor R (1984) Non-specific immunological studies in kidney tranplant recipients with and without cancer. Transplantation 37:368–372
King GN, Healy CM, Glover MT, Kwan JTC, Williams DM, Leigh IM, Thornhill MH. Increased prevalence of dysplastic and malignant lip lesions in renal transplant recipients. (submitted)
Klein G, Klein E (1977) Immune surveillance against virus-induced tumors and non-rejectability of spontaneous tumors: contrasting consequences of host versus tumor evolution. Proc Natl Acad Sci USA 74:2121–2125
Kripke M (1981) Immunological mechanisms in ultra-violet radiation carcinogenesis. Adv Cancer Res 34:69–106
Kripke M, Cox P, Alas L, Yorosh D (1992) Pyrimidine dimers in DNA initiated systemic immunosuppression in UV irradiated mice. Proc Natl Acad Sci USA 89:7516–7520
Leigh IM, Purkis PE, Markey A, Collins P, Neill S, Proby CM, Glover MT. Lane EB (1993) Keratinocyte alterations in skin tumour development. In: Hecker E, Jung EG, Marks F, Tilgen W (eds) Skin carcinogenesis in man and in experimental models. Springer, Berlin Heidelberg New York (Recent results in cancer research, vol 128)
Lutzner MA, Orth G, Dutronquay V, Ducasse MF, Kreis H, Crosnier J (1983) Detection of human papillomavirus type 5 DNA in skin cancers of an immunosuppressed renal allograft recipient. Lancet 2:422–424
Lutzner MA, Blanchet-Bardon C, Orth G (1984) Clinical observations, virologic studies and treatment trials in patients with epidermodysplasia verruciformis, a disease induced by specific papillomaviruses. J Invest Dermatol 83: 18s–25s
Obalek S, Favre, M, Szymanczyk J, Jablonska S, Orth G (1992) Human papillomavirus (HPV) types specific of epidermodysplasia verruciformis detected in warts induced by HPV3 or HPV3-related types in immunosuppressed patients. J Invest Dermatol 98:936–941
Parrish J (1983) Ultraviolet radiation affects the immune system. Pediatrics 71:129–134
Penn I (1988) Tumours of the immunocompromised patient. Annu Rev Med 39:63–73
Pfister H (1984) Biology and biochemistry of papillomaviruses. Rev Physiol Biochem Pharmacol. 99:112–181
Pierceall WE, Goldberg, LH, Ananthaswamy HN (1991) Presence of human papillomavirus type 16 DNA sequences in human nonmelanoma skin cancers. J Invest Dermatol 97:880–884
Price M, Tidman M, Fagg N et al (1988) Distinctive epidermal atypia in immunosuppression-associated cutaneous malignancy. Histopathology 13:89–94

Proby CM, Churchill L, Purkis PE, Glover MT, Sexton CJ, Leigh IM (1993) Keratin 17 expression as a marker for epithelial transformation in viral warts. Am J Pathol 143:1667–1678

Purdie KJ, Sexton CJ, Proby CM, Glover MT, Williams AT, Stables JN, Leigh IM (1993) Malignant transformation of cutaneous lesions in renal allograft patients: a role for HPV? Cancer Res 53:5328–5333

Rudlinger R, Grob R (1989) Papilloma virus and skin cancer in renal allograft recipients. Lancet 1:1132–1133

Scheffner M, Werness BA, Hulbregtae JM et al (1990) The E6 oncoprotein encoded by human papillomavirus types 16 and 18 promotes and degradation of p53. Cell 63:1129–1136

Scheffner M, Munge K, Byrne JC, Howley PM (1991) The state of p53 and retinoblastoma genes in human cervical carcinoma cell lines. Proc Natl Acad Sci USA 88:5523–5527

Sheil AGR (1977) Cancer in renal allograft recipients in Australia and New Zealand. Transplant Proc 9:1133–1136

Shuttleworth D, Marks R, Griffin P, Salaman J (1988) Treatment of cutaneous neoplasia with etretinate in renal transplant recipients. Q J Med 257:717–724

Strickland P (1986) Photocarcinogenesis by near-ultraviolet (UVA) radiation in Sencar mice. J Invest. Dermatol. 87:272–275

Taylor A, Shuster S (1992) Skin cancer after renal transplantation: the causal role of azathioprine. Acta. Derm. Venereol (Stockh) 72:115–119

Werness BA, Levine AJ, Howley PM (1990) Association of human papilloma virus types 16 and 18 E6 proteins with p53. Science 248:76–79

Williams AT, Sexton CJ, Sinclair AL, Purdie KJ, Thomas MS, Hanna NA, Goh BT, Williams DM, Leigh IM (1994) Retention of low copy number human papillomavirus DNA in cultured cutaneous and mucosal wart keratinocytes. J Gen Virol 75:505–511

Yoshikawa T, Rae V, Bruins-Slot W et al (1990) Susceptibility to effects of UVB radiation on induction of contact hypersensitivity as a risk factor for skin cancer in humans. J Invest. Dermatol 95:530–536

Zur Hausen H (1991) Viruses' in human caners. Science 22:1167–1172

Risk of Developing Cutaneous Malignant Melanoma in Atypical-Mole Syndrome: New York University Experience and Literature Review

J. Slade[1–3], T.G. Salopek[1–3,5], A.A. Marghoob[1–4], A.W. Kopf[1–3], and D.S. Rigel[1–3]

[1] Ronald O. Perelman Department of Dermatology, New York University School of Medicine 550 First Avenue, New York, NY 10016, USA
[2] Oncology Section, Charles C Harris Skin and Cancer Pavilion, New York University Medical Center, New York, USA
[3] New York University Melanoma Cooperative Group, New York, USA
[4] Department of Dermatology, State University of New York at Stony Brook, USA
[5] T.G. Salopek is a lecturer at the University of Alberta, Division of Dermatology, Edmonton, Canada and is currently on leave of absence

Abstract

The presence of atypical moles (AM) is considered to be a marker for an increased risk of developing cutaneous malignant melanoma (MM). The extent to which individuals with the atypical-mole syndrome (AMS) are at risk for developing MM is unknown. We present a review of the world literature and of our experience at New York University. We conclude that the presence of AMS in Caucasians significantly increases the risk of developing MM, regardless of geographic location. A further increase in MM risk is noted if there is a personal and/or family history of MM.

Introduction

Dr. William Norris is credited with the first English publication of an entity that in all probability represented the atypical-mole syndrome (AMS) in a melanoma-prone family (Norris 1820). In 1978 Dr. Wallace Clark Jr. and his colleagues heralded the onset of modern research on this disorder with their landmark paper on the "B-K mole" syndrome (Clark et al. 1978). Since Norris' first description of familial melanoma, several different names and definitions have been applied to this syndrome, and these continue to evolve to the present day. Some of these names include the "B-K mole" syndrome (Clark et al. 1978), familial atypical multiple mole melanoma syndrome (FAMMM; Frichot et al. 1977), dysplastic nevus syndrome (DNS; Greene et al. 1980; Elder et al. 1982), large atypical nevus syndrome (LANS; Bondi et al. 1981), Clark's nevus syndrome (Nollet 1986), and "classic" AMS (Kopf et al. 1990).

Recent Results in Cancer Research, Vol. 139

AMS is said to be a marker for an increased risk of developing cutaneous malignant melanoma (MM; Kraemer and Greene 1985; Rigel et al. 1989; Friedman et al. 1991; Tiersten et al. 1991; Halpern et al. 1991; McHenry and MacKie 1993; Marghoob et al. 1994). The precise magnitude of this risk has not been well defined.

Researchers have relied on three different epidemiologic approaches in assessing the risk of developing MM in patients with AMS (Swerdlow and Green 1987). One approach involves simple population comparisons. Another involves prospective cohort studies in which patients with and without AMS are followed for the development of MM. The prospective cohort study is the best and most rigorous method for assessing MM risk, but requires large numbers of patients and many years of follow-up. Hence, it is the most difficult and costly study to conduct. The majority of such studies have been carried out on MM-prone families. The third approach involves retrospective case-control studies, in which the presence or absence of AM in MM patients is contrasted with individuals without MM (controls), and a relative risk (RR) assigned for the presence of that trait. Such studies are troubled with various biases, notably observer bias.

This paper reviews the world literature and the New York University Melanoma Cooperative Group (NYU-MCG) experience on the risk of developing MM in patients with AM and, more importantly, AMS.

Atypical-Mole Syndrome

AMS has been described in a number of different ways and therefore there is no universally accepted definition. However, the definitions are all based on clinical and/or histologic criteria of a common phenotypically distinct mole – the "dysmorphic" or "atypical" melanocytic nevus (MN). "Classic" AMS (Kopf et al. 1990) is defined by the presence of. (a) 100 or more MN; (b) one or more MN, 8 mm or larger in greatest diameter; and (c) one or more MN with clinically atypical features. These atypical MN have some or all of the "ABCD" clinical features of MM (*A*symmetry, *B*order irregularity, *C*olor variability, and *D*iameter greater than 6 mm; Friedman et al. 1985). Table 1 summarizes the criteria for defining the "classic" AMS.

The National Institute of Health (NIH) Consensus Conference has defined AMS as: (a) the occurrence of AM and MM in one or more first- or second-degree relatives; (b) a large number of MN, often greater than 50, some of which are atypical and often variable in size; and (c) MN that demonstrate certain histologic features (National Institutes of Health Consensus Development Conference 1992).

Patients with AMS can be categorized into a risk gradient for developing MM. Kraemer et al. (1983) classified patients with the AMS into risk types for the development of MM as follows: A, sporadic AMS (no MM or AM in blood relatives); B, familial AMS (AM but no MM in blood relatives); C,

Table 1. Clinical characteristics of melanocytic nevi in patients with "classic" atypical-mole syndrome

Feature	Clinical finding
General clinical characteristics of melanocytic nevi	
Number	100 or more
Uniformity	Heterogenous (neighboring nevi differ from each other)
Clinical characteristics of melanocytic nevi	
Size	At least one, 8 mm or more in diameter
Color	Variegate: multiple shades of tan, brown, black, red
Elevation	For its large diameter, its center is only slightly raised
Perimeter	May be irregular; usually fades imperceptibly into surrounding skin
"Shoulder"	Peripheral macular tan zone
Surface	Often mammillated
Symptoms	None
Hypertrichosis	Absent
Erosion/ulceration	Absent

Modified with permission from Tiersten, et al. (1991).

sporadic AMS with MM (no AM or MM in blood relatives); D1, familial AMS with MM (AM and MM in one blood relative); and D2, familial AMS with MM (AM and at least two blood relatives with MM).

More recently, Rigel et al. (1988) divided AMS patients into one of four risk groups based on personal and/or family history of MM. In this classification, one point is given if the patient has had MM and two points are given per family member with MM. The family members must belong to the modified nuclear pedigree which includes siblings, parents, grandparents, aunts, and uncles. The points are totalled and the patient is then classified into one of four risk groups: group 0, 0 points; group I, 1 point; group II, 2 points; and group III, 3 or more points. In both the Rigel and Kraemer classification schemes, the risk of MM increases with the increasing prevalence of MM in the kindred.

New York University Experience

Rigel et al. (1989) prospectively studied 452 white patients with AMS for the occurrence of newly diagnosed MM. All patients were followed by total cutaneous examinations (TCE) every 3–12 months. Sixteen patients developed 18 MM within an average follow-up of 27 months. There were six invasive and 12 in situ MM. The patients were classified into one of four risk groups, as defined by Rigel et al. (1988), and their proclivity to develop MM was compared to a population matched for age, sex, and total months of follow-up taken from the Surveillance, Epidemiology, and End Results

(SEER) data base (Ries et al. 1991). The relative risk (RR) for developing invasive MM in all 452 patients with AMS was calculated to be 53. Only invasive MM were used in the calculation of RR, since the SEER data excludes in situ MM from their data base.

The main bias of this study was the difference in follow-up between the study cohort and the SEER population. The AMS cohort was followed by frequent TCE, whereas no data exist as to what type of cutaneous examinations, if any, were performed in the SEER population.

In the second NYU study, Tiersten et al. (1991) prospectively followed 357 white patients with classic AMS for the development of MM. All patients had total cutaneous photographs (TCP) taken as baselines. These photographs were used in conjunction with subsequent TCE to help detect any changes in existing MN or the appearance of new MN. Seventeen patients developed 18 MM within an average of 32 months of follow-up. There were eight in situ and ten invasive MM. The invasive MM were compared to a SEER population matched for age, sex, and total months of follow-up, as was done in the study by Rigel et al. (1989). The RR for the development of MM in the AMS patients was calculated to be 60.

The main bias in this study was the same as with the Rigel study, namely, that AMS patients were followed by periodic TCE using baseline TBP, whereas the SEER population was not. The results of these two studies are summarized in Table 2.

The third NYU study by Marghoob et al. (1994) compared the risk of developing MM in a population of patients with and without classic AMS. Both cohorts were followed by at least annual TCE. There were 287 white patients with classic AMS and 831 white patients without classic AMS. The medical records of both cohorts were reviewed for the occurrence of newly diagnosed MM starting from the time of their initial visit. The cumulative 10-year life-table risk (Cutler and Ederer 1958) of developing MM was calculated for each cohort (Table 3). Ten of the 287 classic AMS patients developed a newly diagnosed invasive MM, resulting in a 10-year cumulative life-table risk of 10.7%. Only two of the 831 controls developed invasive MM, resulting in a 10-year cumulative life-table risk of 0.62%. The risk of developing MM was significantly higher in the AMS patients ($p < 0.0005$). Furthermore, the cases and controls were classified into risk groups as defined by Rigel et al. (1988). The AMS patients had an increased risk of developing MM, irrespective of their risk group, as compared to controls (Table 3). This is the only study reporting the risk of developing MM in patients with the classic AMS versus controls (without AMS), where both cohorts were followed regularly in the same clinical setting.

The combined results of the three aforementioned NYU studies are summarized in Table 4. The conclusion derived from these studies is that, compared to controls, patients with AMS have a significantly increased risk of developing MM irrespective of risk group. Furthermore, it is important to note that none of the patients in the three NYU studies developed metas-

Table 2. Invasive melanomas found on prospective follow-up of atypical-mole syndrome patients based on the New York University observations by Rigel et al. and Tiersten et al.

Group[a]	Patients (n)		Invasive MM (n)		SEER expected	
	Rigel et al. (1989)	Tiersten et al. (1991)	Rigel et al. (1989)	Tiersten et al. (1991)	Rigel et al. (1989)	Tiersten et al. (1991)
0	281	157	1	4	0.062	0.076
I	66	95	1	4	0.028	0.054
II	69	89	1	1	0.015	0.030
III	36	16	3	1	0.009	0.007
Total	452	357	6	10	0.113 $p < 0.003$	0.167 $p < 0.001$

MM, cutaneous malignant melanoma; SEER, Surveillance, Epidemiology, and End Results.
[a] As defined by Rigel et al. (1988).

Table 3. Ten-year cumulative risk of melanoma in classic atypical-mole syndrome (AMS) cohort versus control cohort[a]

Group[b]	AMS patients (n)	Control patients (n)	10-Year MM risk in AMS	10-Year MM risk in controls	RR	95% Cl
0*	124	679	8.6%	0.2%	39	21.6–74.1
I + II + III**	163	152	11.7%	3.1%	54	32.5–76.9
Total***	287	831	10.7%	0.6%	47	31.8–65.1

Cl, confidence interval; MM, cutaneous malignant melanoma; RR, relative risk.
[a] From Marghoob et al. (1994).
[b] Using the Rigel classification, Rigel et al. (1989).
* $p < 0.005$.
** $p < 0.05$.
*** $p < 0.0005$.

tases, died of MM, or had a MM thicker than 0.88 mm Breslow tumor thickness.

Literature Review

Retrospective Case-Control Studies Assessing the Relative Risk of Developing Cutaneous Malignant Melanoma in Patients With and Without Atypical Nevi

To determine the risk of developing MM in patients with both common acquired nevi and AM, researchers have predominantly relied on retrospective case-control studies (Table 5). This approach identifies MM patients and assesses whether they have quantitative or qualitative MN abnormalities. A RR for developing MM is then assigned, based on the presence of these abnormalities in patients versus age- and sex-matched controls without MM. Early studies were fraught with bias in that they relied on the patients to count their own MN, did not address whether the nevi were atypical or not, or counted MN only on localized body regions (Beral et al. 1983; Holman and Armstrong 1984; Green et al. 1985; Dubin et al. 1986). Recently, it has been demonstrated that nevus counts limited to the arms is one of the least valuable methods for detecting high-risk individuals (Kruger et al. 1992).

A study from Scotland by Swerdlow et al. (1986) demonstrated that color variation and an irregular border in MN resulted in RR for developing MM of 29.7 and 70.4, respectively.

An American study by Holly et al. (1987) found a direct relationship between MM risk and both the total number of MN and the presence of clinically AM. They compared the number of "nondysplastic" (nonatypical)

Table 4. Comparison of melanoma risk in the three New York University studies

Study	Patients (*n*)	Mean follow-up (months)	Invasive MM observed (*n*)	Invasive MM expected (*n*)	RR	95% Cl
Rigel et al. (1989)	452	27.0	6	0.113	53	34.0–82.6
Tiersten et al. (1991)	357	49.0	10	0.167	60	43.0–83.8
Marghoob et al. (1993)						
AMS	287	57.8	10	0.213	47	35.9–66.9
Control	831	88.7	2	1.3	–	–

AMS, atypical-mole syndrome; MM, cutaneous malignant melanoma; RR, relative risk; Cl, confidence interval.

Table 5. Case-control studies assessing relative risk (RR) for developing MM based on the presence or absence of common or atypical nevi

Researchers	Country	Patients (*n*)	Controls (*n*)	RR (Nevi, *n*)	RR (Atypical moles, *n*)
Swerdlow et al. 1986	Scotland	180	197	1.0 (0) 0.8 (1–9) 6.7 (10–24) 10.7 (25–49) 53.9 (≥ 50)	1.0 (0) 5.2 (1–4) 5.7 (≥ 5) 29.7 Color variation 70.4 Irregular edge
Holly et al. 1987	USA (CA)	121	139	1.0 (0–10) 1.6 (11–25) 4.4 (26–50) 5.4 (51–100) 9.8 (>100)	1.0 (0) 3.8 (1–5) 6.3 (≥6)
Roush et al. 1988	Australia	246	134	1.0 (<16) 1.3 (16–30) 1.7 (31–45) 0.8 (≥46)	7.6 (Not adjusted for no. of nevi) 7.7 (Adjusted for no. of nevi)
Garbe et al. 1989	Germany	200	200	1.0 (0–10) 3.1 (11–20) 2.3 (21–40) 7.3 (41–60) 14.7 (>60)	1.0 (0) 11.4 (1–2) 6.1 (≥3)

MacKie et al. 1989	Scotland	280	280	Male 1.0 (<20) 13.9 (≥20) Female 1.0 (<20) 6.7 (≥20)	Male 2.1 (1–2) 4.5 (≥3) Female 2.1 (1–2) 4.4 (≥3)
Grob et al. 1990	France	207	295	1.0 (0–10) 1.2 (11–20) 3.8 (21–40) 3.5 (41–80) 4.1 (81–120) 16.1 (>120)	2.77 (>1) 4.31 Very atypical (>1)
Augustsson et al. 1991	Sweden	121	378	1.0 (1–74) 1.2 (75–149) 2.6 (≥150)	1.0 (0) 2.5 (1–2) 5.6 (≥3)
Halpern et al. 1991	USA (PA)	105	181	1.0 (<25) 6.5 (≥25)	8.8 (Present versus absent)

All controls were age- and sex-matched. In addition, Swerdlow et al. matched for city. The diagnostic criteria for nevi and atypical moles (AM) were similar in all of the studies.

and "dysplastic" (atypical) MN on all body sites in a group of patients with nonfamilial MM and a group of age- and sex-matched controls. There were an average of 97 MN in cases, compared to 36 in the controls. The mean number of AM was ninefold greater in the cases as compared to the controls: 6.3 versus 0.7, respectively. The increased frequency of AM could not be attributed to an increased number of MN, since there were only 2.7-fold more MN in cases versus controls. They found a direct relationship between the number of MN and MM risk, which became apparent when more than 11 MN were present. In terms of AM, the existence of even one AM was associated with an increased risk of MM. The presence of one to five AM resulted in a RR of 3.8.

An Australian study (Roush et al. 1988) determined that *only* AM were associated with an increased risk for MM. They examined the contention that the MM risk in nonfamilial AMS could simply be due to a quantitative abnormality, namely that affected individuals have an increased number of nevi, some of which could progress to MM. The researchers found that the risk for MM due to AM was independent of the total number of nevi present. The RR for MM in individuals with 16 or more MN was significantly elevated at 1.8, but became statistically insignificant once adjusted for the presence of AM (RR, 1.2). They concluded that patients with nonfamilial AMS were at considerably increased risk for MM regardless of total MN counts when compared to controls without melanoma (RR, 7.7).

A study from Germany determined that AM and total number of MN were independent predictors of MM risk (Garbe et al. 1989). Although the presence of AM and the total number of MN were independent variables, the stronger determinant for developing MM was the total number of MN, particularly if more than 40 were present (RR, 7.3). Persons with at least one AM demonstrated a RR of 11.4 for developing MM as compared to individuals without that phenotype.

A study from Scotland by MacKie et al. (1989) wished to identify the relative importance of clinically recognizable risk factors for MM. Of all variables assessed, they found that the total number of MN was the most important determinant of MM risk. The effect of this variable was twice as great in men as compared to women, irrespective of age. The presence of AM imparted a RR of between 2.1 and 4.5, depending on the number of AM seen.

A French study by Grob et al. (1990) showed that the total MN count was the most important predictor of MM risk. Melanoma risk was slightly elevated in subsets of the study population with less than 120 total nevi (RR, 1–4.1). If more than 120 nevi were present, the RR increased to 16.1. The most important variables for MM risk were the total number of nevi, number of nevi between 5 and 10 mm in diameter, and the presence of AM. The presence of AM imparted a RR of between 2.77 and 4.31, depending on the clinical severity of atypia. When each of the above variables was adjusted for the other two factors, the risk of developing MM was found to be dependent on the number of nevi between 5 and 10 mm in diameter, regardless of whether they were clinically atypical or not.

A Swedish study concluded that the presence of AM was a better predictor of MM risk than total number of MN (Augustsson et al. 1991). The average number of MN seen in the patients was 115, almost twice the number seen in the controls (n = 67). The incidence of AM was significantly higher in the cases versus the control group: 56% versus 18%, respectively. They found that the total number of MN had a minimal influence on MM risk. Less than 150 MN resulted in a RR of 1.2, and 150 or more MN resulted in a RR of 2.6. In contrast, the presence of AM resulted in a definite increased MM risk, particularly if more than three AM were present (RR, 5.6). The presence of clinically atypical MN was determined to be as good a prognosticator of MM risk as was histological evidence of atypia.

A second study from the USA demonstrated that both the number of AM and the total number of MN were important determinants of MM risk (Halpern et al. 1991). The average number of MN in the patients was 31.1 and in the controls 9.4. The average number of AM was 8.6 in the patients versus 1.7 in the controls. No increase in MM risk was noted if the total number of MN was less than 25, whereas more than 25 MN imparted a RR of 6.5. The RR for developing MM was estimated to be 8.8 if AM were present and dropped slightly to 6.4 once corrected for the total number of MN present.

In summary, most retrospective case-control studies report a significantly increased risk of developing MM in individuals with AM, and this is independent of other risk factors. The RR for developing MM in association with AM varies from 2.1 to 70.4, and is a consistent finding in white populations, regardless of geographic location.

Risk of Cutaneous Malignant Melanoma in Prospectively Followed Atypical-Mole Syndrome Patients

The evidence for developing MM in the familial form of AMS has been irrefutably documented in the literature. Greene et al. (1985) prospectively studied 401 members of 14 melanoma prone families with dysplastic nevi for the development of MM. They detected 39 new MM in 22 patients over a maximum follow-up of 8 years. The cumulative MM risk was calculated to be 7.2% at 8 years. Between the ages of 20 and 59 years, the actuarial probability of developing MM was 56% in family members with AMS. The RR for developing MM was 148 and 500, respectively, depending on whether there was a prior personal history of MM or not. The life-time risk for developing MM in AMS individuals was determined to be 100%.

Tucker and her colleagues (1993) have recently expanded upon the aforementioned work of Greene et al. They evaluated the risk of developing MM in 23 MM-prone families, which included the 14 kindreds reported by

Greene et al. (1985) and nine additional families accrued in the interim since the first report. Over a total of 259 person-years of follow-up, 47 new MM had developed in 105 family members affected with AMS. The cumulative risk of developing MM by the age of 50 was calculated to be 48.9%, a slight drop from that previously reported (56.0%). The RR for developing a second primary MM in affected members was 229 and this was a time interval-dependent finding (i.e., the consecutive annual RR decreased with the passage of time). The RR for developing MM in family members with AMS who did not have a prior history of MM was 85 times the predicted rate. The life-time risk for developing MM was calculated to be 81.6%, a substantial reduction from the previously calculated life-time risk of 100%.

Vasen et al. (1989) from the Netherlands prospectively followed nine families with the dysplastic nevus syndrome over an average of 57 months. During the study period, 20 new MM had been detected. Unfortunately, no cumulative life-time risk value was reported, but it is quite apparent that this is considerably higher than would be expected in the general population.

McHenry and MacKie (1993) from Scotland followed seven Kraemer DNS type D individuals over 56 person-years. This small group developed four MM over the study period. The RR for developing MM in this group was calculated to be 444. This is in keeping with the RR of 150–500 reported by Greene et al. (1985).

Prospective studies assessing the risk of developing MM in the non-familial form of AMS is less well established. With the exception of the NYU-MCG experience (see above), there have only been three other prospective cohort studies to address this issue (Table 6).

Initial attempts to attribute a RR for developing MM in AMS patients were based on the presumed prevalence of AM in the general population. At best, these results can only be considered estimates of the true risk. Kraemer et al. (1986) calculated the risk of MM in types A and B (AMS with no personal or family history of MM) to be seven times that seen in the general population. This was based on the assumption that the prevalence of AM in the general population was 7%, compared to 50% in MM patients. The cumulative lifetime risk of developing MM was estimated to be 6%. This risk of developing MM is considerably higher than the reported lifetime risk of 1% in the white USA population.

Rhodes et al. (1987) calculated the RR of MM in individuals with the nonfamilial form of AMS to be 27. This was based on the assumption that the prevalence of AM in the general population was 1.8%, compared to 34% in patients with MM.

Halpern et al. (1993) from the USA recently reported on a cohort of 153 prospectively studied patients. Over an average of 61 months of follow-up, 11 new MM were detected in 11 patients. The age-adjusted MM incidence in the study group was 692 per 100000 person-years, which is almost 71 times the estimated MM incidence in the state of Pennsylvania (9.7 per 100000 person-years in 1985). Once adjusted for prior family or personal history of

Table 6. Prospective studies in atypical-mole syndrome (AMS) patients from non-melanoma-prone families

Group/Class	Number of patients	Person-years of follow-up	Relative risk	95% Confidence interval
Marghoob et al.				
Group 0	124	661.3	39	21.7–70.7
Groups I + II + III	163	721.2	54	34.8–84.2
McHenry et al.				
Type A/B[a]	85	583	92	30–216
Type C[a]	24	178	91	11–328
Type D[a]	7	56	444	121–1138
Halpern et al.				
All types	153	1119	71[b]	NA
Schneider et al.				
All types	267	NA	47[c]	5.2–426

NA, not availabe.
[a] Refers to Kraemer classification (Kraemer and Greene 1985).
[b] Values derived from published data in which the malignant melanoma (MM) incidence in the state of Pennsylvania was estimated to be 9.7/100 000 person-years.
[c] Values derived from published data.

MM, the age-adjusted incidence of MM was calculated to be 154 per 100 000 person-years, which is 16 times the MM incidence in their area.

Schneider et al. from the USA prospectively studied 267 individuals with AM over an 8.5-year period (Schneider et al. 1994). Over the study period, five invasive MM were detected. They calculated the RR of MM in AMS individuals to be 47.4.

McHenry from Scotland (McHenry and MacKie 1993) followed 141 individuals, at increased risk of developing MM, over a minimum of 5 years. They showed that the RR of developing MM in the Kraemer DNS types A plus B and type C patients to be 92 and 91, respectively.

In summary, the above prospective studies suggest that individuals with AMS have a markedly increased risk of developing MM. The RR for developing MM in association with AMS varies from 16 to 92.

Conclusion and Recommendations for the Management of Atypical-Mole Syndrome Patients

The authors consider a clinically atypical mole to be a partly macular, partly papular MN with irregular and/or ill-defined borders and color variegation with a mostly tan to brown spectrum, sometimes with a pink background (Table 1). These MN have some or all of the ABCD features of MM (Friedman et al. 1985). We define classic AMS as a triad of: (1) 100 or more

MN; (2) one or more MN 8 mm or larger in greatest diameter; and (3) one or more clinically AM (Kopf et al. 1990).

We recommend that from the outset patients should be classified into one of the risk groups as defined by Rigel et al. (1989) or Kraemer and Greene (1985). We utilize the Rigel classification since the Kraemer classification requires knowing whether or not relatives of the affected patient have AM, which is difficult to verify in most clinical settings. Furthermore, examining all family members is usually impractical. Crijns et al. (1991), in a cross-sectional survey of 156 living family members of 31 probands who were originally classified as having sporadic AMS (type A), found that 60% of the patients with sporadic AMS had one or more relatives with the AMS phenotype. Only 25% of the probands were ultimately shown to be "true" sporadic AM cases. Therefore, the Rigel classification is much more practical to use in a clinical setting.

The superb work on MM-prone families by Tucker, Greene, and their colleagues has shown that affected individuals have a 150- to 500-fold increased risk for developing MM. The lifetime risk for developing MM has been calculated to be 81.6% (Tucker et al. 1993; Greene et al. 1985).

Recent prospective studies on AMS patients, including the NYU-MCG studies, suggests that the RR for developing MM varies from 16 to 92, depending on previous personal and/or family history of MM (McHenry and MacKie 1993; Halpern et al. 1993; Marghoob et al. 1994; Schneider et al. 1994).

Based on review of the literature and our own experience, we have drafted some recommendations regarding the management of patients with AMS. Since the concept of the AMS is in a state of flux, some of these recommendations will change as our understanding of the biology and natural course of the syndrome evolves. For now, the following is our approach to patients who have AMS:

1. All individuals with AMS are routinely screened, at least on an annual basis. The frequency of screening may be increased if the conditions warrant it (e.g., during adolescence and pregnancy).
2. Screening is begun around puberty (Tucker et al. 1993).
3. The entire cutaneous surface is examined every 4–12 months. For examination of the scalp, a hand-held hairdryer is very useful (Rigel et al. 1989; Titus-Ernstoff et al. 1989).
4. We have found baseline TCP, viewed during each examination, to be very helpful in identifying early changes in preexisting MN or newly acquired melanocytic neoplasms. This approach should be considered optional, but if circumstances permit, it is strongly recommended. It has been shown that surveillance in conjunction with photographic documentation is one of the best methods for the detection of early MM, i.e., MM in situ (Slue et al. 1988).

5. Histological confirmation is performed on any lesion suspected of being a MM (Piepkorn et al. 1989). Biopsy techniques which we consider to be acceptable include excision, punch, and deep saucerization (National Institutes of Health Consensus Development Conference 1992). Step-sectioning of the surgical specimen is recommended, since MM can be present in only a focal area of a melanocytic neoplasm.
6. Patients are instructed on the self-skin examination technique. They are instructed to examine their skin every 1–2 months. Patients are also provided with information detailing the early signs of MM (Friedman et al. 1985).
7. Patients are warned of the potential hazards of sun exposure, as it is nevogenic and it has been implicated as an important factor in the pathogenesis of MM (Stefanato et al. 1993; Kopf et al. 1977, 1978, 1985, 1986; Smith et al. 1982; Jung et al. 1986; Elwood et al. 1986). Sun exposure should be minimized through sun avoidance, the use of sun-protective clothing, and the use of broad-spectrum sunscreens with an sun protection factor (SPF) of at least 15.
8. Patient's family members are encouraged to have TCE to determine whether they, too, are at increased risk for MM. It has become apparent that many so-called sporadic AMS patients come from AMS families (Crijns et al. 1991; Albert et al. 1990).

We look forward to a uniformly accepted agreement on the definition of AMS. We concur with the Consensus Conference that the term AMS is an improvement over such terms as DNS or B-K mole syndrome. We continue to espouse public and primary care education regarding the early diagnosis of MM. The potential clinical usefulness of dermoscopy, digital imaging, serum markers, and immunotherapy continue to make AMS a most fruitful area of research.

Acknowledgements. This work was supported by the William Randolph Hearst Malignant Melanoma Fellowship; the Ronald O. Perelman Department of Dermatology, NYU School of Medicine; the Niarchos Fund of the Skin Cancer Foundation; and the Cancer Center Support Core Grant No. P30 CA-16087-16.

References

Albert LS, Rhodes AR, Sober AJ (1990) Dysplastic melanocytic nevi and cutaneous melanoma: markers of increased melanoma risk for affected persons and blood relatives. J Am Acad Dermatol 22:69–75

Augustsson A, Stierner U, Rosdahl I et al (1991) Common and dysplastic naevi as risk factors for cutaneous malignant melanoma in a Swedish population. Acta Derm Venereol (Stockh) 71:518–524

Beral V, Evans S, Shaw H et al (1983) Cutaneous factors related to the risk of malignant melanoma. Br J Dermatol 109:165–172
Bondi EE, Clark WH Jr, Elder D et al (1981) Topical chemotherapy of dysplastic melanocytic nevi with 5% fluorouracil. Arch Dermatol 114:89
Clark WH Jr, Reimer RR, Greene M et al (1978) Origin of familial malignant melanomas from heritable melanocytic lesions–the B-K mole syndrome. Arch Dermatol 114:732–738
Crijns MB, Vink J, Van Hees CLM et al (1991) Dysplastic nevi–occurrence in first- and second-degree relatives of patients with "sporadic" dysplastic nevus syndrome. Arch Dermatol 127:1346–1351
Cutler SJ, Ederer F (1958) Maximum utilization of the life-table method in analyzing survival. J Chronic Dis 8:699–712
Dubin N, Moseson M, Pasternack BS (1986) Epidemiology of malignant melanoma: pigmentary traits, ultraviolet radiation, and the identification of high-risk populations. In: Gallagher RP (ed) Epidemiology of malignant melanoma. Springer, Berlin Heidelberg New York, pp 56–75 (Recent results in cancer research, vol 102)
Elder DE, Greene MH, Guerry D IV et al (1982) The dysplastic nevus syndrome our definition. Am J Dermatopathol 4:455–460
Elwood JM, Williamson C, Stapleton PJ (1986) Malignant melanoma in relation to moles, pigmentation, and exposure to fluorescent and other lighting sources. Br J Cancer 53:65–74
Frichot BC III, Lynch HT, Guirgis HA et al (1977) New cutaneous phenotype in familial malignant melanoma. Lancet 1:864–865
Friedman RJ, Rigel DS, Kopf AW (1985) Early detection of malignant melanoma: the role of physician examination and self-examination of the skin. CA 35:130–151
Friedman RJ, Rigel DS, Kopf AW et al (1991) Dysplastic nevi. In: Friedman RJ et al (eds) Cancer of the skin. Saunders, Philadelphia
Garbe C, Kruger S, Stadler R et al (1989) Markers and relative risk in a German population for developing malignant melanoma. Int J Dermatol 28:517–523
Green A, MacLennan R, Siskind V (1985) Common acquired nevi and the risks of malignant melanoma. Int J Cancer 35:297–300
Greene MH, Clark WH Jr, Tucker MA et al (1980) Precursor naevi in cutaneous malignant melanoma: a proposed nomenclature. Lancet 2:1024
Greene MH, Clark WH Jr, Tucker MA et al (1985) High risk of malignant melanoma in melanoma-prone families with dysplastic nevi. Ann Intern Med 102:458–465
Grob JJ, Gouvernet J, Aymar D et al (1990) Count of benign melanocytic nevi as a major indicator of risk for nonfamilial nodular and superficial spreading melanoma. Cancer 66:387–395
Halpern AC, Guerry D IV, Elder DE et al (1991) Dysplastic nevi as risk markers of sporadic (nonfamilial) melanoma. A case-control study. Arch Dermatol 127: 995–999
Halpern AC, Guerry D IV, Elder DE et al (1993) A cohort study of melanoma in patients with dysplastic nevi. J Invest Dermatol 100:346S–349S
Holly EA, Kelly JW, Shpall SN et al (1987) Number of melanocytic nevi as a major risk factor for malignant melanoma. J Am Acad Dermatol 17:459–468
Holman CDJ, Armstrong BK (1984) Pigmentary traits, ethnic origin, benign nevi, and family history as risk factors for cutaneous malignant melanoma. J Natl Cancer Inst 72:257–266
Jung EG, Bohnert E, Boonen H (1986) Dysplastic nevus syndrome: ultraviolet hypermutability confirmed in vitro by elevated sister chromatid exchanges. Dermatologica 173:297–300
Kopf AW, Bart RS, Rodriguez-Sains RS (1977) Sunlight and malignant melanoma. J Dermatol Surg Oncol 3:45–48

Kopf AW, Lazar M, Bart RS et al (1978) Prevalence of nevocytic nevi on lateral and medial aspects of arms. J Dermatol Surg Oncol 4:153–158

Kopf AW, Lindsay AC, Rogers GS et al (1985) Relationship of nevocytic nevi to sun exposure in dysplastic nevus syndrome. J Am Acad Dermatol 12:656–662

Kopf AW, Gold RS, Rogers GS et al (1986) Relationship of lumbosacral nevocytic nevi to sun exposure in dysplastic nevus syndrome. Arch Dermatol 122:1003–1006

Kopf AW, Friedman RJ, Rigel DS (1990) Atypical mole syndrome. J Am Acad Dermatol 22:117–118

Kraemer KH, Greene MH (1985) Dysplastic nevus syndrome – familial and sporadic precursors of cutaneous melanoma. Dermatol Clin 3:225–237

Kraemer KH, Greene MH, Tarone R et al (1983) Dysplastic naevi and cutaneous melanoma risk. Lancet 2:1076–1077

Kraemer KH, Tucker M, Tarone R et al (1986) Risk of cutaneous melanoma in dysplastic nevus syndrome types A and B. N Engl J Med 315:1615–1616

Kruger S, Garbe C, Buttner P et al (1992) Epidemiologic evidence for the role of melanocytic nevi as risk markers and direct precursors of cutaneous malignant melanoma. J Am Acad Dermatol 26:920–926

MacKie RM, Freudenberger T, Aitchison TC (1989) Personal risk-factor chart for cutaneous melanoma. Lancet 2:487–490

Marghoob AA, Kopf AW, Rigel DS et al (1994) Risk of cutaneous malignant melanoma in patients with "classic" atypical-mole syndrome: a case-control study. Arch Dermatol 130:993–998

McHenry PM, MacKie RM (1993) A prospective study of the value of surveillance in individuals thought to be at increased risk of developing melanoma. Br J Dermatol 129:18

National Institutes of Health Consensus Development Conference (1992) Diagnosis and treatment of early melanoma, vol 10(1), p 12

Nollet DJ (1986) Clark's nevus syndrome. Am J Dermatopathol 8:367

Norris W (1820) Case of fungoid disease. Edinburgh Med Surg J 16:562–565

Piepkorn M, Meyer LJ, Goldgar D et al (1989) The dysplastic melanocytic nevus: a prevalent lesion that correlates poorly with clinical phenotype. J Am Acad Dermatol 20:407–415

Rhodes AR, Weinstock MA, Fitzpatrick TB et al (1987) Risk factors for cutaneous melanoma – a practical method of recognizing predisposed individuals. JAMA 258:3146–3154

Ries LAG, Hankey BF, Miller BA et al (1991) Cancer statistics review 1973–1988. National Cancer Institute, NIH Publ no 91-2789, surveillance epidemiology and end results

Rigel DS, Rivers JK, Friedman RJ et al (1988) Risk gradient for malignant melanoma in individuals with dysplastic nevi. Lancet 1:352–353

Rigel DS, Rivers JK, Kopf AW et al (1989) Dysplastic nevi – markers for increased risk for malignant melanoma. Cancer 63:386–389

Roush GC, Nordlund JJ, Forget B et al (1988) Independence of dysplastic nevi from total nevi in determining risk for nonfamilial melanoma. Prev Med 17/3:273–279

Schneider JS, Moore DH II, Sagebiel RW (1994) Risk factors for melanoma incidence in prospective follow-up: the importance of atypical (dysplastic) nevi. Arch Dermatol 130:1002–1007

Slue W, Kopf AW, Rivers JK (1988) Total-body photographs of dysplastic nevi. Arch Dermatol 124:1239–1243

Smith PJ, Greene MH, Devlin DA et al (1982) Abnormal sensitivity to UV-radiation in cultured skin fibroblasts from patients with hereditary cutaneous malignant melanoma and dysplastic nevus syndrome. Int J Cancer 30:39–45

Stefanato CM, Romero JB, Kopf AW et al (1993) Solar nevogenesis: a surrogate for predicting a rise in incidence of malignant melanoma because of ozone depletion. J Am Acad Dermatol 29:486–487

Swerdlow AJ, Green A (1987) Melanocytic naevi and melanoma: an epidemiological perspective. Br J Dermatol 117:137–146

Swerdlow AJ, English J, MacKie RM et al (1986) Benign melanocytic nevi as a risk factor for malignant melanoma. Br Med J 292:1555–1559

Tiersten AD, Grin CM, Kopf AW et al (1991) Prospective follow-up for malignant melanoma in patients with atypical-mole (dysplastic-nevus syndrome. J Dermatol Surg Oncol 17:44–48

Titus-Ernstoff L, Ernstoff MS, Kirkwood JM et al (1989) Usefulness of frequent skin examination for the early detection of second primary cutaneous melanoma. Cancer Detect Prevent 13:317–321

Tucker MA, Fraser MC, Goldstein AM et al (1993) Risk of melanoma and other cancers in melanoma-prone families. J Invest Dermatol 100:350S–355S

Vasen HFA, Bergman W, Van Haeringen A et al (1989) The familial dysplastic nevus syndrome – natural history and the impact of screening on prognosis – a study of nine families in the Netherlands, vol 25, pp 337–341

II. Malignant Melanoma

Properties of Metastasizing and Nonmetastasizing Human Melanoma Cells

G.N.P. van Muijen[1], E.H.J. Danen[1], T.J. de Vries[1], P.H.A. Quax[2], J.H. Verheijen[2], and D.J. Ruiter[1]

[1] Department of Pathology, University Hospital Nijmegen, P.O. Box 9101, 6500 HB Nijmegen, The Netherlands
[2] Gaubius Laboratory IVVO-TNO, P.O. Box 430, 2300 AK Leiden, The Netherlands

Abstract

Dissemination of tumor cells includes several steps, such as: (a) detachment of tumor cells from the primary tumor, (b) traversement of the basement membrane, and (c) migration into the extracellular matrix. In these processes, at least two important categories of proteins are involved: proteases and adhesion molecules. In this contribution we describe the expression and function of components of the plasminogen activator (PA) system (proteases) and of integrins (cell–matrix adhesion molecules) in a panel of four human melanoma cell lines with different invasive and metastatic capacity. Regarding the components of the PA system, we found differences in expression of urokinase-type PA (uPA) and type 1 and 2 PA inhibitors (PAI-1 and -2) between metastasizing and nonmetastasizing cell lines. Both components were exclusively expressed in the highly invasive and metastatic cell lines. Interestingly, studies on the expression of PA components in fresh human melanocytic lesions, showed expression of these components exclusively in advanced primary melanomas and melanoma metastases. Regarding integrin expression we found elevated levels of VLA-2 and VLA-6 in the highly invasive and metastatic cell lines compared with normal cultured melanocytes and nonmetastatic melanoma cell lines. In addition, increased adhesion of the highly metastatic cell lines to laminin (LM) and collagen (COLL) was observed. Furthermore, reduced adhesion of normal melanocytes and nonmetastatic melanoma cells to LM and CO was mainly due to the fact that the integrins involved in adhesion to these matrix components were present in an inactive state. Finally, differences were observed in expression of integrins involved in adhesion to fibronectin.

Recent Results in Cancer Research, Vol. 139

Introduction

The most important feature of malignancy is the capacity of tumor cells to metastasize. The process of metastasis is very complex and can be subdivided in several steps (Liotta et al. 1983; Juliano 1987; Bastida 1988; Fidler 1989):

1. Outgrowth of the primary tumor, invasive growth into the surrounding tissue, and detachment of neoplastic cells from the primary tumor.
2. Migration of tumor cells or shedding of clumps of tumor tissue into the lymphatics or blood vessels.
3. Embolization and survival of tumor cells in the circulation and adhesion to remote vascular or lymphatic endothelium or the subendothelial basement membrane.
4. Migration through the extracellular matrix and outgrowth at the distant site.

In this process multiple factors are involved, such as molecules involved in DNA repair, oncogenes, tumor suppressor genes, growth factors and their receptors, motility factors, angiogenic factors, transcription factors, signal-transducing proteins, cytokines, extracellular matrix components, proteases, and cell–cell and cell–matrix adhesion molecules. Although each step of the metastatic cascade is crucial for the development of a metastatic lesion, tumor cell metastasis–defined as the ability of tumor cells to detach from the primary tumor, to traverse the basement membrane, and to migrate through the extracellular matrix–marks the transition from benign to malignant behavior. In these processes, basement membrane penetration by proteases involved in degradation of the extracellular matrix and interactions of the tumor cells with their environment through cell adhesion molecules are essential. Therefore, in this chapter we will focus on proteases and cell–matrix adhesion molecules.

At least two major extracellular proteolytic systems are thought to be involved in metastasis formation, those of the metalloproteinases and the plasminogen activation (PA) components of system (Danø et al. 1985; Stetler-Stevenson 1990; Pöllänen et al. 1991; Mignatti and Rifkin 1993). Elevated expression of both proteases, especially collagenase IV and urokinase, and their inhibitors. (TIMP-1 and -2 and PAI-1, respectively) has been found in several types of tumors.

By far the most extensively studied family of basement membrane receptors are the integrins. A number of immunohistochemical studies have demonstrated that changes in integrin expression are associated with tumor progression (Albelda 1993; Paulus et al. 1993). In addition, transfection studies with certain integrins have demonstrated the relevance of these receptors in tumorigenicity and metastasis formation (Giancotti and Ruoslahti 1990; Chan et al. 1991; Felding-Habermann et al. 1992).

Different steps of tumor progression have been defined not only for melanoma, but for almost all other human tumors. In human cutaneous melanoma, several stages in the process of tumor progression have been identified clinically, histopathologically, and immunologically (Clark et al. 1984; Bröcker et al. 1985; Herlyn et al. 1987). All lesions are derived from normal melanocytes and represent sequential steps starting with locally invasive lesions, some of which may develop into tumors with metastatic potential and ultimately metastasize. Because of their superficial location and the simultaneous presence in some patients of lesions representing different stages of tumor progression, melanomas of the skin are preeminently suitable to study tumor progression. Furthermore, many well-characterized human melanoma cell lines have been established.

As extracellular proteolysis and adhesion to extracellular matrix components is essential for tumor cell dissemination, we studied: (a) the expression and biological activity of the plasminogen activation system and (b) the expression and the biological activity of a number of integrins in melanoma cell invasion and metastasis formation. For this study we used a set of four different human melanoma cell lines which were previously extensively characterized with respect to the expression of melanocytic differentiation and progression antigens and their metastatic behavior in nude mice (Van Muijen et al. 1989, 1991a,b).

In this contribution we will not present a comprehensive review of the literature. Instead, we will put emphasis on the discussion of our own work and compare it to recent literature data.

Invasion and Metastasis

Although the expression, role, and activity of molecules involved in invasion and metastasis preferentially should be studied in the human system in order to unravel the complexity of the metastasic cascade in patients, it is profitable to invcstigate the different steps in various in vitro and in vivo model systems separately.

For our purposes we first determined the invasive capacity of a set of four different human melanoma cell lines in vitro using a human amnion basement membrane (Mignatti et al. 1986). After radiolabeling of the tumor cells with ^{125}I-iododeoxyuridine, they were seeded on the amniotic membrane obtained from fresh human placenta. Cells were permitted to invade the basement membrane for a period of 72h. A marked difference in invasion was seen between the cell lines (Fig. 1a). The invasive capacity of the BLM and MV3 cell lines was strongly enhanced as compared to the IF6 and 530 cell lines.

To investigate the biological behavior of the cell lines in vivo, we determined their tumorigenicity and metastatic capacity after inoculation into nude mice. It was found that all four cell lines were tumorigenic (Fig. 1b). After intravenous inoculation, all cell lines except IF6 were capable of developing lung colonies (experimental metastases). After subcutaneous

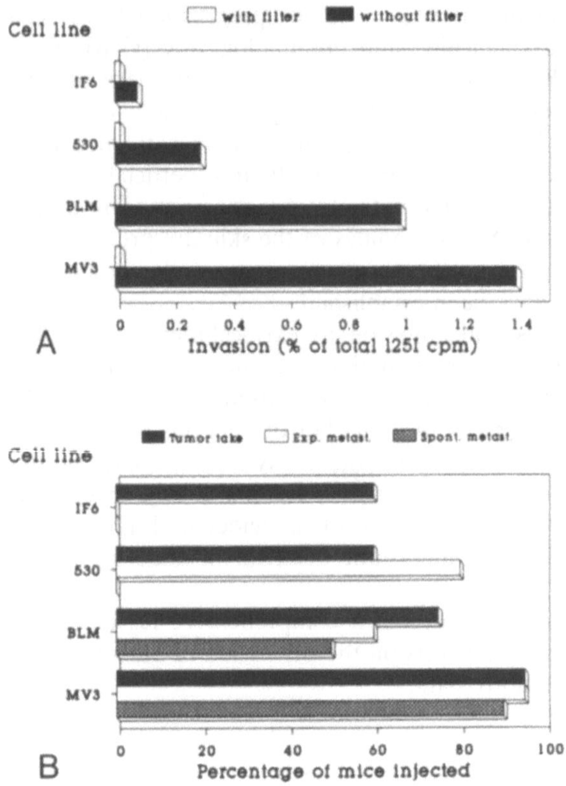

Fig. 1A,B. Invasion and metastasis of human melanoma cell lines. **A** Amnion basement membrane invasion of radiolabeled melanoma cells. The amnion basement membrane was isolated from fresh human placenta. The mean of three combined experiments, each performed in triplicate, is shown. SD, 0.2%. **B** Tumor take and metastasis rate after intravenous (experimental metastasis) or subcutaneous (spontaneous metastases) inoculation into nude mice. At least three groups of five mice each were inoculated with each cell line

inoculation we found that the non- or poorly invasive cell lines IF6 and 530 did not metastasize at all, while the two strongly invasive cell lines BLM and MV3 showed frequent formation of lung metastases as assessed by light microscopical examination at autopsy (Figs. 1b, 2). No metastases were found in other organs or tissues.

In view of this marked difference in invasive and metastatic behavior, these cell lines seemed to be very useful to study possible correlations between their capacity to invade and to form metastases and the involvement of components of the plasminogen activation system and adhesion molecules of the integrin superfamily in these processes.

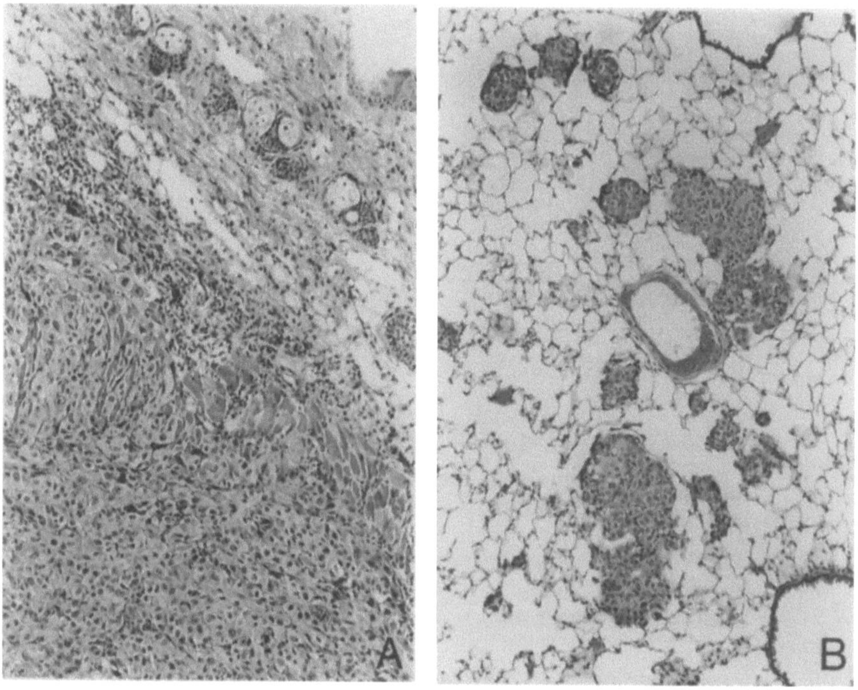

Fig. 2A,B. Histopathology of human melanoma xenografts. **A** Tumor growing at the inoculation site after subcutaneous injection of 2 × 10^6 MV3 cells (×180). **B** Lung metastases developed after subcutaneous inoculation of 2 × 10^6 MV3 cells (×75)

Extracellular Proteolysis

We investigated the expression and activity of the following components of the plasminogen activation system: urokinase-type and tissue-type plasminogen activator (uPA and tPA), type 1 and type 2 plasminogen activator inhibitors (PAI-1 and PAI-2), and the uPA receptor (uPAR). The expression of all plasminogen activation components were analyzed both on the mRNA and protein level (Quax et al. 1991). mRNA analysis was performed qualitatively by northern blot analysis and quantitatively by a dot blot technique (Quax et al. 1990; not shown). Protein analysis was executed on tissue culture supernatants and on cell extracts using commercially available enzyme-linked immunoadsorbent assay (ELISA) kits (Quax et al. 1990). Northern blotting revealed that all four cell lines extensively expressed tPA mRNA, while uPA, PAI-1, and PAI-2 mRNA expression could only be detected in BLM and MV3 cells (not shown). The data of the quantitative mRNA and protein analyses (Fig. 3a; Table 1) corresponded with the northern blotting results, except for PAI-2. Although PAI-2 mRNA was

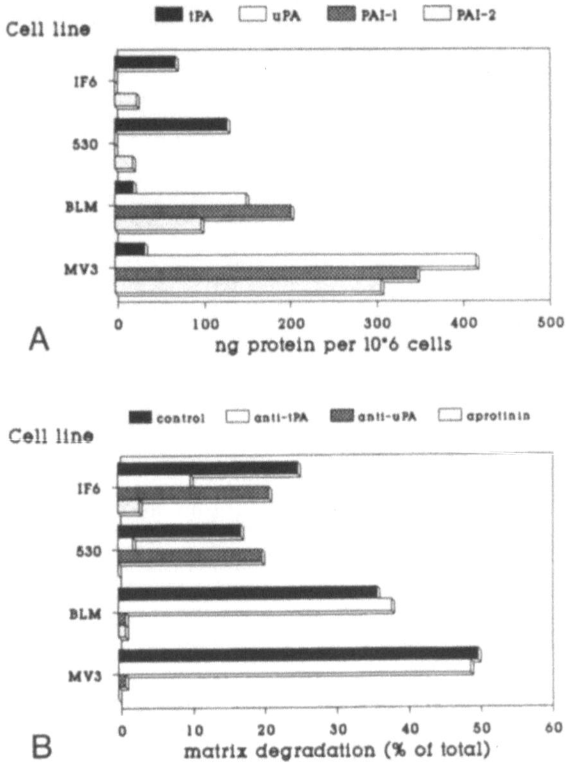

Fig. 3A,B. Analysis of plasminogen activation (PA) components in human melanoma cell lines. **A** Production of tissue-type PA (*tPA*), urokinase-type PA (*uPA*), and PA inhibititors 1 and 2 (*PAI-1* and *PAI-2*) by the cell lines after 24 h. Levels were determined by enzyme-linked immunoabsorbent assays (ELISA) on tissue culture supernatant. **B** Degradation of radiolabeled extracellular matrix by incubation with the different cell lines. Specificity was determined by incubation with aprotinin, anti-tPA, or anti-uPA. Degradation was expressed as percentage of total radioactivity released after trypsin treatment

only detectable in BLM and MV3 cells, the protein could be detected in all cell lines. However, in comparison with IF6 and 530, expression was markedly elevated in BLM and MV3 cells.

uPAR northern blot analysis revealed expression in all four cell lines. A slightly elevated mRNA expression was seen in BLM and MV3 cells (not shown). However, binding assays with ^{125}I-labeled uPA showed that expression on the protein level based on the binding capacity of the receptor was similar in all four cell lines (Table 1).

To analyze the proteolytic capacity and the involvement of the plasminogen activators in matrix degradation, the cell lines were seeded on a ^{3}H-labeled extracellular matrix produced by bovine aortic smooth muscle

Table 1. Expression of plasminogen activator components in human melanoma cell lines and in fresh human melanocytic lesions

	Metastatic capacity[a]	tPA[b]	uPA	PAI-1	PAI-2	uPAR
Cell lines						
IF6	–	++	–	–	+	+
530	–	++	–	–	+	+
BLM	++	+	++	++	++	+
MV3	+++	+	+++	+++	+++	+
Lesions						
NN	–	0[c]	0	0	0	0
AN	–	0	0	0	0	0
ePM	+/–	0	0	0	0	0
aPM	++	20	55	65	55	55
MM	++	35	70	55	50	65

PA, plasminogen activator; tPA, tissue-type PA; uPA, urokinase-type PA; PAI, PA inhibitor; uPAR, uPA receptor; NN, nevocellular nevus; AN, atypical nevus; ePM, early primary melanoma; aPM, advanced primary melanoma; MM, melanoma metastasis.

[a] –, no; +/–, very low; ++, high; +++, very high.

[b] –, no expression; +, weak expression; ++, moderate expression; +++, strong expression.

[c] Total percentage of lesions with immunoreactivity after immunohistochemical staining.

cells, and the release of radioactive matrix fragments was determined. All four cell lines were capable of degrading extracellular matrix in vitro (Fig. 3b). Degradation could almost completely be inhibited by incubation with aprotinin, a plasmin inhibitor, indicating that degradation was plasmin dependent. To determine whether proteolysis was tPA or uPA mediated, incubations were performed in the presence of anti-tPA or -uPA antibodies. While extracellular matrix degradation by IF6 and 530 was inhibited by anti-tPA, no tPA-mediated proteolysis was observed with BLM and MV3. In contrast, no inhibition was seen with IF6 and 530 using anti-uPA, as expected, while treatment of BLM and MV3 with anti-uPA resulted in a complete inhibition of matrix degradation. These data strongly suggested that matrix degradation by poorly invasive, nonmetastatic melanoma cells is tPA mediated and by highly invasive, metastatic melanoma cells is uPA mediated.

From the results of our experiments it was concluded that a highly invasive and metastatic behavior of human melanoma cells in vitro and in vivo is associated with specific expression of uPA and PAI-1, with strongly increased expression of PAI-2 and with uPA-mediated degradation in vitro (Table 1). Furthermore, as no correlation was found with the potency of tumor cells to develop lung colonies after intravenous inoculation into nude mice, we concluded that uPA, PAI-1, and increased levels of PAI-2 play a role in early stages of melanoma metastasis formation, e.g., detachment of tumor cells from the primary tumor.

As little is known about the expression and involvement of the PA system in human cutaneous melanocytic lesions in situ, we recently analyzed a large series of fresh human lesions containing all different stages of melanocytic tumor progression (common nevocellular nevus, atypical nevus, early primary melanoma, advanced primary melanoma, melanoma metastasis) for the occurrence of PA components (Table 1; De Vries et al. 1994). Gene expression was studied on the mRNA level by in situ hybridization and on the protein level by immunohistochemistry; uPA and tPA activity was determined by in situ zymography (Fig. 4). Interestingly, we found that uPA, PAI-1, PAI-2, and uPAR emerge, generally simultaneously, in more than half of the advanced primary melanomas and melanoma metastases, strongly indicating that PA is a late event in melanocytic tumor progression and plays a role in melanoma metastasis formation, which fits with our conclusions from the in vitro and in vivo studies with the melanoma cell lines.

Cell–Matrix Interaction

As adhesion to extracellular matrix components is essential in tumor cell dissemination, we investigated the expression and activity of a great number of integrins during invasion and melanoma metastasis formation.

We started to determine the capacity of our set of human melanoma cell lines and of normal cultured human melanocytes to adhere to various purified extracellular matrix components (Danen et al. 1993). After radiolabeling with ^{51}Cr, the cells where allowed to attach to laminin (LM), fibronectin (FN), and collagen (COLL) types I and IV. In contrast to the melanocytes and the nonmetastasizing cell lines IF6 and 530, the highly metastatic cell lines BLM and MV3 adhered strongly to LM and COLL types I and IV (Fig. 5a). A different pattern was found for adhesion to FN. Most cells exhibited strong binding to FN, including melanocytes. Only 530 cells adhered poorly.

As adhesion of the invasive and highly metastatic cell lines to LM and COLL was markedly increased, we focused on those integrins known to be involved in adhesion to these extracellular matrix components ($\alpha_1\beta_1$, $\alpha_2\beta_1$, $\alpha_3\beta_1$ for COLL; $\alpha_1\beta_1$, $\alpha_2\beta_1$, $\alpha_3\beta_1$, $\alpha_6\beta_1$, $\alpha_6\beta_4$ for LM). Fluorescence-activated cell sorter (FACS) analysis revealed very low expression of $\alpha_1\beta_1$, and no expression of $\alpha_6\beta_4$ on all cells, including melanocytes (Table 2). Expression of $\alpha_3\beta_1$ was found on all cell lines and on melanocytes. Expression of $\alpha_2\beta_1$ and $\alpha_6\beta_1$ was high on the highly invasive and frequently metastasizing cell lines BLM and MV3, whereas melanocytes and the nonmetastasizing cell lines showed a strongly reduced expression.

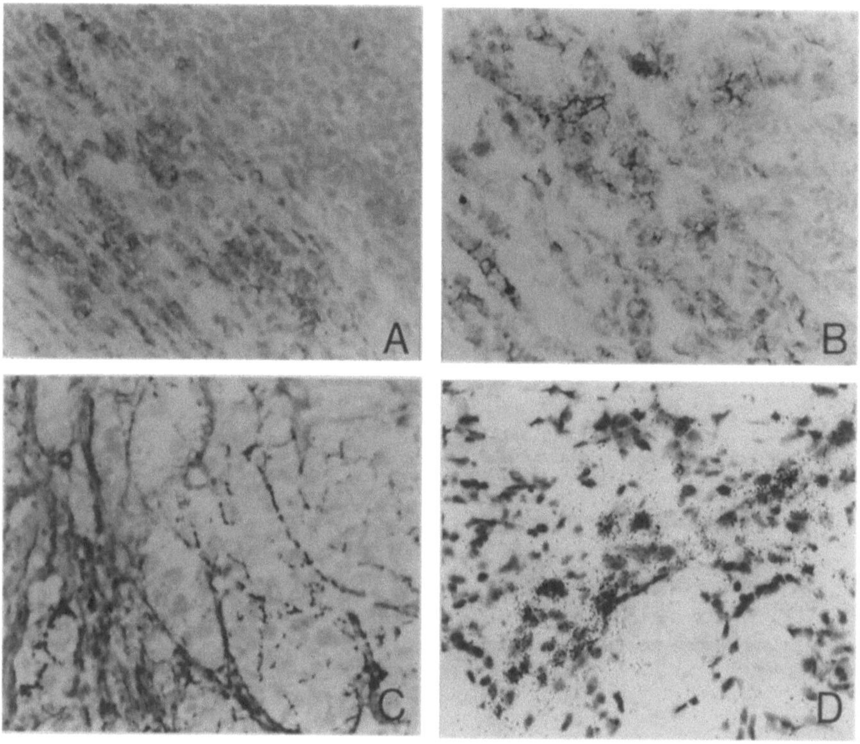

Fig. 4A–D. Microphotographs of sections of fresh human melanocytic lesions after immunohistochemical staining (**A, B, C**) with antibodies or mRNA in situ hybridization (**D**) with probes specific for different components of the plasminogen actvation system. **A–C** are stainings on the same melanoma metastasis lesion. **A** Incubation with anti-urokinase-type plasminogen activator (anti-uPA) antibodies. Note that uPA protein is present on invading tumor cells (×500). **B** Incubation with anti-uPA receptor (-uPAR) antibodies. Note that uPAR is present on invading tumor cells (×500). **C** Incubation with PA inhibitor (PAI)-1 antibodies. Note that PAI-1 is mainly located in the extracellular matrix surrounding tumor cells (×500). **D** mRNA in situ hybridization with a PAI-1 cDNA probe on an advanced primary melanoma. Note that PAI-1 mRNA is expressed by invasive tumor cells (×840)

To determine which of the integrin receptors were specifically involved in attachment to LM and COLL, adhesion inhibition assays were performed with the strongly adhesive cell lines BLM and MV3 using appropriate monoclonal antibodies (MAbs) known to block the receptor adhesion site. These experiments showed that VLA-2 is the major receptor for COLL and that VLA-2 and VLA-6 are the major receptors for LM (Fig. 5b).

In the last few years it has been demonstrated that high-affinity interaction of integrins with their ligands requires activation of the receptor (van Kooyk et al. 1989; Wilkins et al. 1991). In addition, it has recently been shown that antibodies recognizing specific epitopes present on the α- or β-

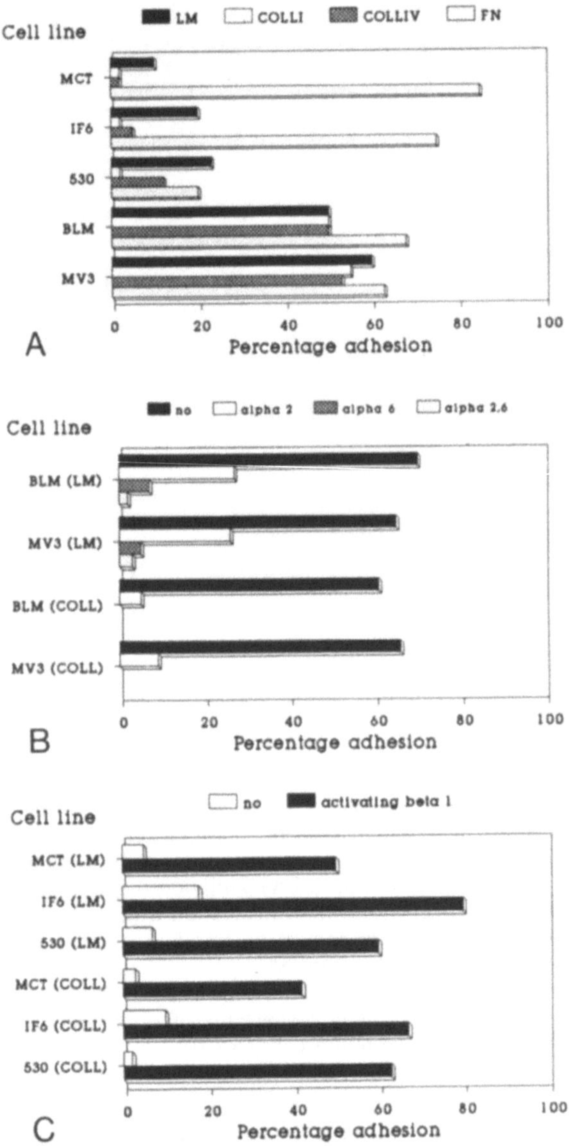

Fig. 5A–C. Adhesion of normal cultured human melanocytes (*MCT*) and human melanoma cell lines to purified extracellular matrix components. SD of triplicate determinations did not exceed 10%. One experiment out of three is shown. **A** Adhesion of radiolabeled cells to laminin (*LM*), collagen types I (*COLL I*) and IV (*COLL IV*), and fibronectin (*FN*). **B** Inhibition of adhesion to LM and COLL I after incubation of the cell lines with monoclonal antibodies specifically blocking α_2- or α_6-integrin-mediated binding. Inhibition assays using COLL IV gave similar results as COLL I. **C** Stimulation of adhesion to LM and COLL I after incubation of the cell lines with a monoclonal β_1-antibody known to be capable of inducing a high-affinity state of β_1 integrins

Table 2. Expression of integrin subunits in human melanoma cell lines

Integrin subunit	Cell line				
	MCT[a]	IF6	530	BLM	MV3
α_1	±	±	±	±	±
α_2	±	±	±	++	++
α_3	++	+	±	++	++
α_4	−	+	+	++	++
α_5	+	+	±	++	++
α_6	±	±	±	++	++
β_1	++	+	+	++	++
β_3	+	+	±	−	−
β_4	−	−	−	−	−
α_V	+	+	+	±	±
α_{IIb}	−	−	−	−	−

MCT, cultured normal human melanocytes.
[a] −, negative; ±, weak expression; +, moderate expression; ++, strong expression.

chain can induce a high-affinity state of various integrins (van de Wiel-van Kemenade et al. 1992). As it was clear from our FACS experiments (Table 2) that melanocytes and nonmetastatic cell lines which did not adhere at all or only very poorly to LM and COLL were not completely negative for those integrins involved in adhesion to these matrix components, we were interested whether the differences in adhesion with the highly metastatic cell lines were only due to quantitative differences in expression of the receptors or may be caused by differences in the activation state. Therefore, adhesion assays with antibodies known to be capable of inducing a high affinity of β_1-integrins were performed. These incubations revealed a markedly increased adhesion of melanocytes and IF6 and 530 cells (Fig. 5c). As no stimulatory effects were obtained with BLM and MV3 cells, we concluded that the number of receptors is less important than the state of activation of the integrins.

Although we did not find a correlation between adhesion of the melanoma cells to FN and their invasive capacity in vitro and metastatic behavior in nude mice, we were interested whether differences in integrin-mediated adhesion to FN between the metastasizing and nonmetastasizing melanoma cells could be observed. As FN contains various binding sites, both arginine-glycine-aspartic acid (RGD) as well as non-RGD, we performed adhesion assays using FN fragments containing different cell attachment sites (not shown). In combination with the results from FACS experiments (Table 2) and adhesion inhibition studies (Fig. 6), we concluded that there are differences in binding to FN between metastatic and nonmetastatic melanoma

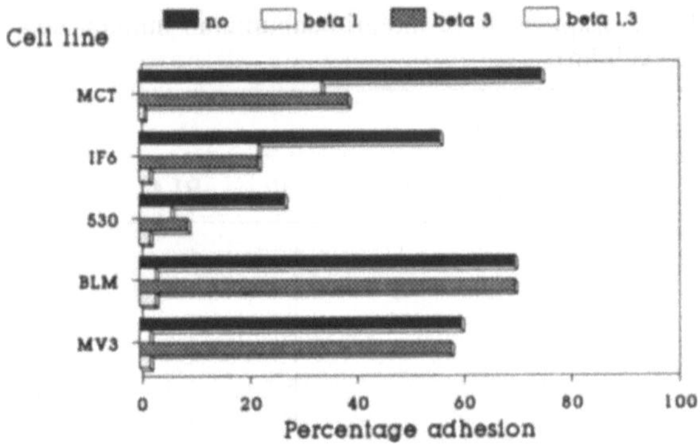

Fig. 6. Inhibition of adhesion to fibronection (FN) after incubation of the cell lines with monoclonal antibodies specifically blocking β_1- or β_3-integrin-mediated binding. SD of triplicate determinations did not exceed 10%. One experiment our of three is shown. *MCT*, normal cultured human melanocytes

cells: (a) adhesion of melanocytes and nonmetastatic melanoma cells to the central cell-binding domain of FN is mediated by VLA-5 and $\alpha_v\beta_3$; (b) adhesion of highly metastatic melanoma cells is exclusively mediated by VLA-5, and (c) all four melanoma cell lines express VLA-4 for binding to the CS-I site of the alternatively spliced IIICS region of FN, while normal melanocytes do not express VLA-4 at all and thus cannot bind to the IIICS region.

Regarding the LM/COLL receptors, we concluded from our experiments that: (a) the level of VLA-2 and VLA-6 expression is strongly increased in highly metastatic melanoma cells; (b) these receptors are present in a low-affinity state on melanocytes and nonmetastatic melanoma cells, whereas they are strongly active on highly metastatic melanoma cells; (c) as a result, highly metastatic melanoma cells show increased adhesion to LM and COLL. Regarding the FN receptors, we concluded that: (a) melanoma cells adhere to the CS-1 site of the V-region of FN via VLA-4, whereas melanocytes do not adhere to this site due do the absence of VLA-4 expression; and (b) there are differences in integrin-mediated adhesion to FN; melanocytes and nonmetastatic melanoma cells adhere via β_1- and β_3-integrins, whereas metastatic melanoma cells exclusively bind via β_1-integrins.

When we compare our data concerning integrin expression on melanocytes and melanoma cell lines in relation to their invasive and metastatic properties with correlations described between integrin expression on human melanoma cells in situ (Fig. 7) and tumor progression, most findings are not conflicting.

Just as in fresh human melanocytic lesions (Bröcker et al. 1985; Klein et al. 1991), we found that increased expression of VLA-2 indicates a high metastatic potential of tumors.

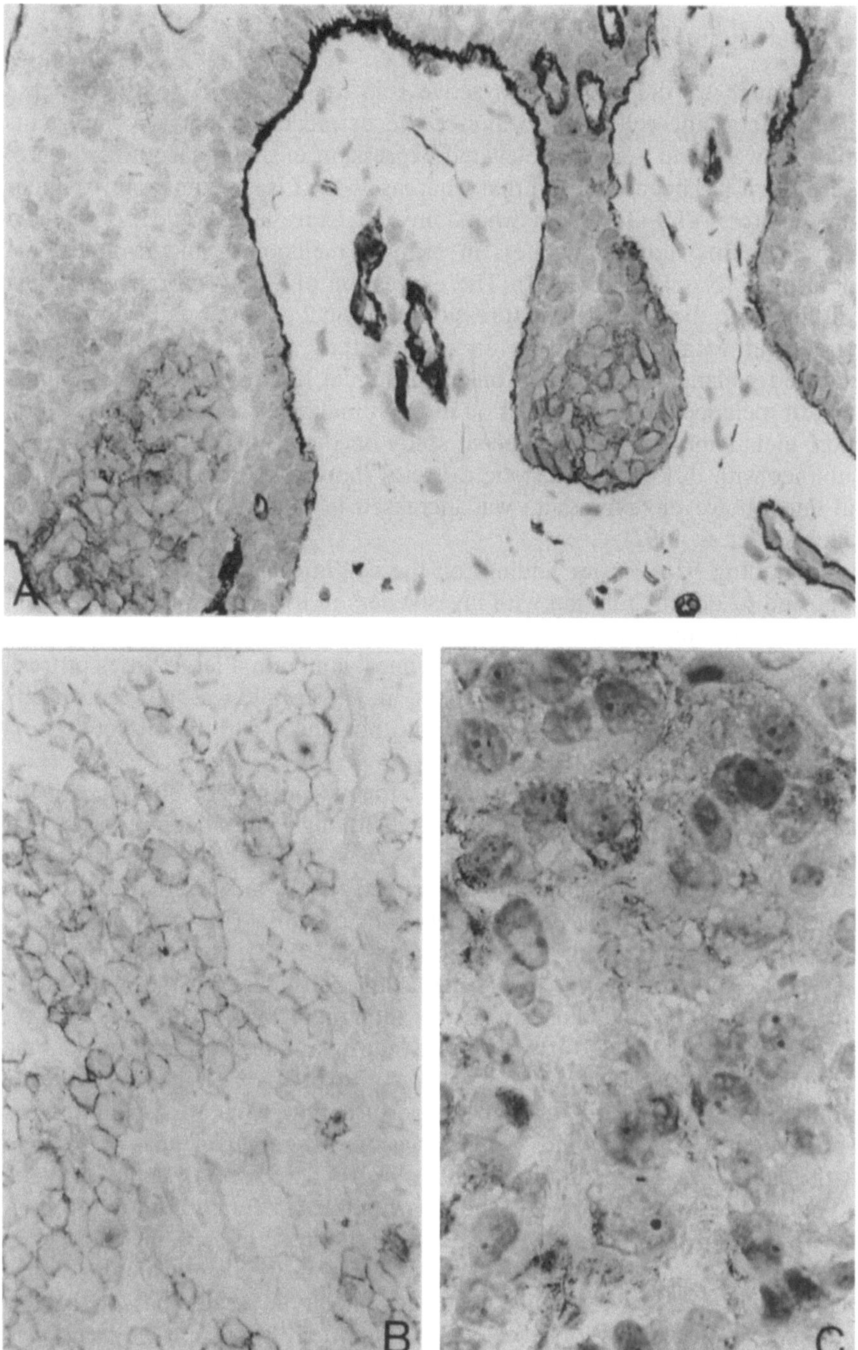

Fig. 7A–C. Microphotographs of sections of fresh human melanocytic lesions after immunohistochemical staining with antibodies directed against different integrin subunits. **A** Nevus nevocellularis stained with anti-α_6 monoclonal antibodies (GoH3; ×200). **B** Advanced primary melanoma stained with anti-α_2 monoclonal antibodies (A1.43; ×400). **C** Melanoma metastasis stained with anti-α_3 monoclonal antibodies (J143; ×400)

Although we did not find an active role for VLA-3 in adhesion of the highly metastatic cell lines to any of the extracellular matrix components studied, we found a slightly elevated expression in the metastatic cell lines. Recently it has been reported that whereas 56% of fresh human nevocellular nevi express VLA-3, a somewhat elevated expression could be detected with increasing tumor thickness in primary melanomas and in melanoma metastates (Natali et al. 1993). The expression of VLA-4 in our melanoma cell lines and the absence of expression in normal cultured melanocytes is in agreement with the results in an earlier study (Albelda et al. 1990) on cultured melanocytic cells and on fresh human lesions: absence in nonmalignant melanocytes and expression in fresh malignant lesions (40%) and on most melanoma cell lines. A recent study on three human A375 melanoma sublines with different metastatic capacity showed expression of VLA-4 on all lines; however, expression was increased in the most metastatic subline (Gehlsen et al. 1992).

Regarding VLA-6, our findings on the cell lines are at variance with the reported α_6 downregulation with invasiveness in fresh human lesions (Natali et al. 1991). However, although we also found a decreased expression of α_6 with progression in an immunohistochemical study on a large series of fresh human melanocytic lesions (Danen et al. 1994a), it was not statistically significant. Albelda et al. (1990) also did not find a correlation between α_6 expression and melanoma progression.

Finally, regarding the expression of the vitronectin receptor $\alpha_v\beta_3$, our data appear to differ from other reports. Although it has been reported that $\alpha_v\beta_3$ expression is often associated with vertical growth phase and melanoma metastasis (Albelda et al. 1990; Danen et al. 1994a,b) and with tumorigenicity, invasive capacity, and/or metastatic potential (Marshall et al. 1991; Felding-Habermann et al. 1992; Gehlsen et al. 1992), we could not detect any $\alpha_v\beta_3$ expression in our highly metastatic cell lines. On the other hand, the nonmetastatic cells did express this integrin. However, in a very recent study (Seftor et al. 1993) it was shown that invasion of a human melanoma cell line with very low $\alpha_v\beta_3$ and high VLA-5 expression could be specifically stimulated after integrin ligation or perturbation with VLA-5 antibodies and not with $\alpha_v\beta_3$ antibodies, while invasion of another melanoma cell line with high $\alpha_v\beta_3$ expression (and also VLA-5 expression) could only be stimulated with $\alpha_v\beta_3$ antibodies and not with VLA-5 antibodies (Seftor et al. 1992). These data strongly indicate that the role of $\alpha_v\beta_3$ in tumor cell invasion can also be fulfilled by VLA-5. Therefore, it is interesting to realize that our $\alpha_v\beta_3$-negative, highly metastatic melanoma cell lines do have a marked VLA-5 expression (Table 2). In addition, in our earlier-mentioned immunohistochemical study (Danen et al. 1994a) on melanocytic lesions, our most striking finding was the emergence of both VLA-5 and $\alpha_v\beta_3$ during tumor progression, especially in advanced primary melanoma and melanoma metastasis. Regarding the VLA-5 receptor, Mortarini et al. (1992) showed that this integrin might not only be involved in melanoma cell invasion, but can also stimulate the proliferation of quiescent melanoma cells.

Conclusions and Future Prospects

In conclusion, a number of studies, including ours, strongly suggest a prominent role for both the PA system and adhesion molecules of the integrin superfamily in the process of melanoma metastasis formation.

In our opinion both our results of in vitro and in vivo studies with human melanoma cell lines as well as the phenotyping of fresh human melanocytic lesions warrant further research. As a result, transfection studies of non-metastasizing, non-uPA-producing melanoma cell lines with uPA cDNA and transfection studies of highly metastatic, uPA-producing cell lines with antisense uPA cDNA are being performed. In addition, we wish to examine whether expression of PA components is a prognostic parameter in melanoma independent of known variables such as the Breslow thickness. Such a new prognostic marker may be helpful in selecting high-risk patients for adjuvant therapy.

Regarding the integrins, we would like to stress that the mere presence of these molecules at the cell surface is not sufficient to explain processes such as anchoring and/or migration, as these molecules may be present in an inactive or low-affinity state. Furthermore, it becomes more and more clear that integrins are not only involved in tumor cell invasion and metastasis by attachment and migration, but that they also may have indirect functions as signaling molecules to initiate or activate other processes (Juliano and Haskill 1993; Mortarini and Anichini 1993; Schwartz 1993). It is likely that future investigations may demonstrate the involvement of the various integrins and their state of activation in specific cell-matrix interactions during tumor growth, invasion, and metastasis formation, thereby yielding new insights into this enigmatic process.

Finally, an impulse for interesting new experiments originates from the recent work done by Seftor and coworkers (1992, 1993), who found that increased invasion of human melanoma cells by ligation or perturbation of $\alpha_v\beta_3$ or VLA-5 integrins with $\alpha_v\beta_3$ or VLA-5 antibodies, respectively, was caused by increased expression and activity of collagenase type IV. These data strongly indicate that synergistic effects of integrins and proteases may be of major importance in tumor cell invasion and dissemination.

Acknowledgements. We would like to thank Dr. R.B. Bankert, Dr. D.A. Cheresh, Dr. C.G. Figdor, Dr. C.E. Klein, Dr. N.L. Kovach, Dr. A. Sonnenberg, Dr. T.S. Springer, Dr. R. Bos, Dr. H.W. Verspaget, and Dr. W.J.M. Tax for kindly providing antibodies; Dr. M. Denijn for her support in performing mRNA in situ hybridization; Dr. P. Mignatti for his help in performing the amnion basement membrane invasion assay; Dr. C.G. Figdor for stimulating discussions; and Mrs. I.M.H.A. Cornelissen and Mr. C.F.J. Jansen for expert technical assistance. Part of this work was supported by the Dutch Cancer Society (NKB) and the EC Concerted Action on melanoma progression.

References

Albelda SM (1993) Biology of disease: role of integrins and other cell adhesion molecules in tumor progression and metastasis. Lab Invest 68:4–17

Albelda SM, Mette SA, Elder DE, Stewart R, Damjanovich L, Herlyn M, Buck C (1990) Integrin distribution in malignant melanoma: association of the β_3 subunit with tumor progression. Cancer Res 50:6757–6764

Bastida E (1988) The metastatic cascade: potential approaches for the inhibition of metastasis. Semin Thromb Hemost 14:66–72

Bröcker E-B, Suter L, Brüggen J, Ruiter DJ, Macher E, Sorg C (1985) Phenotype dynamics of tumor progression in human malignant melanoma. Int J Cancer 36:29–35

Chan BMC, Matsuura N, Takada Y, Zetter BR, Hemler ME (1991) In vitro and in vivo consequences of VLA-2 expression on rhabdomyosarcoma cells. Science 251:1600–1602

Clark WH Jr, Elder DE, Guerry D, Epstein MN, Greene MH, van Horn M (1984) A study of tumor progression: the precursor lesions of superficial spreading and nodular melanoma. Hum Pathol 15:1147–1156

Danen EHJ, van Muijen GNP, van de Wiel-van Kemenade E, Jansen CFJ, Ruiter DJ, Figdor CG (1993) Regulation of integrin-mediated adhesion to laminin and collagen in human melanocytes and in non-metastatic and highly metastatic human melanoma cells. Int J Cancer 54:315–321

Danen EHJ, ten Berge PJM, van Muijen GNP, van't Hof-Grootenboer AE, Bröcker E-B, Ruiter DJ (1994a) Emergence of $\alpha_5\beta_1$ fibronectin- and $\alpha_v\beta_3$ vitronectin receptor expression in melanocytic tumor progression. Histopathology (in press)

Danen EHJ, Jansen CFJ, Ruiter DJ, van Muijen GNP (1994b) Expression of α_v-integrins in human cutaneous melanoma: decreased expression of $\alpha_v\beta_5$ during melanoma progression (submitted)

Danø K, Andreasen PA, Grøndahl-Hansen J, Kristensen P, Nielsen LS, Skriver L (1985) Plasminogen activators, tissue degradation and cancer. Adv Cancer Res 44:139–266

De Vries TJ, Quax PHA, Denijn M, Verrijp KN, Verheijen JH, Verspaget HW, Weidle UH, Ruiter DJ, van Muijen GNP (1994) Plasminogen activators, their inhibitors and urokinase receptor emerge in late stages of melanocytic tumor progression. Am J Pathol 144:71–80

Felding-Habermann B, Mueller BM, Romerdahl CA, Cheresh DA (1992) Involvement of integrin α_v gene expression in human melanoma tumorigenicity. J Clin Invest 89:2018–2022

Fidler IJ (1989) Origin and biology of cancer metastasis. Cytometry 10:673–680

Gehlsen KR, Davis GE, Sriramarao P (1992) Integrin expression in human melanoma cells with differing invasive and metastatic properties. Clin Exp Metastasis 10:111–120

Giancotti FG, Ruoslahti E (1990) Elevated levels of the $\alpha_5\beta_1$ fibronectin receptor suppress the transformed phenotype of chinese hamster ovary cells. Cell 60: 849–859

Herlyn M, Clark WH, Rodeck U, Mancianti ML, Jambrosic J, Koprowski H (1987) Biology of disease: biology of tumor progression in human melanocytes. Lab Invest 56:461–474
Juliano RL (1987) Membrane receptors for extracellular matrix macromolecules: relationship to cell adhesion and tumor metastasis. Biochem Biophys Acta 907: 261–278
Juliano RL, Haskill S (1993) Signal transduction from the extracellular matrix. J Cell Biol 120:577–585
Klein CE, Steinmeyer T, Kaufmann R, Weber L, Bröcker E-B (1991) Identification of a melanoma progression antigen as integrin VLA-2. J Invest Dermatol 96: 281–284
Liotta LA, Rao CN, Barsky SH (1983) Tumor invasion and extracellular matrix. Lab Invest 49:636–649
Marshall JF, Nesbitt SA, Helfrich MH, Horton MA, Polakova K, Hart IR (1991) Integrin expression in human melanoma cell lines: heterogeneity of vitronectin receptor composition and function. Int J Cancer 49:924–931
Mignatti P, Rifkin DB (1993) Biology and biochemistry op proteinases in tumor invasion. Physiol Rev 73:161–195
Mignatti P, Robbins E, Rifkin DB (1986) Tumor invasion through the human amniotic membrane: requirement for a proteinase cascade. Cell 47:487–498
Mortarini R, Anichini A (1993) From adhesion to signalling: roles of integrins in the biology of human melanoma. Melanoma Res 3:87–97
Mortarini R, Gismondi A, Santoni A, Parmiani G, Anichini A (1992) Role of the $\alpha_5\beta_1$ integrin receptor in the proliferative response of quiescent human melanoma cells to fibronectin. Cancer Res 52:4499–4506
Natali PG, Nicotra MR, Cavaliere R, Giannarelli D, Bigotti A (1991) Tumor progression in human malignant melanoma is associated with changes in $\alpha_6\beta_1$ laminin receptor. Int J Cancer 49:168–172
Natali PG, Nicotra MR, Bartolazzi A, Cavaliere R, Bigotti A (1993) Integrin expression in cutaneous malignant melanoma: association of the $\alpha_3\beta_1$ heterodimer with tumor progression. Int J Cancer 54:68–72
Paulus W, Baur I, Schuppan D, Roggendorf W (1993) Characterization of integrin receptors in normal and neoplastic human brain. Am J Pathol 143:154–163
Pöllänen J, Stephens RW, Vaheri A (1991) Directed plasminogen activation at the surface of normal and malignant cells. Adv Cancer Res 50:273–328
Quax PHA, Leeuwen RTJ, Verspaget HW, Verheijen JH (1990) Protein and messenger RNA levels of plasminogen activators and inhibitors analyzed in 22 human tumor cell lines. Cancer Res 50:1488–1494
Quax PHA, van Muijen GNP, Weening-Verhoeff EJD, Lund LR, Dano K, Ruiter DJ, Verheijen JH (1991) Metastatic behavior of human melanoma cell lines in nude mice correlates with urokinase-type plasminogen activator, its type-1 inhibitor, and urokinase-mediated matrix degradation. J Cell Biol 115:191–199
Schwartz MA (1993) Signaling by integrins: implications for tumorigenesis. Cancer Res 53:1503–1506
Seftor REB, Seftor EA, Gehlsen KR, Stetler-Stevenson WG, Brown PD, Ruoslathi E, Hendrix MJC (1992) Role of the $\alpha_v\beta_3$ integrin in human melanoma cell invasion. Proc Natl Acad Sci USA 89:1557–1561
Seftor REB, Seftor EA, Stetler-Stevenson WG, Hendrix MJC (1993) The 72kDa type IV collagenase is modulated via differential expression of $\alpha_v\beta_3$ and $\alpha_5\beta_1$ integrins during human melanoma cell invasion. Cancer Res 53:3411–3415
Stetler-Stevenson WG (1990) Type IV collagenases in tumor invasion and metastasis. Cancer Metastasis Rev 9:289–303
Van de Wiel-van Kemenade E, van Kooyk Y, de Boer AJ, Huijbens RJF, Weder P, van de Kasteele W, Melief CJM, Figdor CG (1992) Adhesion of T and B

lymphocytes to extracellular matrix and endothelial cells can be regulated through the β subunit of VLA. J Cell Biol 117:461–470
Van Kooyk Y, van de Wiel-van Kemenade P, Weber P, Kuijpers TW, Figdor CG (1989) Enchancement of LFA-1-mediated cell adhesion by triggering through CD2 or CD3 on T lymphocytes. Nature 342:811–813
Van Muijen GNP, Cornelissen IMHA, Jansen CFJ, Ruiter DJ (1989) Progression markers in metastasizing human melanoma cells xenografted to nude mice. Anticancer Res 9:879–884
Van Muijen GNP, Cornelissen IMHA, Jansen CFJ, Figdor CG, Johnson JP, Bröcker E-B, Ruiter DJ (1991a) Antigen expression of metastasizing and non-metastasizing human melanoma cells xenografted into nude mice. Clin Exp Metastasis 9:259–272
Van Muijen GNP, Jansen CFJ, Cornelissen IMHA, Smeets DFCM, Beck JLM, Ruiter DJ (1991b) Establishment and characterization of a human melanoma cell line (MV3) which is highly metastatic in nude mice. Int J Cancer 48:85–91
Wilkins JA, Stupack D, Stewart S, Caixia S (1991) β_1 Integrin mediated lymphocyte adherence to extracellular matrix is enchanced by phorbol ester treatment. Eur J Immunol 21:517–522

Protein Patterns of Benign and Malignant Human Melanocytes Show Consistent Changes in Gene Expression

J. Eberle, C. Garbe, G. Kroumpouzos, and C.E. Orfanos

Department of Dermatology, The Free University of Berlin, University Medical Center, Steglitz, Hindenburgdamm 30, 12200 Berlin, Germany

Abstract

For human malignant melanoma, no pattern of oncogene activation has yet been identified which consistently occurs in the malignant cells. In order to better understand the transformation process, we studied the overall gene expression at the protein level in human melanoma cells in vitro by two-dimensional gel electrophoresis. For that, four established cell lines, MEWO, M5, SKMEL13, and IGR39, were used and compared with newly established cultures of normal human melanocytes. Considerable variations in the protein patterns of the different melanoma cell lines were found, whereas the patterns of normal human melanocytes correlated fairly well with each other.

With respect to the expression of single proteins, we identified four major proteins which were consistently found in cultured melanocytes and stringently repressed in the four melanoma cell lines examined. On the other hand, induction of new proteins in the different melanoma cell lines was found to be less stringent and also less uniform. We propose that malignant transformation of melanocytes may be more associated with the suppression of melanocytic proteins rather than with new expression of melanoma specific proteins.

Introduction

Today, a genetic basis for the development of cancer is generally accepted, though many questions still are open. For human malignant melanoma, several oncogenes have been proposed as being involved in the transformation process, but no consistent pattern of oncogene activation has yet been identified (Schrier 1992).

Recent Results in Cancer Research, Vol. 139

Beside the direct identification of activated oncogenes, the malignant phenotype may also be characterized by alterations in the expression of specific proteins. For human malignant melanoma, several tumor-specific antigens have been described and monoclonal antibodies were created (Houghton et al. 1982, 1987; Holzwann et al. 1987). The use of antibodies for the detection of specifically expressed proteins, however, is limited to some extent, because of their preference to bind antigens at the surface or the membrane of the target cells; if one intends to get an overview of all changes in the protein expression of tumor cells the technique of two-dimensional protein gel electrophoresis can be used (Tracy et al. 1982; Hanash et al. 1985). For human melanoma cells, such a comparison has already been performed between a metastatic and a nonmetastatic cell line (Easty et al. 1991), but a comparison between benign and malignant melanocytes has not yet been reported.

The present investigation is based on the comparison of four established melanoma cell lines (MC) and several newly established cultures of normal human melanocytes (NHM). The cell line phenotype was examined with respect to morphology, growth behavior, and antigen expression. Analysis of the protein patterns was performed in order to obtain an overview of the variations in gene expression between normal and malignant melanocytes.

Materials and Methods

Cell Lines and Culture Conditions

Melanoma cell lines SKMEL13 (Livingston et al. 1985), MEWO (Bean et al. 1975), IGR39 (Aubert et al. 1980), and M5 (Leyva et al. 1983) were cultured in Dulbecco's Modified Eagle medium containing 4.5 g D-glucose/l (Gibco, Paisly, Scotland). The medium was supplemented with 10% fetal calf serum (Biochrom, Berlin, Germany) and antibiotics (Biochrom).

NHM were derived from human foreskin after trypsin digestion (Eisinger and Marco 1982) and cultured in MCDB 153 (Biochrom, Berlin, Germany) The following supplements were given (Krasagakis et al. 1991): 2 m*M* Ca^{2+}, 5 μg insulin/ml (Sigma, St. Louis, USA), 10 μg human transferrin/ml (Sigma), 0.4% v/v whole bovine pituitary extract (Clonetics Inc., San Diego, USA), 2 ng bovine basic fibroblast growth factor/ml (Boehringer Mannheim, Germany). 1 n*M* cholera toxin (Calbiochem, La Jolly, USA), and 50 μM hydrocortisone (Serva, Heidelberg, Germany). With subculturing, 10% fetal calf serum was added to NHM cultures for 24 h and then replaced by serum-free medium. Before harvesting, usually three to four passages were performed with 10^6 cells (MC) or 2×10^6 (NHM) per 75 cm^2 flask.

Characterization of Phenotypic Parameters

Doubling times were determined in six-well plates (Falcon, Berlin, Germany), into which equal numbers of cells were seeded. Every second day, two wells were harvested and cell numbers were counted with a hemacytometer. Multilayer growth was determined by a phase-contrast microscope (Olympus, FRG). The plating efficiency of cell lines was determined by cell seeding in twofold serial dilution steps in 96-well culture plates (Falcon), beginning with 10^4 cells/ml (Sauvaigo et al. 1986). After 15 days, cell attachment was monitored microscopically. For determining melanin content (Friedmann and Gilchrest 1987), cells were grown in Dulbecco's Modified Eagle medium supplemented with 10% serum and 2 m*M* L-tyrosine. Confluent fibroblast cultures were used as negative controls and all MC values were corrected for the fibroblast value. Immunological markers were determined with the alkaline phasphatase and monoclonal anti-alkaline phosphatase (APAAP) technique (Cordell et al. 1984). Two melanoma-specific antibodies were used: HMB45 (Gown et al. 1986), purchased at (Enzo, New York, USA), and NKI-C3 (Vennegoor et al. 1985), purchased at (Monosan, Amsterdam, Netherlands).

Protein Extraction

For protein extraction, cells were harvested from a 75-cm^2 flask at 70%–80% confluence. Fresh medium had been applied 24 h before harvesting. After briefly washing the cell layer with 10 ml phosphate-buffered saline (PBS) without Ca^{2+}, Mg^{2+} (Seromed, Berlin, Germany), cells were scraped with a rubber policeman, transferred to a centrifugation tube, and centrifuged at 4000 *g* for 5 min. Lysis was performed according to a protocol designed by Celis and Bravo (1984): cells were resuspended in the cold in a buffer containing TRIS-Cl (20 m*M*) and $CaCl_2$ (2 m*M*) by a narrow-gauge needle. Then sodium dodecyl sulfate (SDS) was added to a final concentration of 0.3%, followed by ribonuclease (RNaseA) and deoxyribonuclease (DNaseI) with concentrations of 50 μg/ml and 100 μg/ml, respectively. The sample was left on ice until the solution was no longer viscous and was then lyophilized.

Protein Gel Electrophoresis

Protein extracts were analysed by two-dimensional gel electrophoresis (O'Farrel 1975). The isoelectric focusing (first dimension) was performed as a tube gel with some modifications for the pH gradient (Chambers et al. 1985). In the second dimension, the proteins were separated in a polyacrylamide/SDS gel (Sambrook et al. 1989). Acrylamide was used in a concentration of 12.5% and bisacrylamide in a ratio of 1:200. The protein gels were stained with silver nitrate (Silver Stain Kit, Richmond, USA) according to the instructions of the supplier. Molecular weight and isoelectric points were determined according to the parallel separation of a two-dimensional marker (BioRad, München, Germany).

Results

Phenotypic Characterization of Melanoma Cell Lines

The aim of the present study was to identify differences in gene expression between melanoma cells (MC) and normal human melanocytes (NHM). In order to mainly identify differences of some general importance for melanoma cells, four distinct cell lines of different origin and phenotype were used for this comparison. In vitro, the best morphological similarity to NHM was seen with the cell line MEWO, which was dendritic, while the MC lines M5 and IGR39 had a more epithelioid-like shape and SKMEL13 represented an intermediate morphology (Fig. 1). In order to better characterize the MC lines used, several phenotypical markers were determined (Table 1). Under the applied growth conditions, measurable melanin pigment was found only in SKMEL13 and M5 cells. Three cell lines expressed both melanoma antigen markers HMB45 (Gown et al. 1986) and NKI-C3 (Vennegoor et al. 1985), while IGR39 was only positive for NKI-C3. The proliferation rates during logarithmic growth were determined to be 32–34 h, similar for all four cell lines. Vertical growth after reaching confluence was observed at the cell lines M5 and MEWO. The highest plating efficiency (Sauvaigo et al. 1986) was found for M5 cells, which were able to attach to microtiter vials even when only a single cell was given, while the other cell lines needed on an average eight cells per vial to attach (Table 1).

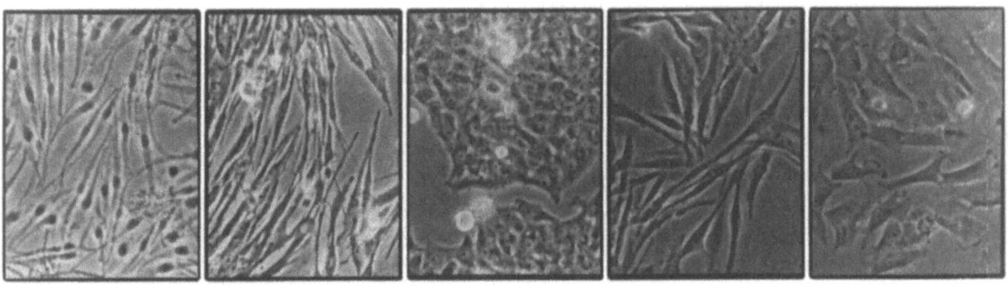

Fig. 1. Morphology of normal human melanocytes (NHM) and melanoma cell (MC) lines. The morphologies of four MC lines, MEWO, M5, SKMEL13 and IGR39, are shown in comparison to a culture of NHM

Table 1. Characteristics of melanoma cell lines

Cell line	Reference	Tumor	Immunoreactivity for antigens		Melanin content ($\mu g/10^6$ cells)	Doubling time (h)	Vertical growth[a]	Plating efficiency[b]
			HMB45	NKI-C3				
M5	Leyva et al. (1983)	Metastasis pigmented	+	+	1	34	+	1
SKMEL13	Livingston et al. (1985)	Metastasis	+	+	2.5	32	−	8
IGR39	Aubert et al. (1980)	Primary pigmented	−	+	0	32	−	8
MEWO	Bean et al. (1975)	Metastasis pigmented	+	+	0	34	+	8

[a] Ability to build up multiple cell layers after reaching confluence.
[b] Number of cells necessary for attachment in microtiter vials.

Two-Dimensional Protein Gel Electrophoresis

In order to identify changes in the gene expression of melanoma cells as compared to normal human melanocytes, we analysed the protein patterns of the human MC lines SKMEL13, M5, MEWO, and IGR39 by two-dimensional gel electrophoresis. The patterns were compared to those of three NHM cultures, which were derived from three different foreskins (Fig. 2). For internal control, two gels of independently grown cultures of each of the two cell lines M5 and MEWO were performed.

For evaluation, the protein spots of all gels were categorized according to four intensity values: no (0), weak (1), medium (2), and strong expression (3), and the subsequent analysis was restricted to major proteins expressed in at least one of the cell lines with values of 2 or 3. Evaluation of the gels from the three NHM cultures revealed 69 major proteins (NHM proteins) and further analysis of the MC gels identified 40 additional proteins (MC proteins). Thus, 109 expression values were obtained for every cell culture, reflecting its expression of major proteins. Based on these expression values, we were able to compare the protein patterns of the different cell lines. In order to get one comparable value for each two cell lines representing all differences between them, the following calculations were performed: the expression values for each protein spot of two cell lines were compared with each other and differences were summed up; these sums of differences were calculated as percentages of the maximal possible difference two cell lines could ever have, which was 327 (109 analysed proteins multiplied by the highest expression, 3), and the finally resulting percentages were designated "dissimilarity values" (Table 2).

The calculated dissimilarity values revealed a relatively high similarity for the three melanocyte protein patterns with 5% deviation on average. The dissimilarity values for independently grown duplicates of the cell lines MEWO and M5 were within the same range (5%) and provided a basis for estimating internal error and reproducibility. Much higher dissimilarity, however, was observed when different MC lines were compared to each other (12% – 20%). The comparison of MC with NHM revealed a relatively high similarity between MEWO and NHM (average value, 11%), while M5 was the most dissimilar, with 21% on average (Table 2; Fig. 2).

The search for specifically regulated proteins revealed four proteins uniformly repressed in the MC tested (nos. 59, 62, 70, and 71; Table 3; Fig. 2). Their repression seemed to be regulated very stringently since they were not detectable in the gels of the four MC lines, whereas three of them (no. 59, 62, and 71) were uniformly found in all NHM cultures tested, and the fourth protein (no. 70) was expressed in two of three NHM cultures. The search for MC-induced proteins revealed two major proteins (nos. 28 and 102). However, their expression was found to be less stringently regulated, since they were also found in NHM to a weaker extent. The molecular

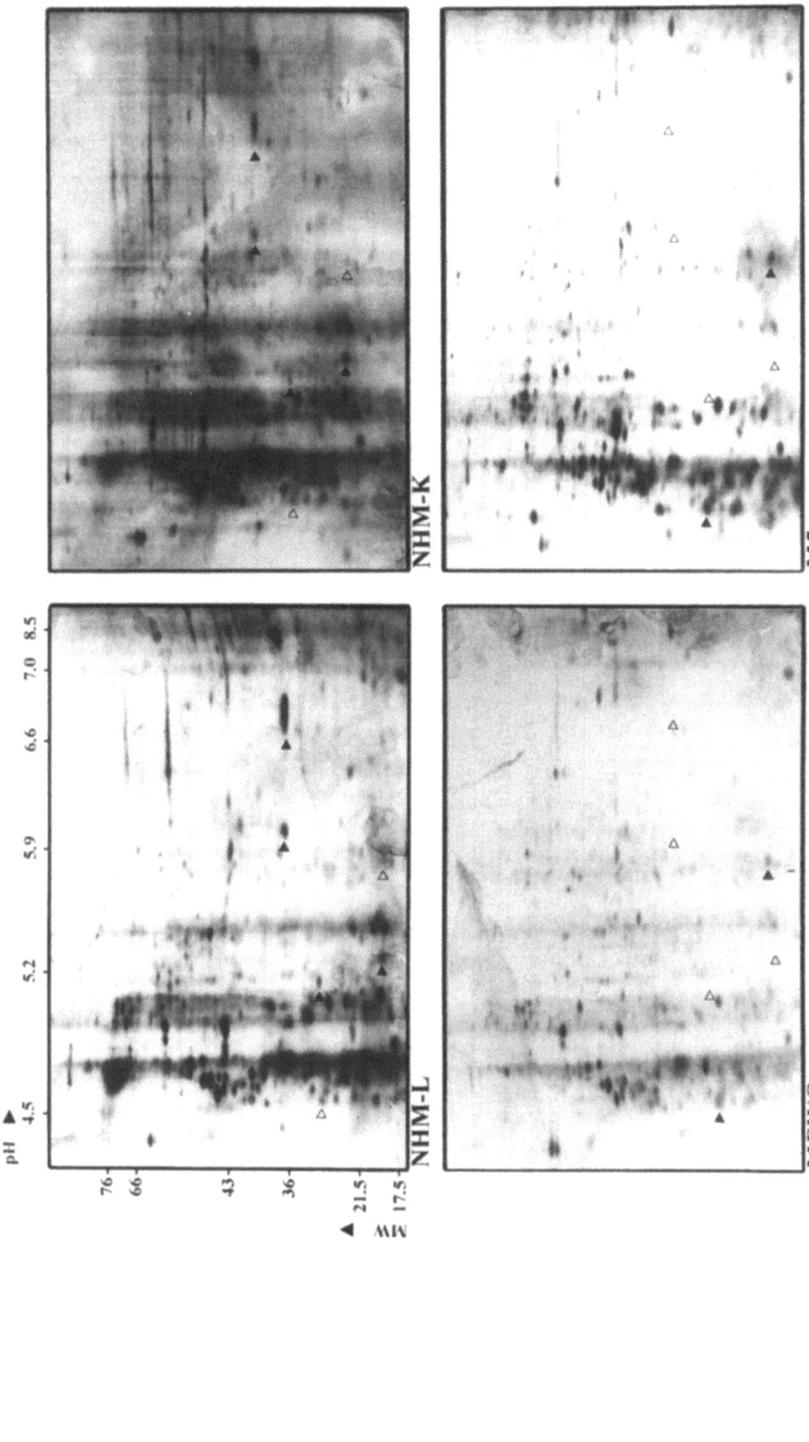

Fig. 2. Protein gels of normal human melanocytes (NHM) and melanoma cell (MC) lines M5 and MEWO. The two-dimensional protein patterns of two melanocyte cultures (NHM-L and NHM-K) and two MC lines (MEWO and M5) are shown. The molecular mass (*MW*, in kDa) and pH values are given for NHM-L. Proteins which were identified as specifically regulated in MC are indicated by *open triangles* (no or weak expression) and *filled triangles* (strong expression), respectively. Their numbers, from left to right, are: 28, 59, 62, 102, 70, 71 (see Table 2)

Table 2. Dissimilarity values of the protein pattern for normal human melanocytes (NHM) and melanoma cell (MC) lines[a]

	NHM-K	NHM-L	NHM-P	MEWO-I[b]	MEWO-II[b]	M5-I[b]	M5-II[b]	SKMEL13
NHM-L	4	–	–	–	–	–	–	–
NHM-P	6	5	–	–	–	–	–	–
MEWO-I[b]	11	13	12	–	–	–	–	–
MEWO-II[b]	10	12	9	5	–	–	–	–
M5-I[b]	21	21	20	17	17	–	–	–
M5-II[b]	21	22	21	17	17	5	–	–
SKMEL13	15	18	16	15	13	19	20	–
IGR39	17	19	17	12	16	20	20	20

[a] Dissmilarity values of the protein pattern are given in percentages of the maximal possible difference two cell lines could ever have: 0% dissimilarity would mean that two cell lines show an identical expression of the 109 major proteins analysed, whereas 100% dissimilarity would mean that two cell lines do not have any mojor protein in common. Each dissimilarity value results from the comparison of two protein gels. Three NHM cultures (-L, -P, -K) and four MC lines (SKMEL13, M5, IGR39, MEWO) were examined.

[b] For the MC lines MEWO and M5, two independent cultures each were analysed: (I, II).

Table 3. Specifically regulated proteins

Protein			Expression in NHM[a]			Expression in MC[b]					
No.	Molecular mass (kDa)	Isoelectric points (pH)	NHM-K	NHM-L	NHM-P	MEWO-I	NEWO-II	M5-I	M5-II	SKMEL13	IGR39
59	29	5.1	1	2	1	0	0	0	0	0	0
62	21	5.3	2	2	1	0	0	0	0	0	0
70	38	6	2	2	0	0	0	0	0	0	0
71	38	6.8	2	3	1	0	0	0	0	0	0
28	28	4.6	1	1	1	2	1	2	2	1	2
102	21	5.8	1	1	1	2	2	2	2	1	2

NHM, normal human melanocyte; MC, melanoma cell.

[a] Expression values in three NHM cultures (NHM-K, -L, -P). The expression was classified as weak, medium, and strong (values 1, 2, 3). No detectable expression is indicated by 0.

[b] For the MC lines MEWO and M5, two independent cultures each were analysed: (-I, -II).

weight of all six identified proteins was relatively low, ranging between 20 and 40 kDa (Fig. 2; Table 3).

Discussion

The present investigation has demonstrated consistent changes in the protein expression of melanoma cells in vitro as compared to normal human melanocytes. The analysis of the protein patterns by two-dimensional gel electrophoresis revealed far-reaching congruence for different NHM cultures, whereas the four examined MC lines showed rather great heterogeneity. Of the 109 analysed major proteins, four NHM proteins were found to be generally and stringently repressed in the MC lines. On the other hand, the induction of new MC-specific proteins appeared to be less stringent and uniform, as the two major proteins, which were identified as induced in MC, were also expressed to a weaker extent in NHM. Thus, as far as the major proteins were concerned, the malignant phenotype was clearly characterized by a general loss of proteins rather than by the uniform induction of new proteins.

Roughly 6% of the major proteins were found to be consistently regulated in MC, compared to more than 50% of the proteins which were found to be induced or repressed irregularly in one or the other cell line. If we expect a similar ratio also among the weaker-expressed proteins, a large number of consistently regulated proteins may be expected in MC.

Previous examinations of specific gene expression in MC have mainly focused on two groups of proteins and genes. The first group consisted of oncogenes, tumor-suppressor genes, and growth factors (Albino 1992; Schrier 1992; Shih and Herlyn 1993), which are of major importance for the characterization of any type of cancer, as they are known to be directly involved in the transformation process and/or growth control. For the oncogene c-*myc*, overexpression in melanoma cells in vitro was reported (Cheah et al. 1984; Versteeg et al. 1988). Of the group of growth factors, basic fibroblast growth factor (bFGF) and transforming growth factor-$\beta 2$ (TGF-$\beta 2$) have been detected to be induced or constitutively expressed in MC, in contrast to NHM (Albino 1992; Albino et al. 1991; Rodeck et al. 1991).

For further analysis of specific protein expression in MC, a number of tumor-specific antigens have been identified by the use of (monoclonal) antibodies. Furthermore, some of these antibodies have been used for the cloning and characterization of their associated genes. Among the group of antigens increasingly expressed with tumor progression, the intercellular adhesion molecule 1 (ICAM-1) molecule (Johnson et al. 1989) and the transferrin-related protein P97 were identified (Rose et al. 1986). The antigen ME491, associated with early stages of melanoma, was characterized as a membrane protein (Hotta et al. 1988), and for the antigen MUC18, seemingly correlated with poor clinical prognosis, a similarity to the immunoglobulin superfamily was identified (Lehmann et al. 1989).

The search for melanoma-specific antigens predominantly has focused on upregulated proteins. A large number of such antigens have now been identified (Houghton et al. 1982, 1987; Holzmann et al. 1987). On the other hand, few investigations have been published identifying antigens which are downregulated in MC. One example is the differentiation marker K.1.2.58, a cytoplasmatic glycoprotein (Suter et al. 1985). Therefore, our findings may stimulate a complementary approach focusing on the identification of downregulated melanocyte proteins and/or genes.

In interpreting our findings we have to be aware of the different levels at which gene regulation may occur which parallel the general course of gene expression: transcription regulation (Dynan 1989), RNA processing (Chou et al. 1987), and RNA stability (Cleveland 1988) result in an altered steady state level of the mRNA, whereas later regulation types such as translation regulation (Hinnebusch 1988) and regulation of the protein stability do not directly affect the mRNA level.

Considering these different levels, it cannot be directly deduced that all protein variations observed in this investigation result from an altered mRNA expression. Nevertheless we suggest that the majority of specifically regulated proteins can be traced back to genes which are regulated at their transcriptional level. Such genes can directly be cloned by the technique of "differential screening," a strategy which is based on the detection of variant mRNA levels of specifically regulated genes, represented in a gene library (Sambrook et at. 1989). Taking into account the fact that we predominantly found uniform regulation of NHM proteins which were repressed in MC, the use of a NHM gene library enriched with such genes may be the best choice.

Not all of the identified major proteins and of the expected high number of regulated minor proteins can be expected to exert a basic role within the transformation process. Most of them might be a result rather than a necessary condition of the transformation state itself. Nevertheless, the cloning and further characterization of their associated genes will help to better understand the character of human melanoma cells and the phenomenon of malignant transformation of melanocytes.

Acknowledgements. This work was partially supported by the Deutsche Forschungsgemeinschaft and by the Maria Sonnenfeld Gedächtnisstiftung.

References

Albino AP (1992) The role of oncogenes and growth factors in progressive melanomagenesis. Pigment Cell Res [Suppl] 2:199–218

Albino AP, Davis BM, Nanus DM (1991) Induction of growth factor RNA expression in human malignant melanoma: markers of transformation. Cancer Res 51:4815–4820

Aubert C, Rouge F, Galdino JR (1980) Tumorigenicity of human malignant melanocytes in nude mice in relation to their differentiation in vitro. J Natl Cancer Inst 64:1029–1040

Bean MA, Bloom BR, Heberman RB, Old LJ, Oettgen HF, Klein G, Terry WD (1975) Cell-mediated cytotoxicity for bladder carcinoma: evaluation of a workshop. Cancer Res 35:2902–2913

Celis and Bravo (1984) Two-dimensional gel electrophoresis of proteins, 1 st edn. Academic, London

Chambers JAA, Degli Innocenti F, Hinkelammert K, Russo VEA (1985) Electrophoresis 6:339–348

Cheah MS, Wallace CD, Hoffman RM (1984) Hypomethylation of DNA in human cancer cells: a site-specific change in the c-myc oncogene. J Natl Cancer Inst 73:1057–1065

Chou T-B, Zachar Z, Bingham PM (1987) Developmental expression of a regulatory gene is programmed at the level of splicing. EMBO J 6:4095–4104

Cleveland DW (1988) Autoregulated instability of tubulin mRNAs. TIBS 13:339–343

Cordell JL, Falini B, Erber WN, Ghosh AK, Abdulaziz Z, MacDonald S, Pulford KA, Stein H, Mason DY (1984) Immunoenzymatic labeling of monoclonal antibodies using immune complexes of alkaline phosphatase and monoclonal antialkaline phosphatase (APAAP complexes). J Histochem Cytochem 32: 219–229

Dynan WS (1989) Modularity in promoters and enhancers. Cell 58:1–4

Easty D, Hart IR, Patel K, Seymour C, Yacoub M, Domscheit A, Gunther S, Postel W, Gorg A, Dunn MJ (1991) Changes in protein expression during melanoma differentiation determined by computer analysis of 2-D gels. Clin Exp Metastasis 9:221–230

Eisinger M, Marco O (1982) Selective proliferation of normal human melanocytes in vitro in the presence of phorbol ester and cholera toxin. Proc Natl Acad Sci USA 79:2018–2022

Friedmann PS, Gilchrest BA (1987) Ultraviolet radiation directly induces pigment production by cultured human melanocytes. J Cell Physiol 133:88–94

Gown AM, Vogel AM, Hoak D, Gough F, McNutt MA (1986) Monoclonal antibodies specific for melanocytic tumors distinguish subpopulations of melanocytes. Am J Pathol 123:195–203

Hanash SM, Gagnon M, Seeger RC, Baier L (1985) Analysis of neuroblastoma cell proteins using two-dimensional electrophoresis. Advances in neuroblastoma research. Liss, New York, pp 261–268

Hinnebusch AG (1988) Mechanisms of gene regulation in the general control of amino acid biosynthesis in Saccharomyces cerevisiae. Microbiol Rev 52:248–273

Holzmann B, Bröcker EB, Lehmann JM, Ruiter DJ, Sorg C, Riethmüller C, Johnson JP (1987) Tumor progression in human malignant melanoma: five stages defined by their antigenic phenotypes. Int J Cancer 39:466–471

Hotta H, Ross AH, Huebner K, Isobe M, Wendeborn S, Chao MV, Ricciardi RP, Tsujimoto Y, Croce CM, Koprowski H (1988) Molecular cloning and characterization of an antigen associated with early stages of melanoma tumor progression. Cancer Res 48:2955–2956

Houghton AN, Eisinger M, Albino AP, Cairncross JG, Old LJ (1982) Surface antigens of melanocytes and melanomas. Markers of melanocyte differentation and melanoma subsets. J Exp Med 156:1755–1766

Houghton AN, Real FX, Davis LJ, Cordon-Cardo C, Old LJ (1987) Phenotypic heterogeneity of melanoma. Relation to the differentiation program of melanoma cells. J Exp Med 164:812–829

Johnson JP, Stade BG, Holzmann B, Schwäble W, Riethmüller G (1989) De novo expression of intercellular adhesion molecule 1 in melanoma correlates with increased risk of metastasis. Proc Natl Acad Sci USA 86:641–644

Krasagakis K, Garbe C, Krüger S, Orfanos CE (1991) Effects of interferons on cultured human melanocytes in vitro: interferon-beta but not -alpha or -gamma inhibits proliferation and all interferons significantly modulate the cell phenotype. J Invest Dermatol 97:364–372

Lehmann JM, Riethmuller G, Johnson JP (1989) MUC18, a marker of tumor progression in human melanoma, shows sequence similarity to the neural cell adhesion molecules of the immunoglobulin superfamily. Proc Natl Acad Sci USA 86:9891–9895

Leyva A, Kraal I, Lankelma J, Delamarre JFM, Pinedo HM (1983) High uridine phosphorylase activity in human melanoma tumor. Anticancer Res 3:227–232

Livingston PO, Albino AP, Chung TJC, Real FX, Houghton AN, Oettgen HF, OLD LJ (1985) Serological response of melanome patients to vaccines prepared from VSV lysates of autologous and allogeneic cultured melanoma cells. Cancer Res 55:713–720

O'Farrel (1975) High resolution two-dimensional gel electrophoresis of proteins. J Biol Chem 250:4007–4021

Rodeck U, Melber K, Kath R, Menssen HD, Varello M, Atkinson B, Herlyn M (1991) Constitutive expression of multiple growth factor genes by melanoma cells but not normal melanocytes. J Invest Dermatol 97:20–26

Rose TM, Plowman GD, Teplow DB, Dreyer WJ, Hellstrom KE, Brown JP (1986) Primary structure of the human melanoma-associated antigen p97 (melanotransferrin) deduced from the mRNA sequence. Proc Natl Acad Sci USA 83:1261–1265

Sambrook J, Fritsch EF, Maniatis T (1989) Molecular cloning, 2nd edn. Cold Spring Harbour Lab Oratory, New York

Sauvaigo S, Fretts RE, Riopelle RJ, Lagarde AE (1986) Autonomous proliferation of MeWo human melanoma cell lines in serum-free medium: secretion of growth-stimulating activities. Int J Cancer 37:123–132

Schrier PI (1992) Melanoma genetics and cytogenetics. Clin Dermatol 10:31–39

Shih IM, Herlyn M (1993) Role of growth factors and their receptors in the development and progression of melanoma. J Invest Dermatol 100:196S–203S

Suter L, Brüggen J, Bröcker EB, Sorg C (1985) A tumor-associated antigen expressed in melanoma cells with lower malignant potential. Int J Cancer 35:787–791

Tracy RP, Word LE, Currie RM, Young DS (1982) Patterns for normal colon mucosa and colon adenocarcinoma compared by two-dimensional gel electrophoresis. Clin Chem 28:915–919

Vennegoor C, Calafat J, Hageman P, van Buitenen F, Janssen H, Kolk A, Rumke P (1985) Biochemical characterization and cellular localization of a formalin-resistant melanoma-associated antigen reacting with monoclonal antibody NKI/C3. Int J Cancer 35:287–295

Versteeg R, Noordermeer IA, Krüse-Wolters KM, Ruiter DJ, Schrier PI (1988) C-myc downregulates class I HLA expression in human melanomas. EMBO-J 170: 621–635

Mutation and Expression of TP53 in Malignant Melanomas

J. Weiss[1], M. Heine[2], K.C. Arden[3], B. Körner[1], H. Pilch[2], R.A. Herbst[3], and E.G. Jung[1]

[1] Department of Dermatology, University of Heidelberg, 68135 Mannheim, Germany
[2] Department of Pathology, University of Heidelberg, 68135 Mannheim, Germany
[3] Ludwig Institute for Cancer Research, San Diego Branch, 9500 Gilman Drive, San Diego, CA 92093-0660, USA

Abstract

Mutations of the TP53 gene are the most common genetic alterations in human malignancies. Overexpression of the p53 protein has been reported in high frequencies in all types of skin cancer. To determine the role of TP53 in the pathogenesis of malignant melanoma, we investigated the expression of p53 in 12 cell lines and 145 primary and metastatic lesions by immunohistochemistry. Overexpression of p53 was predominantly detected in the cytoplasm of the cells in 96 (66%) tumor and 12 (93%) cell lines. In contrast to findings in other tumor types, in melanomas immunoreactive cells were found in clusters or as scattered single cells. In primary melanomas, the frequency of p53 overexpression did not correlate with tumor thickness. Nucleotide sequencing of TP53 genes of 24 melanoma tumors/cell lines demonstrated point mutations in seven samples, all coding for mutant p53 protein species. The frequency of TP53 alterations of 20%–30% is lower than in other skin tumor types. Notably, immunohistochemistry was not a suitable method to distinguish overexpression of wild-type p53 from mutant species, since cell lines/tumors with TP53 mutations did not show distinctive staining patterns. The mutation pattern in six out of seven lesions was similar to that caused by ultraviolet light damage. This finding may be regarded a further indication for a pathogenetic role of UV light damage in at least a subgroup of malignant melanomas.

Introduction

The TP 53 gene on chromosome 17p13.1 encodes a nuclear protein (p53) which is implicated in cell proliferation and tumor progression. Whereas the wild-type form has tumor-suppressive properties, various mutations appear to inactivate these capabilities (Levine et al. 1991; Hollstein et al. 1991).

Recent Results in Cancer Research, Vol. 139

There is increasing evidence that mutations in the TP53 gene are among the most common somatic genetic alterations in human cancers (Hollstein et al. 1991). Loss of wild-type p53 protein and expression of mutant forms have been demonstrated in a high proportion of malignant tumors of the colon (Campo et al. 1991), breast (Coles et al. 1992), and brain and in lower frequency in cancers of the liver, bladder, esophagus, and head and neck as well as in sarcomas (Hollstein et al. 1991). Germline mutations of the locus also predispose to Li-Fraumeni syndrome, a heritable cancer syndrome (Malkin et al. 1990).

Functions of p53 Protein

Many p53-mediated activities have been identified; however, the full functional role of this protein is still under intensive investigation (Oren 1992; Zambetti and Levine 1993). This protein is centrally involved in the regulation of the cell cycle. Binding of p53 to a specific site detected in the promoter regions of several genes induces a downregulation of transcription (Ginsberg et al. 1991a), and genes that lack this p53-binding motif seem to be stimulated by p53 (Klein 1993). Based on these observations, Zambetti and Levine (1993) predicted a model for the function of wild-type p53 in tumor suppression that includes the downregulation of growth-promoting genes such as *fos* and *jun* and an induction of genes involved in negative growth control and perhaps in differentiation. Increased nuclear concentrations due to a stabilization of wild-type p53 have been observed as a consequence of stress to the cells such as ultraviolet (UV) light, ionizing irradiation, and mutagens (Kastan et al. 1991; Maltzman and Czyzyk 1984). These noxious agents induce a halt of DNA synthesis and subsequently a growth arrest, which ultimately can cause cells to undergo programmed cell death (Shaw et al. 1992; Zambetti and Levine 1993). These functions appear to be crucial for DNA repair mechanisms and thereby for maintaining DNA stability and genome integrity. Reflecting this important function, Lane (1992) designated p53 as the "guardian of the genome."

While p53 function is not mandatory for the development of normal tissues (Donehower et al. 1992), the transfection of wild-type p53 expression vectors into malignant lymphoma cells has been shown to induce differentiation and programmed cell death (Yonish-Rouach et al. 1991). Finally, the p53 protein seems to be involved in the control of senescence, since the loss of the function of wild-type protein is correlated with the emergence of immortalized cell lines at least in fibroblasts (Harvey and Levine 1991).

Regulation of p53 Function

The p53 protein is highly active and has a half-life of only a few minutes (Levine et al. 1991). Physiologic concentrations of p53 are therefore very low; peak levels in the late G1-S phase of the cell cycle are barely detectable by immunohistochemical methods (Shaulski et al. 1990). Immunostaining with anti-p53 antibodies, indicating an overexpression of the protein, can be due to increased transcription, but more commonly to alterations in the metabolic pathway of p53 (Zambetti and Levine 1993). The occurrence of DNA damage leads to increased steady state levels of wild-type p53, which appear to cause a growth arrest. The precise mechanisms for stabilizing a functionally active p53 are not known yet (Kastan et al. 1991). Likewise, binding to various proteins such as hsc70, the oncoproteins E1B and E6, and also to S100 protein impairs the metabolism of p53 and is associated with a stabilization but also an inactivation of the protein (Baudier et al. 1992; Zambetti and Levine 1993; Vousden 1993). Conformation of the p53 protein has been found to be crucial for its stability and therefore half-life, but also its functional activity (Oren 1992). This has led to speculations that a switch to an aberrant conformation may be a possible mechanism for the regulation of p53 activity (Milner 1991). Most mutant p53 species are characterized by an altered conformation which causes an increased stability and thereby a prolonged half-life, but also a functional deficiency (Oren 1992). However, the hypothesis that overexpression of p53 protein is an indicator for the presence of mutant protein species which lack the capabilities of wild-type p53 cannot be upheld in light of recent data (Barnes et al. 1992; Campbell et al. 1993b). Several mutant p53 protein species have been described which are overexpressed, but show at least some functional activity, and also others which are not detectable by immunohistochemistry with the anti-p53 antibody PAb 240, but have lost all their functions (Halevy et al. 1990; Dittmer et al. 1993; Zambetti and Levine 1993).

Mutation of TP53 are not the only mechanisms at work to inactivate p53 function. Since p53 appears to act in the nucleus, a reduction of its nuclear concentrations by nuclear exclusion, either by an insufficient nuclear transport or by retaining p53 in the cytoplasm bound to other proteins, has the same effect as the expression of inactive mutant p53 species (Moll et al. 1992).

Anti-p53 Antibodies

Several anti-p53 antibodies are currently commercially available. The monoclonal antibodies DO-1, DO-7, and PAb 1801 bind to denaturation resistant epitopes in the N-terminal region of the p53 protein and can be used for both paraffin-embedded and frozen specimens (Vojtesek et al. 1992). In contrast, the monoclonal anti-p53 antibody PAb 240 binds to a denaturation sensitive epitope which is not accessible in p53 with wild-type conformation (Stephen and Lane 1992). However, denaturation of wild-type protein as well as many TP53 mutations appear to effect a change in protein conformation, thereby exposing the PAb 240 epitope. Wild-type conformation of p53 is very sensitive to denaturation, and even mild fixation procedures in immunohistochemistry may alter the native p53 conformation (Gannon et al. 1990). As a result, the specificity of PAb 240 for mutant proteins is not reliably retained when used for immunostaining. However, some immunoprecipitation procedures do not impair protein conformation. This renders PAb 240 suitable for the detection of a variety of mutant p53 species when used in immunoprecipitation. The polyclonal antibody CM-1 is commonly used for immunohistochemistry of paraffin-embedded tissues (Midgley et al. 1992).

Expression of p53 in Nonmelanomatous Skin Cancers

Recent reports have shown a high frequency of overexpression of p53 protein not only in squamous cell carcinomas of the skin (SCC) and basal cell carcinomas (BCC; Campbell et al. 1993b; Moles et al. 1993; Ziegler et al. 1993), but also in normal skin, in particular after UV irradiation (Hall et al. 1993). However, there is increasing evidence that immunostaining, regardless of the anti-p53 antibody used, does not necessarily indicate the presence of mutant p53 protein species (Campbell et al. 1993b). The frequencies of TP53 mutations detected in BCC ranged from 10% (Campbell et al. 1993b) to 65% (Ziegler et al. 1993) and in SCC and Bowen's disease from 15% (Campbell et al. 1993a) to 58% (Brash et al. 1991). Analyses of mutation spectra in these tumors demonstrated a different pattern of mutations when compared to those commonly found in internal malignancies. In nonmelanoma skin cancers, cytosine to thymidine transitions at dipyrimidine sites were the most frequent type of point mutations (Ziegler et al. 1993). This type of genetic alteration has been shown to be associated with UV light damage (Miller 1985).

Expression of p53 in Melanoma Cell Lines

Expression of p53 and characteristic immunostaining patterns elicited by different anti-p53 antibodies are readily detectable in cultured melanoma cells (Fig. 1). Using three different monoclonal anti-p53 antibodies (Mab DO-1, PAb 240, PAb 1801) for immunocytochemistry (immunofluorescence method), typical qualitative immunoreactions were observed in 12 out of 13 cell lines which were established from primary and metastatic malignant melanomas (Weiss et al. 1993). The visual estimates of staining frequencies are shown in Table 1. The signals were seen in both the nuclei and the cytoplasm of the melanoma cells, although qualitative variations were apparent. Figure 1 shows representative examples of two mutated cell lines (WM852 and WM164) stained with the three different monoclonal anti-p53 antibodies.

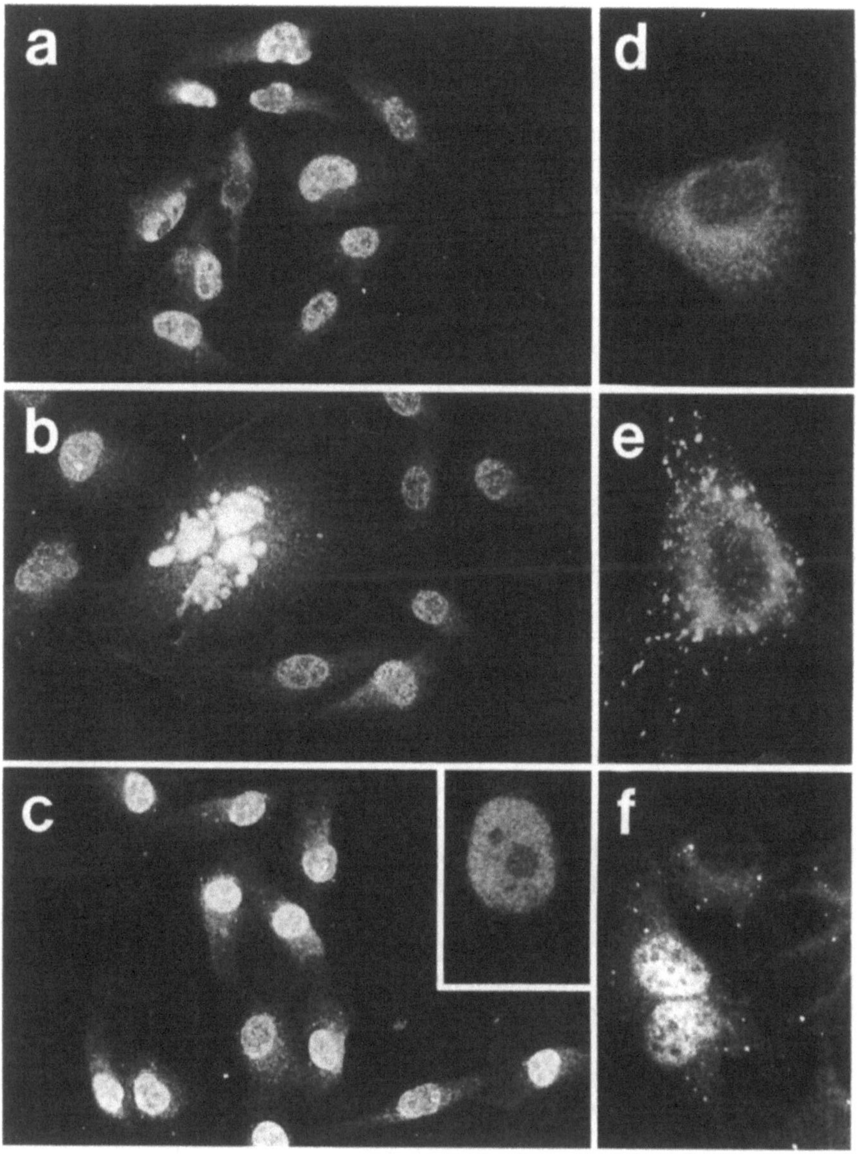

Fig. 1 a–f. Nuclear and cytoplasmatic staining patterns of p53 detected by monoclonal antibodies (MAb) PAb 240 (**a,d**), Do-1 (**b,e**), and PAb 1801 (**c,f**) in two melanoma cell lines with TP53 mutations. Shown are immunoreactions in WM852 (**a–c**) and in WM164 (**d–f**). The inset (**c**) gives an example of an immunostained nucleus with negative nucleoli

Table 1. Overexpression of p53 protein detected by different monoclonal antibodies (MAb) (Given are visual estimates of stained cells: −, negative; (+), single cells; +, 5%–25%; ++, 25%–50%; +++, >50% are positive. In four of the cell lines, TP53 mutations (*mut*) were detected, whereas the others had wild-type sequence (*wt*) in the regions examined.)

Melanoma cell line	TP53 sequence	Nuclear immunoreactivity			Cytoplasmic immunoreactivity		
		DO-1	PAb 240	PAb 1801	DO-1	PAb 240	PAb 1801
WM 8	wt	+	+	+	++	++	++
WM 9	wt	(+)	(+)	−	+++	+++	++
WM 46	wt	++	++	+	++	+++	+++
WM 115	wt	+	+	+	+++	++	++
WM 164	mut	(+)	+	+	+++	+++	+
WM 239	wt	(+)	(+)	−	+++	+++	+
WM 266	wt	+	+	(+)	+++	+++	+++
WM 373	n.d.	+	+	(+)	++	++	−
WM 793	wt	−	+	−	−	(+)	−
WM 852	mut	+++	+++	+++	+	+	+
WM 983A	mut	+++	+++	++	++	+++	+
WM 983B	mut	+	+	++	+++	+++	++
WM 1158	wt	(+)	(+)	(+)	(+)	(+)	−

In nuclei the immunoreactions were found to be distributed uniformly, with the exception of the obviously negative nucleoli (Fig. 1c). Remarkably, positively stained cells were not randomly distributed in the cultures, but often seen in clusters. The highest frequencies of nuclear reactivity were observed in cells in the exponential growth phase. In highly confluent cultures, the number of positive cells was markedly reduced. At least in a subgroup of melanoma cells, this finding is likely to be due to increased levels of wild-type p53 in the G1-S phase of the cell cycle (Shaulski et al. 1990). Likewise, nuclear immunoreactivity was frequently detected in less firmly attached melanoma cells and in cells with multiple nuclei and micronuclei (Fig. 1b). Permanent overexpression of p53 induces growth arrest and ultimately programmed cell death (apoptosis; Shaw et al. 1992), which may explain these observations.

In contrast to cell lines derived from other tumor types, melanoma cell lines showed cytoplasmic immunoreactivity with high frequency. Interestingly, although each of the different anti-p53 antibodies detected p53 protein in the same cell lines, they did so with distinct cytoplasmic staining patterns (Fig. 1). It is known that the p53 protein is bound to various cellular proteins that can impair the binding of particular antibodies in different ways (Levine et al. 1991; Zambetti and Levine 1993). Variations in the intracellular distribution of these binding proteins might therefore result in the different staining patterns. The most pronounced cytoplasmic staining signals were seen with MAb DO-1; PAb 1801, on the other hand, elicited distinct but very discrete signals. Remarkably, Bartek et al. (1990) reported in a breast cancer cell line an immunoreaction with PAb 240 almost identical to the staining pattern we found in melanoma cell lines with PAb 1801. This raises the possibility that staining patterns of the particular anti-p53 antibodies might be tumor specific. The high frequency of cytoplasmic p53 overexpression in our melanoma cells is in contrast to the findings of Volkenandt et al. (1991). Performing immunocytochemistry with PAb 1801 in nine different melanoma cell lines, they found nuclear overexpression of p53 in one of them, but failed to detect any signals located in cytoplasm. However, the discrete cytoplasmic immunoreactions produced by this antibody, which are often barely detectable, may be an explanation of this discrepancy.

It can not be ruled out completely that the cytoplasmic signals are due to some unspecified cross-reactivity. One antibody, PAb 240, has been reported to show cross-reactivity with an unknown 70-kDa protein in various cell lines (Stephen and Lane 1992). We therefore performed immunoprecipitations of p53 in these cells lines, but failed to detect specific prepitates other than p53. Nonetheless, the ability of several antibodies directed against different epitopes of the protein to produce qualitatively similar data would argue that these results are not due to some undefined cross-reactive proteins. The immunoprecipitation data with PAb 1801 and antibody DO-1, which showed a good correlation between p53 detected and the observed staining frequencies, also strongly supports this conclusion.

Mutations in TP53 are reported to effect a predominantly nuclear overexpression of p53 protein in cell lines established from colon carcinomas (Nigro et al. 1989; Campo et al. 1991), although distinct mutant p53 proteins have been shown to cause cytoplasmic immunoreactivity (Ginsberg et al. 1991b). Moll et al. (1992) found nuclear immunoreactivity in breast cancer to be commonly associated with TP53 alterations, whereas mutations could not be detected in tumors showing predominantly cytoplasmic staining. Nucleotide sequencing in our melanoma cell lines showed that four out of 13 expressed mutant p53 species. Neither immunostainign with the "mutant-specific" antibody PAb 240 nor the staining patterns with differences in cytoplasmic or nuclear reactivity were sufficient to distinguish melanoma cell lines with mutant p53 from those with wild-type p53. Interestingly, PAb 240 immunoprecipitated p53 protein exclusively in mutant melanoma cell lines.

Expression of p53 in Primary and Metastatic Malignant Melanomas

Expression of p53 protein was examined by immunohistochemistry in 113 primary and 32 metastatic lesions of malignant melanomas. Since the tissue was paraffin embedded, we used the polyclonal anti-p53 antibody CM-1 for immunostaining. (The antibody was a kind gift from Dr. D.P. Lane,

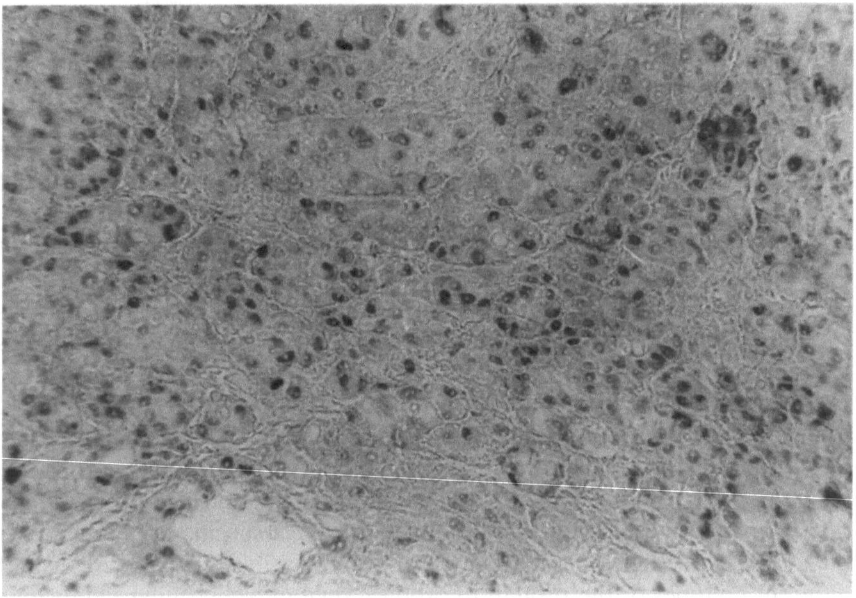

Fig. 2. Nuclear immunoreactivity in a primary melanoma with wild-type TP53 sequence. Immunostaining was performed with CM-1 using the alkaline phosphatase method. The section is not counterstained

Dundee, Scotland). This antibody reliably identifies p53 protein in formaldehyde-fixed tissue (Midgley et al. 1992).

Immunoreactivity was detected in 80 (71%) primary melanomas. Similar to findings in melanoma cell lines, the staining signals were found predominantly in the cytoplasm of the tumor cells. Immunoreactivity in this cellular compartment was seen in 65 (58%) tumors, whereas 37 (33%) showed nuclear immunostaining. In 22 (19%) melanomas, immunoreactions were present in both cellular compartments. Table 2 summarizes the results of immunostaining in these primary malignant melanomas.

Similar to findings in internal malignancies, overexpression of p53 protein is detectable in circumscribed areas rather than uniformly in the whole melanoma. Positive cells, particularly those with cytoplasmic immunoreactivity, were frequently seen in clusters. Occasionally, immunostaining was restricted to morphologically distinct clones of melanoma cells. Interestingly, cells with cytoplasmic reactivity were frequently detected in the shoulders of the melanomas in the dermoepidermal junction. It is tempting to speculate that this phenomenon is an equivalent to findings in melanoma cultures, in which cells in the exponential growth phase showed the highest frequencies of p53 overexpression. Nevertheless, the functional role of a cytoplasmic overexpression of p53 in malignant melanoma remains unclear. Since there are reports that p53 binds to various proteins, e.g., S-100 protein (Baudier

Table 2. Frequencies of immunostaining with the polyclonal anti-p53 antibody CM-1 in primary and metastatic malignant melanomas

	Immunoreactivity							
	Cytoplasm		Nucleus		Cytoplasm/ nucleus		Negative	
	(*n*)	(%)	(*n*)	(%)	(*n*)	(%)	(*n*)	(%)
Primary melanomas (*n* = 113)	43	38	15	13	22	19	33	30
SSM (*n* = 70)	32	46	5	7	14	20	19	27
LMM (*n* = 23)	5	22	6	26	1	4	11	48
ALM (*n* = 8)	2	25	3	37	1	13	2	25
NM (*n* = 12)	4	33	1	8	6	50	1	8
Metastatic melanomas (*n* = 32)	8	25	6	19	2	6	16	50
In-transit metastasis (*n* = 3)	1	33	0	0	0	0	2	67
Lymph node metastasis (*n* = 26)	7	27	4	15	2	8	13	50
Visceral metastasis (*n* = 3)	0	0	2	67	0	0	1	33

SSM, superficial spreading melanomas; LMM, lentigo maligna melanomas; ALM, acrolentiginous melanomas; NM, nodular melanomas

et al. 1992), it may be hypothesized that tumor cells in the shoulders of the melanomas express particular proteins which bind to p53 and thus retain it in the cytoplasm.

The number of melanoma cells showing nuclear overexpression of p53 was usually low; however, distinct patterns of immunoreactivity were identified. In the majority of cases, positive cells were randomly distributed over the tumor, comprising only a few cells. Interestingly, binucleated cells were frequently seen, paralleling the findings in melanoma cell lines. Clusters or extended areas of cells showing nuclear p53 overexpression were observed only infrequently.

In both qualitative and quantitative respect, our findings are similar to results reported by Stretch et al. (1991). They detected immunoreactivity to PAb 240 in 45 (85%) out of 53 primary and metastatic melanoma lesions. In their series, 29 of the tumors expressing detectable levels of p53 did so with combined nuclear and cytoplasmic staining, and eight each showed nuclear or cytoplasmic reactions only. Likewise, Bartek et al. (1991) found an overexpression of p53 protein in 35 (92%) out of 40 melanomas. Lassam et al. (1993) and Cristofolini et al. (1993) reported frequencies in melanomas of 7% and 27%, respectively. In the latter reports, the lower frequencies of immunoreactivity are explained by the fact that only nuclear overexpression of p53 protein was evaluated. In Japanese patients, Yamamoto and Takahashi (1993) detected nuclear staining in 38% of the melanomas examined. This could indicate that the frequency of nuclear p53 overexpression is influenced by possibly different pathogenetic factors.

Interestingly, our data suggest that the frequency and the pattern of immunoreactivity is correlated with the histologic melanoma subtype. Superficial spreading melanomas (SSM) are characterized by a high rate of cytoplasmic immunoreactivity, which was seen in 46 (66%) tumors. Nuclear immunostaining was detected either isolated or combined with cytoplasmic signals in 21 (27%) cases. This is in contrast to findings in lentigo maligna melanomas (LMM), in which only six (26%) out of 23 tumors showed staining in cytoplasm and seven (30%) in nuclei. The difference in cytoplasmic reactivity of both melanoma subtypes was statistically significant ($p < 0.002$; Fisher's exact test). Due to small numbers of acrolentiginous (ALM) and nodular (NM) melanomas, statistical analysis was impaired; however, the nuclear staining frequency in NM was shown to be significantly higher than that found in SSM ($p < 0.05$; Fisher's exact test). Our observations in NM confirm results of Akslen and Morkve (1992), who detected nuclear immunostaining in 29 out of 30 tumors.

The analysis of staining frequencies after stratification in thin melanomas with a Breslow thickness of less than 1 mm and thicker tumors did not show any differences (Table 3). A separate calculation for the SSM subtype did not reveal differences either (data not shown). Stretch et al. (1991) and Lassam et al. (1993) reported that in metastatic lesions immunostaining was more frequent than in primary lesions and confirmed this observation by statistical analysis. The latter result suggested that p53 overexpression might be a late event in melanoma development associated with melanoma progression. However, in our series of melanomas we could not confirm the aforementioned observation. Nuclear staining frequencies in metastatic lesions revealed results which were not statistically different from those in primary tumors. Notably, the frequency of cytoplasmic staining was significantly lower in metastatic lesions ($p < 0.01$; Fisher's exact test). Likewise, Akslen and Morkve (1992) reported lower rates of nuclear

Table 3. Frequency of immunostaining with CM-1 in primary malignant melanomas with a tumor thickness of less than 1 mm and thicker tumors

Melanoma thickness	Immunoreactivity							
	Cytoplasm		Nucleus		Cytoplasm/nucleus		Negative	
	(*n*)	(%)	(*n*)	(%)	(*n*)	(%)	(*n*)	(%)
<1 mm ($n = 56$)	20	36	9	16	9	16	18	32
>1 mm ($n = 57$)	23	40	6	11	13	23	15	26

immunoreactivity in melanomas of progressed stages. Our data of similar staining frequencies in both thin, thick, and metastatic melanomas suggest that overexpression of p53 protein is an early event in melanoma pathogenesis and cannot be regarded as a progression marker in this tumor type. Notably, immunoreactivity to p53 antibodies is not restricted to malignant melanocytic tumors (McGregor et al. 1992; Yamamoto and Takahashi 1993; Cristofolini et al. 1993) but also seen in benign nevi. Confirming these reports we have observed overexpression of p53 protein in a small percentage of dysplastic and Spitz' nevi (data not shown). This strongly indicates that, unlike in other tumor types (Hall et al. 1991), the detection of p53 overexpression cannot be considered a diagnostic marker distinguishing benign and malignant melanocytic tumors.

Overexpression of p53 protein in melanoma cells does not indicate the presence of mutant protein species. We performed nucleotide sequencing analyses in two primary and ten metastatic melanomas and detected mutations in three lesions. Staining patterns of tumors with TP53 alterations were not distinct from lesions expressing wild-type TP53. Two visceral metastases in one patient (M.W., Table 4) carried identical point mutations. However, only in the colon metastasis was nuclear staining detected, whereas the brain tumor was not immunoreactive. A lymph node metastasis in a different patient (B.M.), in which a missense point mutation in TP53 was detected, showed nuclear overexpression of p53. In the primary lesion, in which we found extended areas of cells with similar morphology and staining pattern, sequencing analysis revealed wild-type sequence in corresponding codons. These observations confirm findings in melanoma cell lines as well as in nonmelanoma skin cancer (Campbell et al. 1993b) that immunostaining is not a reliable method for the detection of mutant p53 species. Assumptions regarding TP53 mutation rates based on immunohistochemistry should therefore be interpreted with caution.

TP53 Mutations in Malignant Melanomas

To date, only limited analyses of TP53 mutations in cutaneous malignant melanomas have been published (Volkenandt et al. 1991; Castresana et al. 1993; Dockhorn-Dworniczack et al. 1993; Weiss et al. 1994), with conflicting results. Volkenandt et al. (1991) performed nucleotide sequencing in nine melanoma cell lines and detected a C-T transition in a cytosine dimer in one of them. In a series of 49 malignant melanomas, only one mutated tumor was detected, showing a stop sequence in codon 100 and an additional guanosine to adenosin transversion in codon 290 (Dockhorn-Dworniczack et al. 1993). (Castresana et al. (1993) examined 51 primary melanomas but failed to detect any mutations in exons 5–8 of the TP53 genes. We performed nucleotide sequencing of TP53 exons 5–9 in 12 primary and metastatic melanomas as well as in 12 melanoma cell lines derived from 20

Table 4. Point mutations in TP53 genes of malignant melanomas, resulting amino acid changes in p53 proteins, and patterns of immunostaining with CM-1 in these lesions

Cell line/tumor	Mutated codon	Base change	Amino acid change	Staining pattern
Cell lines				
WM 164	220	TAT-TGT	Tyr-Cys	C++/N(+)
WM852	241	TCC-TTC	Ser-Phe	C(+)/N+++
WM983A	278	CCT-TTT	Pro-Phe	C++/N++
WM983B	278	CCT-TTT	Pro-Phe	C++/N+
Tumors				
Lymph node (B.M.)	177	CAC-CAT	none (His)	C(+)/N++
	178	CAT-TAT	His-Tyr	
Brain metastasis (M.W.)	245	GGC-GG/AC	Gly-Asp/Gly	Negative
Colon metastasis (M.W.)	245	GGC-GG/AC	Gly-Asp/Gly	C−/N+

C, cytoplasmic; N, nuclear.

patients (Weiss et al. 1994). These areas are reported to harbor more than 90% of the point mutations in a variety of malignancies (Hollstein et al. 1991). Point mutations were detected in three tumors and four cell lines representing five patients, thus indicating mutations occurred in 25% of the melanoma samples (Table 4). The cell lines WM983A and WM983B (samples 3, 4) were established from primary and subsequent metastatic lesions from the same patient and, as expected, identical alterations were found in these two samples. In the two visceral metastases in patient M.W. (samples 6, 7) identical base substitutions were detected, indicating a common origin of these tumor cells. Due to tumor-infiltrating lymphocytes both wild-type and mutant sequence was detected in the affected codon. Interestingly, we could not find mutations in a preceding lymph node metastasis of the aforementioned patient (the primary tumor was not available for analysis) or in the primary melanoma of patient B.M. (SSM; Breslow thickness, 2.8 mm; Clark's level 4) from which the lymph node metastasis (sample 5) originated. Table 4 summarizes point mutations detected in TP53, resulting amino acid changes in p53 proteins, and results of immunohistochemistry in the tumors.

The mutation frequency of 25% detected in our series of melanomas is in contrast to the findings of Castresana et al. (1993) and of Dockhorn-Dworniczack et al. (1993), who reported only one TP53 alteration in 100 malignant melanomas. The discrepancy is unclear. It may be speculated that different approaches for the analysis of mutations could have influenced results. We performed direct nucleotide sequencing of individually polymerase chain reaction (PCR)-amplified exons, a method which is tedious in tumors in which only DNA extracted from formaldehyde-fixed tissue is available. In contrast, both Castresana et al. (1993) and Dockhorn-Dworniczack et al. (1993) screened TP53 exons by SSCP (single strand conformation polymorphisms) analyses before performing nucleotide sequencing. There is evidence that this rapid method does not detect all mutations present (Sheffield et al. 1993). Furthermore, in many melanomas the extraction of a pure tumor cell population is very difficult. Separation of melanoma cells from overlaying keratinocytes and surrounding infiltrates in primary lesions in particular in thin tumors or from infiltrating lymphocytes in lymph node metastases is frequently not feasible. Therefore, it is likely that TP53 mutations in clones of cells which may have distinct morphological or immunohistological features are likely to be missed in sequencing analyses due to a low number of mutant cells and/or the contamination with cells carrying wild-type TP53 alleles. Whether or not this is true for the lesions in our patients M.W. and B.M. remains a point of speculation.

Six of the seven point mutations detected in our series occurred in cytosine–guanosine base pairs which were substituted by thymidine–adenosine pairs. All six were seen in dipyrimidine sites in highly conserved domains of TP53. This pattern of mutation is characteristic of that caused by UV light damage (Miller 1985; Brash et al. 1991). The sites in TP53 which are most susceptible to UV damage are not known. However, analyses of the mutation patterns in nonmelanoma skin cancers which arose in sun-exposed body areas and therefore were likely to be due to UV damage revealed particular sites in TP53 which seem to be preferentially affected (UV mutation hotspots; Ziegler et al. 1993). Most of the sites were different from those found in internal malignancies, in which substitutions of cytosines adjacent to guanosines (CpG sites) were frequent alterations (Coles et al. 1992; Hollstein et al. 1991). It is noteworthy that in our melanomas none of the cytosine transitions detected occurred in CpG sites, but four of the samples (numbers 3, 4, 6, 7,) showed alterations in the same UV light mutation hotspots reported for nonmelanoma skin cancers (Ziegler et al. 1993).

Melanoma metastases and cell lines with TP53 mutations showed evidence for a loss of genetic material in 17p. In many malignancies tumor suppressor genes including TP53 have been found to be inactivated by point mutations in one allele and the subsequent loss of the remaining wild-type allele (Bishop 1987; Baker et al. 1989; Bhatia et al. 1993). Polymorphism analyses of 17p markers revealed in all three melanoma metastases with TP53 mutations allelic loss (loss of heterozygosity) in this locus (Weiss et al. 1994). For the mutated melanoma cell lines, no corresponding normal tissue was available for analysis. However, we detected single alleles in a panel of several adjacent highly polymorphic 17p markers, indicating also loss of genetic material. In contrast, all other tumor samples as well as all melanoma cell lines with wild-type TP53 sequences were shown to be heterozygous in the TP53 locus. It is noteworthy that allelic loss for 17p is not the only mechanism at work in the inactivation of TP53 in cutaneous malignancies. Although not detected in our series of melanomas, independent mutations of both TP53 alleles were frequently observed in basal cell carcinomas of the skin (Ziegler et al. 1993).

The majority of our samples with TP53 alterations were derived from metastatic melanomas (numbers 1, 2, 4–7). However, the UV-like pattern of mutations in TP53 genes might indicate that these alterations occurred in primary lesions. This assumption is in accordance with findings in Bowen's disease, in which TP53 mutations precede invasive tumor formation (Campbell et al. 1993a). Very interesting in this respect is the patient from whom the lymph node metastasis (sample 5) was derived. Nucleotide sequencing of the primary tumor showed wild-type sequence of TP53 exon 5. Nevertheless, this finding is puzzling, since the observed pattern of mutation, a CC-TT transition, strongly suggests that the genetic damage was caused by UV light and therefore occurred in the primary tumor. Sidransky et al. (1992) were able to show clonal outgrowth of TP53 mutant tumor cells in progressive stages of gliomas. It is likely that this mechanism of tumor progression may also be at work in malignant melanomas and other cancer types.

Summary and Conclusion

The present study and reports from many other authors give evidence for an altered expression of its gene product, the p53 protein, in tumors of melanocytic origin. Overexpression of p53 appears to be an early event in melanoma development, since the frequency of p53 immunoreactivity does not correlate with tumor thickness. It is noteworthy that an altered expression of this tumor suppressor protein is not restricted to malignant lesions; immunostaining with anti-p53 antibodies is therefore not a reliable diagnostic marker for distinguishing those from benign nevi. However, it has still to be established whether overexpression of p53 protein in malignant melanomas is indicative for the prognosis of the patients.

The present data demonstrate a high rate of cytoplasmic immunoreactivity in malignant melanoma, which has not been detected in this degree in other tumor types. Further research is warranted to clarify this phenomenon, which may be specific for melanocytic tumors. The elucidation of the different staining frequencies in melanoma subtypes and of the cytoplasmic p53 overexpression in tumor cells located in the shoulders of the melanomas might lead to the identification of other tumorigenic mechanisms at work in melanoma development.

Findings in melanoma cell lines and in malignant melanomas in this study as well as similar observations in nonmelanoma skin cancers give evidence that immunoreactivity to anti-p53 antibodies is not indicative for the presence of mutant p53 protein forms. Sequencing studies of large series of unscreened malignant melanomas are warranted to establish the frequency of TP53 alterations in this tumor type in order to determine the clinical impact of mutations in particular for the prognosis of the patients. Since the initial transforming melanoma gene has not been characterized yet, the confirmation of genetic alterations likely to be due to UV damage in TP53 may give further evidence for a pathogenetic role of sunlight in melanoma development. Additionally, understanding how the multitude of p53 actions can be mediated at the molecular level promises important insights into complex biological problems and therapeutic options for the treatment of melanoma patients.

References

Akslen LA, Morkve O (1992) Expression of p53 protein in cutaneous melanoma. Int J Cancer 52:13–16

Baker SJ, Fearon ER, Nigro JM, Hamilton SR, Preisinger AC, Jessup JM, van Tuinen P, Ledbetter DH, Barker DF, Nakamura Y, White R, Vogelstein B (1989) Chromosome 17 deletions and p53 gene mutations in colorectal carcinomas. Science 244:217–220

Barnes DM, Hanby AM, Gillett CE, Mohammed S, Hodgson S, Bobrow LG, Leigh IM, Purkis T, MacGeoch C, Spurr NK, Bartek J, Vojtesek B, Picksley SM, Lane

DP (1992) Abnormal expression of wild type p53 protein in normal cells of a cancer family patient. Lancet 340:259–263
Bartek J, Iggo R, Gannon JV, Lane DP (1990) Genetic and immunochemical analysis of mutant p53 in human breast cancer cell lines. Oncogene 5:893–899
Bartek J, Bartkova J, Vojtesek B, Staskova Z, Lukas J, Rejthar A, Kovarik J, Midgley CA, Gannon JV, Lane DP (1991) Aberrant expression of the p53 oncoprotein is a common feature in a wide spectrum of human malignancies. Oncogene 6:1699–1703
Baudier J, Delphin C, Grunwald D, Khochbin S, Lawrence JJ (1992) Characterization of the tumour suppressor protein p53 as a protein kinase C substrate and a S100b binding protein. Proc Natl Acad Sci USA 89:11627–11631
Bhatia K, Goldschmits W, Gutierrez M, Gaidano G, Dalla-Favera R, Magrath I (1993) Hermi- or homozygosity: a requirement for some but not other p53 mutant proteins to accumulate and exert a pathogenetic effect. FASEB J 7:951–956
Bishop JM (1987) The molecular genetics of cancer. Science 235:305–311
Brash DE, Ziegler JA, Simon JA, Lin A, McKenna GJ, Baden HP, Halperin AJ, Ponten J (1991) A role for sunlight in skin cancer: UV induced p53 mutations in squamous cell carcinoma. Proc Natl Acad Sci USA 88:10124–10128
Campbell C, Quinn AG, Ro YS, Angus B, Rees JL (1993a) p53 mutations are common and early events that precede tumor invasion in squamous cell neoplasia of the skin. J Invest Dermatol 100:746–748
Campbell C, Quinn AG, Angus B, Rees JL (1993b) The relation between p53 mutations and p53 immunostaining in non-melanoma skin cancer. Br J Dermatol 129:235–241
Campo E, Calle-Martin O, Miquel R, Palacin A, Romero M, Fabregat V, Vives J, Cardesa A, Yague J (1991) Loss of heterozygosity of p53 gene and p53 protein expression in human colorectal carcinomas. Cancer Res 51:4436–4442
Castresana JS, Rubjo MP, Vazquez JJ, Idoate M, Sober AJ, Seizinger BR, Barnhill RL (1993) Lack of allelic deletion and point mutation as mechanisms of p53 activation in human malignant melanoma. Int J Cancer 55:562–565
Coles C, Condie A, Chetty U, Steel CM, Evans HJ, Prosser J (1992) p53 mutations in breast cancer. Cancer Res 52:5291–5298
Cristofolini M, Boi S, Girlando S, Zumiani G, Cristofolini P, Dalla Plam P, Barbaresch M (1993) p53 protein expression in nevi and melanomas. Arch Dermatol 129:739–743
Dittmer D, Pati S, Zambetti G, Chu S, Teresky AK, Moore M, Finlay C, Levine AJ (1993) p53 gain of function mutations. Nature Gen 4:42–45
Dockhorn-Dworniczack B, Yandell DW, Merritt V, Böcker W, Poremba C (1993) p53 mutation in malignant melanoma. 84rd annual meeting of the American Association of Cancer Research, Orlando. Proc Am Assoc Cancer Res 34:658
Donehower LA, Harvey M, Slagle BL, McArthur MJ, Montgomery CA, Butel JS, Bradley A (1992) Mice deficient for p53 are developmentally normal but susceptible to spontaneous tumors. Nature 356:215–221
Gannon JV, Greaves R, Iggo R, Lane DP (1990) Activating mutations in p53 produce a common conformational effect. A monoclonal antibody specific for the mutant form. EMBO J 9:1595–1602
Ginsberg D, Mechta F, Yaniv M, Oren M (1991a) Wild-type p53 can down-modulate the activity of various promoters. Proc Natl Acad Sci USA 88:9979–9983
Ginsberg D, Michael-Michalovitz D, Ginsberg D, Oren M (1991b) Induction of growth arrest by a temperature sensitive p53 mutant is correlated with increased nuclear localization and decreased stability of the protein. Mol Cell Biol 11: 582–585
Halevy O, Michalovitz D, Oren M (1990) Different tumor-derived p53 mutants exhibit distinct biological activities. Science 250:113–116

Hall PA, Ray A, Lemoine NR, Midgley CA, Krauz T, Lane DP (1991) p53 immunostaining is a marker of malignancy in diagnostic cytopathology. Lancet 338:513
Hall PA, McKee PH, Menage HP, Dover R, Lane DP (1993) High levels of p53 protein in UV-irradiated normal human skin. Oncogene 8:203–207
Harvey D, Levine AJ (1991) p53 alteration is a commmon event in the spontaneous immortalization of primary BALB/c murine embryo fibroblasts. Genes Dev 5:2375–2385
Hollstein M, Sidransky D, Vogelstein B, Harris CC (1991) p53 mutations in human cancers. Science 253:49–53
Kastan MB, Onyekwere O, Sidransky D, Vogelstein B, Craig RW (1991) Participation of p53 protein in the cellular response to DNA damage. Cancer Res 51: 6304–6311
Klein G (1993) Genes that can antagonize tumor development. FASEB J 7:821–825
Lane DP (1992) p53 the guardian of the genome. Nature 358:15–16
Lassam NJ, From L, Kahn HJ (1993) Over-expression of p53 is a late event in the development of malignant melanoma. Cancer Res 53:2235–2238
Levine AJ, Momand J, Finlay CA (1991) The p53 tumour suppressor gene. Nature 351:453–456
Malkin D, Li FP, Strong LC, Fraumeni JF, Nelson CE, Kassel J, Gryka MA, Bischoff FZ, Tainsky MA, Friend SH (1990) Germline p53 mutations in a familial syndrome of breast cancer, sarcomas and other neoplasias. Science 254:1233–1238
Maltzman W, Czyzyk L (1984) UV irradiation stimulates levels of p53 cellular tumor antigen in nontransformed mouse cells. Mol Cell Biol 4:1689–1694
McGregor JM, Yu CCW, Levison DAL, MacDonald DM (1992) Aberrant expression of p53 tumour suppressor protein in malignant melanoma and dysplastic naevi. 22nd annual meeting of the European Society of Dermatological Research ESDR, London, p 166
Midgley CA, Fisher CJ, Bartek J, Vojtesek B, Lane DP, Barnes DM (1992) Analysis of p53 expression in human tumours: an antibody raised against p53 expressed in E.coli. J Cell Sci 101:183–189
Miller HJ (1985) Mutagenic specificity of ultraviolet light. J Mol Biol 182:45–68
Milner J (1991) p53 in the normal control of cell proliferation. Curr Opin Cell Biol 3:282–286
Moles JP, Moyret C, Guillot B, Jeanteur P, Guilhou JJ, Theillet C, Basset-Seguin N (1993) p53 gene mutations in human epithelial skin cancers. Oncogene 8:583–588
Moll UM, Riou G, Levine AJ (1992) Two distinct mechanisms alter p53 in breast cancer: mutation and nuclear exclusion. Proc Natl Acad Sci USA 89:7262–7266
Nigro JM, Baker SJ, Preisinger AC, Jessup JM, Hostetter R, Cleary K, Bigner SH, Davidson N, Baylin S, Devilee P, Glover T, Collins FS, Weston A, Modali R, Harris CC, Vogelstein B (1989) Mutations in the p53 gene occur in diverse human tumour types. Nature 342:705–708
Oren M (1992) p53: the ultimate tumor suppressor gene? FASEB J 6:3169–3176
Shaw P, Bovey R, Tardy S, Sahli R, Sordat B, Costa J (1992) Induction of apoptosis by wild-type p53 in a human colon-tumor-derived cell line. Proc Natl Acad Sci USA 89:4495–4499
Shaulski G, Ben-Zeev A, Rotter V (1990) Subcellular distribution of the p53 protein during the cell cycle of Balb/c 3T3 cells. Oncogene 5:1707–1711
Sheffield VC, Beck JS, Kwitek AE, Sandstrom DW, Stone EM (1993) The sensitivity of single-strand conformation polymorphism analysis for the detection of single base substitutions. Genomics 16:325–332
Sidransky D, Mikkelsen T, Schwechheimer K, Rosenblum M, Cavenee WK, Vogelstein B (1992) Clonal expansion of p53 mutant cells is associated with brain tumour progression. Nature 355:846–847

Stephen CW, Lane DP(1992) Mutant conformation of p53: precise epitope mapping using a filamentous phage epitope library. J Mol Biol 225:577–583
Stretch JR, Gatter KC, Ralfkiaer E, Lane D, Harris AL (1991) Expression of mutant p53 in melanoma. Cancer Res 51:5976–5979
Vojtesek B, Bartek J, Midgley CA, Lane DP (1992) An immunochemical analysis of the human nuclear phosphoprotein p53. New monoclonal antibodies and epitope mapping using recombinant p53. J Immunol Methods 151:237–244
Volkenandt M, Schlegel U, Nanus DM, Albino AP (1991) Mutational analysis of the human p53 gene in malignant melanoma. Pigment Cell Res 4:35–40
Vousden K (1993) Interactions of human papillomavirus transforming proteins with the products of tumor suppressor genes. FASEB J 7:872–879
Weiss J, Schwechheimer K, Cavenee WK, Herlyn M, Arden KC (1993) Mutation and expression of the p53 gene in malignant melanoma cell lines. Int J Cancer 53:693–699
Weiss J, Cavenee WK, Herbst RA, Jung EG, Arden KC (1994) Point mutations and allelic loss in the TP53 locus of malignant melanomas. Arch Dermatol Res 286: 417–419
Yamamoto M, Takahashi H (1993) Immunohistochemical detection of the p53 oncoprotein in tumours of melanocytic origin. Virchows Arch [A] 422:127–132
Yonish-Rouach E, Resnitzky D, Lotem J, Sachs L, Kimchi A, Oren M (1991) Wild-type p53 induces apoptosis of myeloid leukaemic cells that is inhibited by interleukin 6. Nature 352:345–347
Zambetti GP, Levine AJ (1993) A comparison of the biological activities of wild-type and mutant p53. FASEB J 7:855–865
Ziegler A, Leffell DJ, Kunala S, Sharma HW, Gailani M, Simon JA, Halperin AJ, Baden HP, Shapiro PE, Bale AE, Brash DE (1993) Mutation hotspots due to sunlight in the p53 gene of nonmelanoma skin cancers. Proc Natl Acad Sci USA 90:4216–4220

Production of Cytokines by Human Melanoma Cells and Melanocytes

S. Krüger-Krasagakes[1], K. Krasagakis[2], C. Garbe[2], and T. Diamantstein[1]

[1] Department of Immunology, University Medical Center Steglitz, The Free University of Berlin, Hindenburgdamm 30, 12200 Berlin, Germany
[2] Department of Dermatology, University Medical Center Steglitz, The Free University of Berlin, Hindenburgdamm 30, 12200 Berlin, Germany

Abstract

Experimental animal models have shown that various cytokines, depending on their specific properties, may support growth and metastasis of tumor cells or even lead to tumor rejection. The analysis of expression of cytokine genes by melanoma cell lines indicated that melanoma cells constitutively produce both autostimulatory and inhibitory cytokines. Using reverse transcriptase polymerase chain reaction analysis, simultaneous expression of several cytokines, including interleukin-1 beta ($IL\text{-}1_{\beta}$), IL-6, IL-8, tumor necrosis factor-α, and granulocyte-macrophage colony-stimulating factor, by melanoma cells was found. The same cytokine transcripts were detected in melanocytes, suggesting that cells of the melanocytic lineage express a specific pattern of cytokines in vitro. All these cytokines are known to be able to stimulate effector cells of the host. Additionally, production of mRNA for IL-10, a cytokine with potential immunosuppressive properties, was detected in melanoma cells and melanocytes. These and other cytokines are likely to be involved in the immune response to cancer and at this time it is unknown what the net effects of multiple cytokines are on the outcome of the host response to tumor.

Introduction

Several lines of evidence suggest that melanoma patients develop an immune response to their tumor, and rare cases of spontaneous regressions have been reported. This is supported by recent data reporting on the isolation of specific T cell clones (Topalian et al. 1989) and the successful cloning of a tumor-specific antigen, MAGE-1 (Van den Ende et al. 1992), from melanoma. The clinical course of melanomas reveals a biologically aggressive tumor with a poor response to various treatment regimens.

Recent Results in Cancer Research, Vol. 139

This contradiction suggests that various immunological mechanisms may determine the outcome of an antitumoral reactivity. Recent experimental work in animal models has shown that several parameters may contribute to the process of tumor rejection, such as the constitutive production of soluble mediators by tumor cells, e.g., cytokines, the expression of surface molecules by tumor cells (major histocompatibility complex or adhesion molecules), and the type of mononuclear tumor cell infiltrate.

During the last decade the analysis of the growth properties and immune response to transplanted tumor cells overexpressing a cytokine gene has been a useful approach for studying the predominant in vivo effects of cytokines. In this setting, several cytokines of the interleukin (IL) family including IL-1, IL-2, IL-4, Il-6, IL-7, and IL-10 induced a host-dependent tumor destruction (see Table 1). Local expression of cytokines such as transforming growth factor beta (TGF-β) or tumor necrosis factor alpha (TNF-α), however, even augmented the metastatic spread. During the last few years immunotherapeutical treatment protocols for melanoma have been developed using IL-2 alone or in combination with lymphokine-activated killer (LAK) cells. The overall response rate to these therapies was only moderate and it cannot be excluded that the microenvironment of the tumor prevents an effective antitumoral response. In this context, the knowledge of which cytokines are spontaneously produced by melanoma cells is crucial for better understanding the biology of the tumor and for the development of treatment strategies. We therefore analyzed the constitutive expression of cytokine gene mRNA in a panel of 13 melanoma cell lines in comparison to seven normal human melanocyte cultures using the very sensitive method of reverse transcriptase polymerase chain reaction (RT-PCR) analysis. So far only one study reports on the constitutive production of several lymphokines in a panel of melanoma cell lines (Colombo et al. 1991). It is not known, however, whether the production of cytokines by melanoma cells is a property of the melanocytic lineage rather than a transformation-associated phenomenon.

Material and Methods

Cell Culture

Thirteen established human melanoma cell lines (Bro, A375, NKI-4, SKMel-28, MeWo, IGR-39, Mel-57, O-Mel-II, Mel-2a, SKMel-13, SKMel-19, IGR-37, and M5; Eberle et al. 1993, and references therein) were grown in Dulbecco's modified Eagle's medium (DMEM) supplemented with 10% fetal calf serum (FCS), 2 m*M* glutamine, and antibiotics. Normal human melanocytes (StNM-1, StNM-7, StNM-8, Lei-1, Mel-4, Mel-5, and Mel-6) were obtained from trypsin-digested foreskin and cultured according to standard protocols in a selective medium: MCDB 153 medium (Biochrom,

Table 1. Tumor cell-targeted cytokine gene transfer in animal models

Effective		No effect		Negative effect	
Interleukin-1	(Douvdevani et al. 1992)	Interleukin-5	(Krüger-Krasagakes et al. 1993)	TGF-β	(Torre-Amione et al. 1990)
Interleukin-2	(Fearon et al. 1990; Gansbacher et al. 1990b)	M-CSF	(Dorsch et al. 1993)	TNF-α	(Qin et al. 1993)
Interleukin-4	(Golumbek et al. 1991; Trepper et al. 1989)	GM-CSF	(Dranoff et al. 1993)		
Interleukin-6	(Sun et al. 1992)				
Interleukin-7	(Hock et al. 1991)				
Interleukin-10	(Richter et al. 1993)				
IFN-γ	(Gansbacher et al. 1990a; Watanabe et al. 1989)				
TNF-α	(Asher et al. 1991; Blankenstein et al. 1991)				
G-CSF	(Colombo et al. 1991)				
JE/MCP-1	(Rollins and Sunday 1991)				
IP-10	(Luster and Leder 1993)				

G(M)-CSF, granulocyte (-macrophage) colony-stimulating factor; IFN-γ, interferon gamma; IP-10, interferon-inducible protein 10; MCP-1, monocyte chemoattractant protein 1; TGF-β, transforming growth factor beta; TNF-α, tumor necrosis factor alpha.

Berlin, Germany) was supplemented with 2 ng/ml basic fibroblast growth factor (Boehringer, Mannheim, Germany), 0.4% v/v bovine pituitary extract (Clonetics, San Diego, CA), 10 μg/ml transferrin (Sigma, Deisenhofen, Germany), 1 nM cholera toxin (Calbiochem, La Jolla, USA), 5 μg/ml insulin (Sigma), 50 μM hydrocortisone (Serva, Heidelberg, Germany), and 2 mM Ca^{2+}. When preconfluent, cells were trypsinized, and snap frozen pellets were stored at −80°C until used.

Reverse Transcriptase Polymerase Chain Reaction Analysis

For RT-PCR analysis, cell pellets were homogenized and total cellular RNA was isolated using the guanidium thiocyanate/cesium chloride method. cDNA was synthesized from 3 μg RNA using random primer and MMLV reverse transcriptase according to the supplier's (Gibco/BRL, Gaithersburg, MD) recommendations. A cDNA equivalent of 0.5 ng RNA was amplified in a 50 μl reaction mix containing 250 μM of each dNTP, 200 nM primers, 2.5 μl tenfold PCR buffer (Perkin Elmer/Cetus, Emeryville, CA), and 0.5 U Taq polymerase (Perkin Elmer). The mixture underwent 30–40 cycles (1 min denaturation at 94°C, 1 min annealing at 60°C, 1 min extension at 72°C). Each experiment included a positive control (cDNA of IL-2-stimulated LAK cells) and negative controls consisting in reaction mix without cDNA or sample RNA that had not been reverse transcribed. Specificity of amplification products was verified by restriction analysis with two enzymes indicative for the expected amplified sequence (data not shown). Electrophoresis of 20 μl PCR reaction or digestion product on 1.5% agarose gel containing ethidium bromide was performed to evaluate amplification and size of the generated fragments in comparison to the 1-kb DNA standard (Gibco/BRL). Primer sequences were taken from Yamamura et al. (1991) and crossed intron–exon boundaries.

Results

To examine whether melanocytic cells constitutively express mRNA for different cytokines, we screened 13 human melanoma lines and seven normal human melanocyte cultures for cytokine transcripts by the sensitive RT-PCR technique. A total of 3 μg total cellular RNA was reverse transcribed and cDNA were amplified during 30–40 cycles using specific oligonucleotide primers. Contamination of the preparations with genomic DNA was excluded using sample RNA that had not been reverse transcribed into cDNA as templates for the PCR analysis (data not shown). For quantitation of mRNA expression, 30, 33, 36, and 40 PCR cycles were performed.

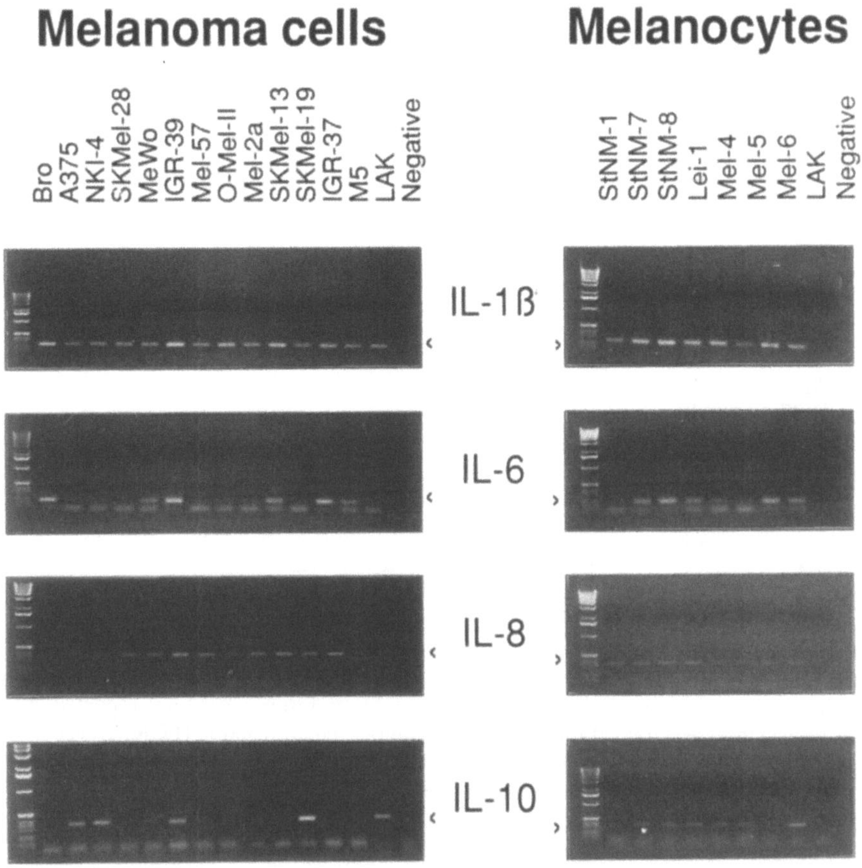

Fig. 1. Expression of interleukin *(IL)-1*$_\beta$, *IL-6*, *IL-8*, and *IL-10* mRNA in a panel of melanoma cell line and melanocyte cultures by reverse transcriptase polymerase chain reaction (RT-PCR). The ethidium bromide-stained gel with the PCR amplification products after 36 cycles is shown. A molecular weight marker is run on the *left lane* of each gel. Cytokine amplification products are shown with *arrows*. The faster migrating bands in IL-6 and IL-10 gels represent primer dimers

Melanoma cells and melanocytes showed the same pattern of cytokine gene expression. Figure 1 shows ethidium bromide-stained agarose gels loaded with PCR products of all IL which were found positive in melanoma cells and melanocytes after 36 PCR cycles. IL-1$_\beta$, IL-6, IL-8, and IL-10 were variably expressed in different cell lines. While mRNA for IL-1$_\beta$ and IL-8 was found more or less in every melanoma line; only seven out of 13 cell lines expressed mRNA for IL-6, and four out of 13 mRNA for IL-10 (see Table 2). All cell lines which had transcripts for IL-6 or IL-10 also produced biologically active IL-6 and IL-10 protein, as determined by enzyme-linked immunosorbent assays (ELISA) and bioassays (data not shown; Krüger-

Table 2. Cytokine gene expression in melanoma cell lines and melanocyte cultures

Cell line	Origin	IL-1β	IL-6	IL-8	IL-10	TNF-α	GM-CSF
Bro	PT	++	+++	+/−	−	−	++
A375	PT	+	−	+	+	−	−
NKI-4	n.r.	+	−	+	++	−	−
SKMel-28	M	+	−	+	−	−	−
MeWo	M	+	+	+	−	+	−
IGR-39	PT	+++	+++	++	++	−	++
Mel-57	PT	+	−	+	−	−	−
O-Mel-II	M	++	+/−	+/−	−	−	−
Mel-2a	M	+	−	+	−	+/−	−
SKMel-13	M	++	++	+	−	+	−
SKMel-19	M	+	−	+	+++	+/−	−
IGR-37	M	++	+++	+	−	−	++
M 5	M	+	+	+/−	−	+/−	−
StNM-1	NS	+	+/−	+	+/−	+/−	+/−
StNM-7	NS	++	+	+	+	+/−	+/−
StNM-8	NS	++	++	+	+	+/−	+/−
Lei-1	NS	+	+	+	+	+	+
Mel-4	NS	+	+	+	+	+	+
Mel-5	NS	+/−	+/−	+	+	+	+
Mel-6	NS	+	++	+	+/−	+	+

IL, interleukin; TNF, tumor necrosis factor; GM-CSF, granulocyte-macrophage colony-stimulating factor; PT, primary tumor; M, metastasis; n.r., not reported; NS, normal skin. +++, detectable after 30 polymerase chain reaction (PCR) cycles; ++, detectable after 33 PCR cycles; +, detectable after 36 PCR cycles; +/−, detectable after 40 PCR cycles; −, not detectable after 40 PCR cycles.

Krasagakes et al., submitted). Gene expression for IL-2, IL-3, IL-4, IL-5, and IL-7 was detected neither in melanoma cells nor in melanocytes. Similarly, interferon-γ was not detected in both cell types. Moreover, TNF-α mRNA was detected in two out of 13 cell lines and at weak levels in three out of 13 cell lines investigated. Gene expression for granulocyte-macrophage colony-stimulating factor (GM-CSF) was found only in a minority of melanoma lines (three out of 13). This variable cytokine gene expression among the different melanoma cell lines did not correlate with the stage of disease, since the panel analyzed included cell lines obtained from primary and from metastatic melanomas (see Table 2).

In contrast, the seven malanocyte cultures showed a more homogeneous pattern of cytokine gene expression. All seven cultures analyzed expressed mRNA for $IL\text{-}1_{\beta}$, IL-6, IL-8, and IL-10, although mostly at lower levels than melanoma cells (Fig. 1). Transcripts for TNF-α and GM-CSF, however, were very weak in melanocytes; only four out of seven cultures had clearly detectable PCR products after 36 PCR cycles on the ethidium bromide-stained agarose gels.

Discussion

In the present study we have analyzed the pattern of cytokine gene expression in a panel of 13 melanoma cell lines and seven melanocyte cultures. We used the method of RT-PCR in order to detect even low amounts of cytokine mRNA. The same pattern of cytokine gene expression was found in melanoma cell lines and melanocyte cultures. We have detected mRNA for IL-1_{β}, IL-6, IL-8, IL-10, TNF-α, and GM-CSF, but not for IL-2, IL-3, IL-4, IL-5, IL-7, or interferon-γ. This suggests that the expression of multiple cytokines by melanoma cells is rather a property of the melanocytic lineage and not a consequence of the transformation process of the cells, as was assumed previously (Rodeck et al. 1991). The reported limited expression of cytokines by cultured melanocytes is probably due to the lower sensitivity of the detection methods used. Using the very sensitive method of RT-PCR we detected low, but significant, expression of several lymphokines by melanocytes. At least in the case of IL-6, melanocytes could also translate the transcribed cytokine into protein, since IL-6 bioactivity was detected in supernatants of melanocyte cultures (data not shown). Significant differences have been found in the level of expression of these cytokines not only between melanocytes and melanoma cells, but also among the different melanoma cell lines. Such differences may be important, since the biological effects of cytokines are greatly dependent on the concentrations of the molecule.

IL-1_{β} was detected in all melanoma cell lines and melanocyte cultures which were examined in our series of experiments, and almost same levels of expression were found in the two cell types. With the exception of a congress presentation by Mitzutani et al. (1991), this is, to our knowledge, the first report describing production of IL-1_{β} mRNA by melanocytes in culture. In contrast, several studies have reported on the constitutive production of either IL-1_{α} and/or IL-1_{β} mRNA and protein by melanoma cell lines (see Table 3). The biological effects of IL-1 secretion by melanoma cells are complex. In vitro, IL-1 has been reported to directly augment or suppress melanoma cell proliferation (Lachman et al. 1986; Bennicelli et al. 1989). In vivo, IL-1 exerts pleiotropic effects, and the role of melanoma-derived IL-1 is still unclear, since it could either enhance or suppress tumorigenicity of melanoma cells. On the one hand, IL-1 has been reported to induce systemic immune suppression in mice upon intraveneous injection (Robertson et al. 1987) and to enhance metastatic spread when coinjected with human melanoma cells in nude mice (Giavazzi et al. 1990). In support of the latter finding, Burrows et al. (1991) reported that melanoma-derived IL-1 mainly induces expression of intercellular adhesion molecule 1 (ICAM-1) on melanoma cells and that treatment of melanoma cells with an anti-IL-1 antibody not only decreased the level of ICAM-1 expression, but also lowered their adherence to cultured endothelium. Alternatively, the secretion of IL-1 by melanoma cells could also act immunostimulatory by its

Table 3. Constitutive production of cytokines by human melanoma cell lines

Cytokine	Melanoma cells		References
	mRNA	Protein	
IL-1_α	+	+/++	Armstrong et al. 1992; Bennicelli et al. 1989; Burrows et al. 1991; Colmbo et al. 1992; Köck et al. 1989; Rodeck et al. 1991
IL-1_β	++	n.d.	Armstrong et al. 1992; Colombo et al. 1992; Rodeck et al. 1991
IL-6	++	++	Armstrong et al. 1992; Colombo et al. 1992
IL-8	++	++	Colombo et al. 1992; Förster et al. 1991; Schadendorf et al. 1993; Zachariae et al. 1991
MGSA	++	++	Chevenix-Trench et al. 1990; Richmond and Thomas 1988; Richmond et al. 1988; Rodeck et al. 1991
IL-10	++	++	Gastl et al. 1993
TNF-α	++	++	Colombo et al. 1992; Lugassy and Escade 1991
G-CSF	+	–	Colombo et al. 1992
GM-CSF	+	+	Armstrong et al. 1992; Sabatini et al. 1990

IL, interleukin; MGSA, melanoma growth-stimulatory activity; TNF, tumor necrosis factor; G(M)-CSF, granulocyte (-macrophage) colony-stimulating factor; n.d., not determined.

potential to activate other lymphoid cells, as has been shown in other tumor systems (Douvdevani et al. 1992).

In the present investigation IL-6 mRNA was detected in seven out of 13 melanoma cell lines and seven out of seven melanocyte cultures. However, high levels of IL-6 were detected only in three melanoma cell lines. These results were confirmed at the protein level using an IL-6-specific bioassay and neutralizing antibodies. Expression of IL-6 mRNA by melanocytes has not been previously reported, but production of IL-6 mRNA and protein has been shown in some melanoma cell lines in previous investigations (see Table 3). While IL-6 is inhibitory for melanocytes, both antiproliferative (Morinaga et al. 1989) as well as growth-stimulatory effects (Lu and Kerbel 1993) have been reported on melanoma cells. Its role in host antitumor responses has not been completely elucidated. IL-6 appears to serve as an inducer of B cell maturation and proliferation and of T cell maturation and cytotoxicity (Kishimoto 1985; Lotz et al. 1988). It has been shown to enhance B cell lymphoma growth directly (Lee et al. 1989). In contrast, IL-6 administration to mice bearing fibrosarcomas or colon carcinomas has reduced tumor growth and metastatic colony formation (Mule et al. 1990). Additionally, a clear antitumor effect has been shown in a syngeneic animal model where B16-derived murine melanoma cells transfected with human IL-6 cDNA demonstrated slower tumor growth in vivo (Sun et al. 1992). Possible mechanisms for this included increased expression of receptor for matrix proteins and an apparent inhibition of neovascularisation in the IL-6-transfected tumors.

Similar to our findings, IL-8 mRNA production by melanoma cells has been reported either constitutively (Colombo et al. 1992; Schadendorf et al. 1993) or upon IL-1 stimulation (Zachariae et al. 1991). Up to now, IL-8 production by melanocytes has been reported only after cytokine stimulation (Zachariae et al. 1991). In our series of experiments we were able to detect constitutive IL-8 mRNA expression in melanocytes. This may be due to differences in the culture conditions of the cells or even to the different sensitivity of the detection method (Northern Blotting versus RT-PCR). It has been reported that melanocytes and melanoma cells express transcripts for another related cytokine, namely melanoma growth-stimulatory activity (MGSA; Richmond et al. 1983; Chevenix-Trench et al. 1990), a factor with 50% homology to IL-8 (Richmond et al. 1988). Experimental findings suggest that IL-8 (Schadendorf et al. 1993; Förster et al. 1991) and MGSA (Lawson et al. 1987) may function as autocrine growth factors for melanoma cells. Besides its growth-promoting activity on melanoma cells, IL-8 acts as an immunostimulator by its chemotactic activity for neutrophils (Yoshimura et al. 1987) and T lymphocytes (Larsen et al. 1989). In addition, IL-8 can induce haptotactic migration of melanoma cells and thereby increase their motility (Wang et al. 1990).

In the present study we were able to detect IL-10 mRNA in several melanoma cell lines. These results are in line with the observation by Gastl et al. (1993). Also melanocytes expressed IL-10 mRNA in vitro; however, the levels were significantly lower than in the melanoma cells, and no IL-10 protein could be detected. Originally, IL-10 was found to be expressed by various normal and malignant cell types of hematopoietic origin (De Waal-Malefyt et al. 1992). IL-10 has been shown to dampen the immune response by downregulating the secretion of several cytokines by T cells and monocytes (Vieira et al. 1991; De Waal-Malefyt et al. 1991a) and by reducing antigen-specific activation of T lymphocytes by diminishing antigen-presenting capacity of monocytes (De Waal-Malefyt et al. 1991b). Recent studies on IL-10 expression in tissues have shown the presence of IL-10 in ovarian carcinoma biopsies (Pisa et al. 1992). Moreover, we found selective expression of IL-10 mRNA in tissues of primary melanomas and melanoma metastases in comparison to normal skin (Krüger-Krasagakes et al., submitted). The biological relevance of IL-10 secretion by carcinoma cells remains unknown, but there is accumulating evidence from in vitro systems that IL-10 may play an important role not only in the suppression of T cell-mediated responses, but also as an anti-inflammatory mediator in vivo (Richter et al. 1993).

In our study, TNF-α mRNA was expressed in six of 13 melanoma cell lines. Other investigators have shown TNF-α production by melanoma cells at the protein level (Colombo et al. 1992; Lugassy and Escade 1991). Additionally, we have found low levels of TNF-α mRNA in cultured melanocytes. Apparently, melanocytes do not synthesize TNF-α in vivo, since immunoelectron microscopic examination of normal skin did not reveal presence of TNF-α in melanocytes (Kolde et al. 1992). In contrast to melanocytes, where it has been shown that TNF-α is a potent growth inhibitor, only some melanoma cell lines are susceptible to TNF in terms of cytostatic activity (Zouboulis et al. 1990; Colombo et al. 1992) and modulation of cell surface antigens and adhesion molecules (Mortarini et al. 1990). Moreover, TNF has been shown to possess cytotoxic properties and therefore may select for melanoma cells with enhanced malignancy in vitro (Zouboulis et al. 1990). With regard to in vivo effects of TNF-α, opposite effects have been observed with different tumor cell lines: suppression of local tumor growth (Blankenstein et al. 1991) as well as enhancement of metastasis formation (Qin et al. 1993). The role of TNF-α as a modulator of melanoma growth and metastasis remains to be further investigated.

We have shown that three of 13 melanoma cell lines and four of seven melanocyte cultures investigated expressed GM-CSF mRNA. Another two melanoma lines have been shown to produce GM-CSF mRNA and protein (Armstrong et al. 1992; Sabatini et al. 1990), but no reports exist on the production of GM-CSF in melanocytes. Originally, GM-CSF was described as promoting the differentiation and maturation of hematopoietic precursors to mature granulocytes, macrophages, and dendritic cells (Sieff et al. 1985). While the biologic consequences of GM-CSF production by melanoma cells are unclear, immunization experiments with GM-CSF-transduced tumor cells revealed an induction of long-lasting systemic immunity, but no effect on the primary tumor mass (Dranoff et al. 1993).

Conclusion

Our study revealed that mRNA of several cytokines with potent antiproliferative effects and immunostimulatory properties are simultaneously produced by melanoma cells and melanocytes, including IL-1, IL-6, IL-8, TNF-α, and GM-CSF. The production of multiple cytokines by melanocytes in culture suggest a possible role as an immunocompetent cell. Although production of cytokines in resting melanocytes in vivo is rather unprobable, its potential for production of immunomodulating cytokines under certain conditions is given. Possibly, the constitutive production of cytokines by melanoma cells reflects a genetically determined property of activated melanocytic cells and not necessarily a transformation-related phenomenon. This assumption is supported by the PCR data showing a common cytokine pattern gene expression for IL-1, IL-6, IL-8, TNF-α, and GM-CSF between melanocytes and melanoma cells. Other cytokines with activating properties for immune cells such as IL-2 and interferon-γ as well as chemotactic cytokines important for recruitment of host effector cells, e.g., IL-4 and IL-5, were not detected in melanocytic cells. The production of IL-10, a cytokine with potent immunosuppressive properties, by several melanoma cell lines underscores the fact that mediators may be present in melanoma lesions, which may induce local immunosuppression. Our findings support the notion that a complex cytokine network is involved in the immune regulation of melanoma growth and development. The net effect of multiple cytokines on the outcome of the host response to melanoma is presently unknown and not predictable from in vitro data. Further investigations on the presence and biological significance of these cytokines in melanoma lesions are necessary.

References

Armstrong CA, Tara DC, Hart CE, Köck A, Luger TA, Ansel JC (1992) Heterogeneity of cytokine production by human malignant melanoma cells. Exp Dermatol 1:37–45

Asher AL, Mule JJ, Kasid A, Restifo NP, Salo JC, Reichert CM, Jaffe G, Fendly B, Kriegler M, Rosenberg SA (1991) Murine tumor cells transduced with the gene for tumor necrosis factor alpha. J Immunol 146:3227–3234

Bennicelli JL, Elias J, Kern J, Guerry D (1989) Production of interleukin 1 activity by cultured human melanoma cells. Cancer Res 49:930–935

Blankenstein T, Qin Z, Überla K, Müller W, Rosen H, Volk H-D, Diamantstein T (1991) Tumor suppression after tumor cell targeted tumor necrosis factor alpha gene transfer. J Exp Med 173:1047–1052

Burrows FJ, Haskard DO, Bart IR (1991) Influence of tumor-derived interleukin 1 on melanoma-endothelial cell interactions. Cancer Res 51:4768–4775

Chevenix-Trench G, Martin NG, Ellem KAO (1990) Gene expression in melanoma cell lines and cultured melanocytes: correlation between level of c-src-1, c-myc and p53. Oncogene 5:1187–1193

Colombo MP, Ferrari G, Stoppacciaro A, Parenza M, Rodofo M, Mavilio F, Parmiani G (1991) Granulocyte colony-stimulating factor gene transfer suppresses tumorigenicity of a murine adenocarcinoma in vivo. J Exp Med 173:889–897

Colombo MP, Maccalli C, Mattei S, Melani C, Radrizzani M, Parmiani G (1992) Expression of cytokine genes, including IL-6, in human malignant melanoma cell lines. Melanoma Res 2:181–189

De Waal-Malefyt R, Abrams J, Bennet B, Figdor CG, De Vries J (1991a) Interleukin 10 (IL-10) inhibits cytokine synthesis by human monocytes: an autoregulatory role of IL-10 produced by monocytes. J Exp Med 174:1209–1220

De Waal-Malefyt R, Haanen J, Spits H, Roncarolo M-G, Te Velde A, Figdor C, Johnson K, Kastelein R, Yssel H, De Vries JE (1991b) Interleukin 10 (IL-10) and viral IL-10 strongly reduce antigen-specific human T-cell proliferation by diminishing the antigen-presenting capacity of monocytes via downregulation of class II major histocompatibility complex expression. J Exp Med 174:915–924

De Waal-Malefyt R, Yssel H, Roncarolo M-G, Spits H, De Vries J (1992) Interleukin-10. Curr Opin Immunol 4:314–320

Dorsch M, Hock H, Kunzendorf U, Diamantstein T, Blankenstein T (1993) Macrophage colony-stimulating factor gene transfer into tumor cells induces macrophage infiltration but not tumor suppression. Eur J Immunol 23:186–190

Douvdevani A, Huleihel M, Zoller M, Segal S, Apte RN (1992) Reduced tumorigenicity of fibrosarcomas which constitutively generate IL-1 alpha either spontaneously or following IL-1 alpha gene transfer. Int J Cancer 51:822–830

Dranoff G, Jaffee E, Lazenby A, Golumbek P, Levitsky H, Brose K, Jackson V, Hamada H, Pardoll D, Mulligan RC (1993) Vaccination with irradiated tumor cells engineered to secrete murine granulocyte-macrophage colony-stimulating factor stimulates potent, specific, and long-lasting anti-tumor immunity. Proc Natl Acad Sci USA 90:3539–3543

Eberle J, Krasagakis K, Garbe C, Orfanos CE (1993) Proliferation and morphology of melanoma cells and benign melanocytes under varying culture conditions. Melanoma Res 3:107–112

Fearon ER, Pardoll DM, Itaya T, Golumbek P, Levitsky HI, Simons JW, Karasuyama H, Vogelstein B, Frost P (1990) Interleukin 2 production by tumor cells bypasses T helper function in the generation of an antitumor response. Cell 60:397–403

Förster E, Kirnbauer R, Urbanski A, Köck A, Luger TA (1991) Human melanoma cells produce interleukin 8 which functions as an autocrine growth factor. J Invest Dermatol 96:608

Gansbacher B, Bannerjii R, Daniels B, Zier K, Cronin K, Gilboa E (1990a) Retroviral vector-mediated interferon-gamma gene transfer into tumor cells generates potent and long lasting antitumor immunity. Cancer Res 50:7820–7825

Gansbacher B, Zier K, Daniels B, Cronin K, Bannerjy R, Gilboa E (1990b) Interleukin 2 gene transfer into tumor cells abrogates tumorigenicity and induces protective immunity. J Exp Med 172:1217–1224

Gastl GA, Abrams JS, Nannes DM, Oosterkamp R, Silver J, Liu F, Chen M, Albino AP, Bander NH (1993) Interleukin-10 production by human carcinoma cell lines and its relationship to interleukin 6 expression. Int J Cancer 55:96–101

Giavazzi R, Garofalo A, Bani MR (1990) Interleukin 1-induced augmentation of experimental metastases from a human melanoma in nude mice. Cancer Res 50:4771–4775

Golumbek PT, Lazenby AJ, Levitsky HI, Jaffee LM, Karasuyama H, Baker M, Pardoll DM (1991) Treatment of established renal cancer by tumor cells engineered to secrete interleukin 4. Science 254:713–716

Hock H, Dorsch M, Diamantstein T, Blankenstein T (1991) Interleukin 7 induces $CD4^+$ T-cell dependent tumor rejection. J Exp Med 174:1291–1298

Kishimoto T (1985) Factors affecting B cell growth and differentiation. Annu Rev Immunol 3:133–157

Köck A, Schwarz T, Urbanski A, Peng Z, Vetterlein M, Micksche M, Ansel JC, Kung HF, Luger TA (1989) Expression and release of interleukin-1 by different human melanoma cell lines. J Natl Cancer Inst 81:36–42

Kolde G, Schulze-Osthoff K, Meyer H, Knop J (1992) Immunohistological and immunoelectron microscopic identification of TNF alpha in normal human and murine epidermis. Arch Dermatol Res 284:154–158

Krüger-Krasagakes S, Li W, Richter G, Diamantstein T, Blankenstein T (1993) Eosinophils infiltrating interleukin 5 gene transfected tumors do not suppress tumor growth. Eur J Immunol 23:992–995

Krüger-Krasagakes S, Krasagakis K, Garbe C, Schitt E, Hüls C, Blankenstein T, Diamanstein T (1994) Expression of interleukin 10 in human melanoma (submitted for publication)

Lachman LB, Dinarello CA, Llansa ND, Fidler IJ (1986) Natural and recombinant human interleukin 1-β is cytotxic for human melanoma cells. J Immunol 136: 3098–3102

Larsen CG, Anderson AO, Appella E, Oppenheim JJ, Matsushima K (1989) The neutrophil-activating protein (NAP-1) is also chemotactic for T-lymphocytes. Science 243:1464–1466

Lawson DH, Thomas HG, Roy RGB, Gordon DS, Chawla RK, Nixon DW, Richmond A (1987) preparation of a monoclonal antibody to melanoma growth-

stimulatory activity released into serum-free culture medium by Hs0294 malignant melanoma cells. J Cell Biochem 34:169–185
Lee C, Biondi A, Wang XH, Iscove NN, de Sousa J, Aarden LA, Wong GG, Clark SC, Messner HA, Minden MD (1989) A possible autocrine role for interleukin-6 in two lymphoma cell lines. Blood 74:798–804
Lotz M, Jirik F, Kabouridis R, Tsoukas C, Hirano T, Kishimoto T, Carson DA (1988) BSF-2/IL-6 is a costimulant for human thymocytes and T lymphocytes. J Exp Med 167:1253–1258
Lu C, Kerbel RS (1993) Interleukin 6 undergoes transition from paracrine growth inhibitor to autocrine stimulator during melanoma progression. J Cell Biol 120:1281–1288
Lugassy C, Escade JP (1991) Immunolocation of TNF-a/Cachectin in human melanoma cells: studies on co-cultivated malignant melanoma. J Invest Dermatol 96:238–242
Luster AD, Leder P (1993) IP-10, a -C-X-C- chemokine, elicits a potent thymus-dependent antitumor response in vivo. J Exp Med 178:1057–1065
Mizutani H, Miwa N, Mizutani T, Kupper TS (1990) Melanocytes produce IL-1 beta and contain IL-1 beta convertase activity: a potential in vivo mechanism for paracrine conversion of keratinocyte pro-IL-1-beta. J Invest Dermatol 94: 556A
Morinaga Y, Suzuki H, Takatsuki F (1989) Contribution of IL-6 to the antiproliferative effect of IL-1 and tumor necrosis factor on tumor cell lines. J Immunol 143:3538–3542
Mortarini R, Belli F, Parmiani G, Anichini A (1990) Cytokine-mediated modulation of HLA-class II, ICAM-1, LFA-3 and tumor-associated antigen profile of melanoma cells. Comparison with anti-proliferative activity by rIL-1 beta, rTNF-alpha, rIFN-gamma, rIL-4 and their combinations. Int J Cancer 45:334–341
Mule JJ, McIntosh JK, Jablons DM, Rosenberg SA (1990) Antitumor activity of recombinant interleukin 6 in mice. J Exp Med 17:629–636
Pisa P, Halapi E, Pisa EK, Gerdin E, Hising C, Bucht A, Gerdin B, Kiessling R (1992) Selective expression of interleukin 10, interferon-gamma, and granulocyte-macrophage colony-stimulating factor in ovarian cancer biopsies. Proc Natl Acad Sci USA 89:7708–7712
Qin Z, Krüger-Krasagakes S, Kunzendorf U, Hock H, Diamantstein T, Blankenstein T (1993) Expression of tumor necrosis factor by different tumor cell lines results either in tumor suppression or augmented metastasis. J Exp Med 178:355–360
Richmond A, Thomas HG (1988) Melanoma growth stimulatory activity: isolation from human melanoma tumors and characterization of tissue distribution. J Cell Biol 36:185–198
Richmond A, Lawson DH, Nixon DW, Stewens JS, Chawia RK (1983) Extraction of a melanoma growth-stimulatory activity from culture medium conditioned by the Hs0294 human melanoma cell line. Cancer Res 43:2106–2112
Richmond A, Balentien E, Thomas HG, Flaggs G, Barton DE, Spiess J, Bordoni R, Francke U, Derynck R (1988) Molecular characterization and chromosomal mapping of melanoma growth stimulatory activity, a growth factor structurally related to β-thromboglobulin. EMBO J 7:2025–2033
Richter G, Krüger-Krasagakes S, Hein G, Hüls C, Schmitt E, Diamantstein T, Blankenstein T (1993) Interleukin 10 transfected into Chinese hamster ovary cells prevents tumor growth and macrophage infiltration. Cancer Res 53:4134–4137
Robertson B, Gahring L, Newton R, Daynes R (1987) In vivo administration of interleukin 1 to normal mice depresses their capacity to elicit contact hypersensitivity responses: prostaglandins are involved in this modification of immune function. J Invest Dermatol 88:380–387

Rodeck U, Melber K, Kath R, Menssen H-D, Varello M, Atkinson B, Herlyn M (1991) Constitutive expression of multiple growth factor genes by melanoma cells but not normal melanocytes. J Invest Dermatol 97:20–26

Rollins BJ, Sunday ME (1991) Suppression of tumor formation in vivo by expression of the JE gene in malignant cells. Mol Cell Biol 11:3125–3131

Sabatini M, Chavez J, Mundy GR, Bonewald LF (1990) Stimulation of tumor necrosis factor release from monocytic cells by the A375 human melanoma via granulocyte-macrophage colony-stimulating factor. Cancer Res 50:2673–2678

Schadendorf D, Möller A, Algermissen B, Worm M, Sticherling M, Czarnetzki BM (1993) IL-8 produced by human malignant melanoma cells in vitro is an essential autocrine growth factor. J Immunol 151:2667–2675

Sieff CA, Emerson SG, Donahue RE (1985) Human recombinant granulocyte-acrophage colony-stimulating factor: a multilineage hematopoietin. Science 230:1171–1173

Sun WH, Kreisle RA, Phillips AW, Ershler WB (1992) In vivo and in vitro characteristics of interleukin 6-tranfected B16 melanoma cells. Cancer Res 52:5412–5415

Tepper RI, Pattengale PK, Leder P (1989) Murine interleukin 4 displays potent anti-tumor activity in vivo. Cell 57:503–512

Topalian SL, Solomon D, Rosenberg SA (1989) Tumor-specific cytolysis by lymphocytes infiltrating human melanomas. J Immunol 142:3714–3719

Torre-Amione G, Beauchamp RD, Koeppen H, Park BH, Schreiber H, Moses HL, Rowley DA (1990) A highly immunogenic tumor transfected with a murine transforming growth factor type $\beta 1$ cDNA escapes immune surveillance. Proc Natl Acad Sci USA 87:1486–1490

Van den Ende B, Knuth A, Boon T (1992) A gene encoding an antigen recognized by cytolytic T lymphocytes on a human melanoma. Science 254:1643–1647

Vieira P, De Waal-Malefyt R, Dang M-N, Johnson KE, Kastelein R, Fiorentino DF, De Vries JE, Roncarolo M-G, Mosman TR, Moore KW (1991) Isolation and expression of human cytokine-synthesis-inhibitory-factor cDNA clones: homology to Epstein-Barr virus open reading frame BCRF1. Proc Natl Acad Sci USA 88:1172–1176

Wang JM, Tarabolett G, Matsushima K, Van Damme J, Mantovani A (1990) Induction of haptotactic migration of melanoma cells by neutrophil activating protein/interleukin-8. Biochem Biophys Res Commun 169:165–170

Watanabe Y, Kuribayashi K, Miyatake S, Nishihara K, Nakayama E-I, Taniyama T, Sakata T-A (1989) Exogenous expression of mouse interferon-gamma cDNA in mouse neuroblastoma C1300 cells results in reduced tumorigenicity by augmented anti-tumor immunity. Proc Natl Acad Sci USA 86:9456–9460

Yamamura M, Uvemura K, Deans RJ, Weinberg K, Rea TH, Bloom BR, Modlin RL (1991) Defining protective responses to pathogens: cytokine profiles in leprosy skin. Science 254:277–279

Yoshimura T, Matsushima K, Tanaka S, Robinson EA, Appella E, Oppenheim JJ, Leonard EJ (1987) Purification of a human monocyte-derived neutrophil chemotactic factor that shares sequence homology with other host defence cytokines. Proc Natl Acad Sci USA 84:9233–9237

Zachariae COC, Thestrup-Pedersen K, Matsushima K (1991) Expression and secretion of leukocyte chemotactic cytokines by normal human melanocytes and melanoma cells. J Invest Dermatol 97:593–599

Zouboulis CC, Schröder K, Garbe C, Krasagakis K, Krüger S, Orfanos CE (1990) Cytostatic and cytotoxic effects of recombinant tumor necrosis factor-alpha on sensitive human melanoma cells in vitro may result in selection of cells with enhanced markers of malignancy. J Invest Dermatol 95:223S–230S

Growth Control of Melanoma Cells and Melanocytes by Cytokines

K. Krasagakis, C. Garbe, Ch.C. Zouboulis, and C.E. Orfanos

Department of Dermatology, University Medical Center Steglitz,
The Free University of Berlin Hindenburgdamm 30, 12200 Berlin, Germany

Abstract

Aberrant proliferation of tumor cells characterizes cancer growth. Investigations of cellular growth control mechanisms have contributed to our understanding of carcinogenesis and to the identification of compounds with specific antitumor activity. Many cytokines have been found to act on melanoma tumors, either produced by the tumor cells themselves or by infiltrating host cells. Purified cytokines allowed direct comparison of the growth response between normal human melanocytes and malignant melanoma cells. The present paper summarizes results of a series of our own experiments not yet published and data from a review of the recent literature. Proliferation of normal human melanocytes is enhanced by several cytokines, including basic fibroblast growth factor (bFGF), melanoma growth stimulatory activity (MGSA), hepatocyte growth factor (HGF), and mast cell growth factor (MGF). Melanoma cells are additionally stimulated by epidermal growth factor (EGF)/transforming growth factor alpha (TGF-α) and nerve growth factor (NGF). Tumor necrosis factor alpha (TNF-α), transforming growth factor beta 1 (TGF-β_1), and interleukin (IL)-6 are all potent inhibitors of melanocyte growth, but they are less effective on melanoma cells or even stimulate their growth. Interferon (IFN)-α and IFN-γ inhibited proliferation of melanoma cells but not of melanocytes, whereas IFN-β showed antiproliferative effects in both cell types. These findings suggest an alteration in growth control mechanisms during melanocyte transformation and possibly play a role in melanoma pathogenesis.

Introduction

Recent advances in culture techniques allow growth of normal and malignant cells in vitro and provide the facilities for studying the mechanisms that

Recent Results in Cancer Research, Vol. 139

control their proliferation. Growth of normal cells is regulated by polypeptides that act via specific cellular receptors. These substances are called cytokines and include the growth factors which modulate the proliferation of nonimmune cells, whereas another group, the lymphokines, is involved in the regulation of immune cells. Experiments of the last decade have showed that alterations in cytokines and their receptors may play a central role in the uncontrolled proliferation of tumor cells in vitro, and such cytokine aberrations are possibly responsible for regulation of tumor growth in vivo.

Mode of Cytokine Action

Cells regulate their own growth as well as the growth of other cells by secreting cytokines which act by several ways (Todaro 1988). The most common modes of cell regulation are summarized in Fig. 1. In *endocrine* cell regulation, the cytokines are brought through blood vessels into the circulation and act at a distant site. In the case of *paracrine* growth regulation, the action of the cytokine is local. The producer cell affects neighboring cells by secreting the particular cytokine which binds to specific receptors. The *autocrine* mechanism of growth is mainly utilized by tumor cells. Tumor cells have the ability to produce cytokines with growth stimulatory properties and at the same time to express specific receptors for these cytokines. In this way they induce an autostimulatory feedback mechanism designated as autocrine growth of tumor cells. Recently, two other cytokine-mediated autostimulatory pathways have been described: the term "intracrine" is used when the cytokine interacts intracellularly with the receptor, and the term "juxtacrine" when the cytokine does not leave the producing cell, but may interact with the receptor on the cell membrane.

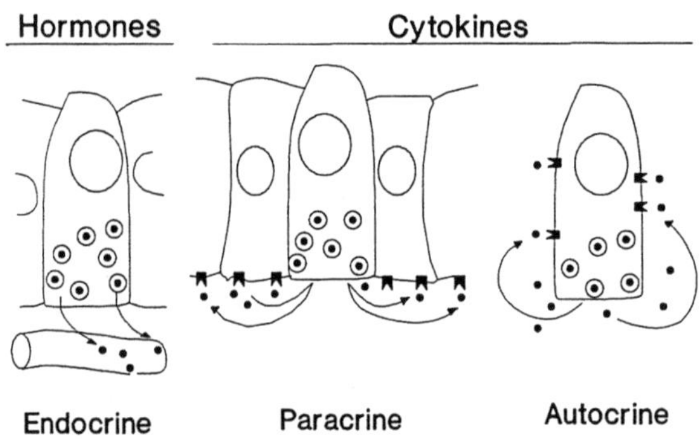

Fig. 1. Three modes of cell regulation (endocrine, paracrine, autocrine) by hormones and cytokines (modified from Todaro 1988)

Cytokines and Melanoma Oncogenesis

Both growth factors and lymphokines are possibly involved in melanocyte oncogenesis. A circulating factor with transforming properties has been isolated from the urine of melanoma patients (Kim et al. 1985). In addition, the transformation of murine melanocytes with *neu* oncogene, which codes a growth factor receptor, made them tumorigenic (Dotto et al. 1989). In contrast, the transfection of murine melanoma cells with the IL-6 gene resulted in suppression of tumor growth in vivo (Sun et al. 1992). The effects of cytokines on tumor growth in vivo are extremely complex. Cell culture systems have been used in order to study the regulation of tumor cells by all these substances. The questions which arise are what mechanisms underlie the escape of melanoma cells from growth control and whether melanoma cells have an altered production and/or response to growth-regulatory cytokines. In the following, our results and data from the literature on autocrine or paracrine regulation of melanoma cells in comparison to melanocytes are summarized.

Growth Factors

Autocrine Growth Control

In vitro experiments indicate that production of autocrine growth factors is involved in the abnormal growth regulation of melanoma cells. Normal human melanocytes require the presence of tumor promoter 12-O-tetradecanoylphorbol acetate (TPA) for growth in culture (Eisinger and Marco 1982). This tumor promoter possibly stimulates melanocyte proliferation through the induction of autocrine growth factors, since conditioned medium from TPA-treated melanocytes stimulated DNA synthesis in quiescent melanocytes and melanoma cells (Arita et al. 1992). Metastatic melanoma cells do not require mitogens such as TPA for growth in culture; conditioned medium from melanoma cells possesses mitogenic properties (Sauvaigo et al. 1986).

We investigated the response of melanoma cells to endogenous growth factor stimulation in serum-free media in vitro in a series of experiments. Therefore, conditioned medium from StML-11 melanoma cell line was prepared through incubation of 2.5×10^6 cells with 50 ml serum-free Dulbecco's modified Eagle's medium (DMEM)/Ham's F12 medium (normal medium, NM) for 48 h. Conditioned medium containing autocrine factors was added at various dilutions to melanoma cell monolayers, and accumulation of endogenous growth factors in supernatants of untreated control cultures was prevented by daily medium change. Figure 2 shows that conditioned medium of the StML-11 melanoma cell line dose-dependently stimulated the growth of the same cell line. This growth stimulation was more prominent in sparse

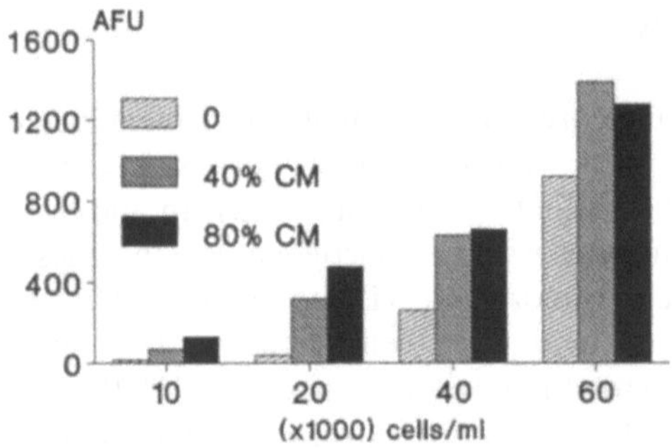

Fig. 2. Cell density-dependent effect of conditioned medium (*CM*) on the proliferation of StML-11 melanoma cell line. Cells were cultured in microtiter plates in serum-free Dulbecco's modified Eagle's medium (DMEM)/Ham's F12 medium for 8 days. Parallel cultures were maintained in this normal medium (NM) and in 40% or 80% CM. Daily medium change was performed. Cell proliferation was evaluated on day 8 by a fluorometric microassay using the substrate 4-methylumbelliferyl heptanoate (MUH; Zouboulis et al. 1991) and recorded as absolute fluoresence units (*AFU*)

monolayers (1307% of the controls at 2×10^4 cells/ml, $p < 0.001$) than in dense cultures (152% of the controls at 4×10^4 cells/ml, $p < 0.001$). The decreased response in higher cell densities may be explained by a high enough concentration of autocrine growth factors secreted in dense cultures even in a short period of time, so that exogenous addition of cytokines does not result in further stimulation of cell proliferation. This effect was also seen in experiments with the addition of certain growth factors (epidermal growth factor, EGF; basic fibroblast growth factor, bFGF; transforming growth factor beta, TGF-β; nerve growth factor, NGF). Stimulation of melanoma cell proliferation by these substances was demonstrated after withdrawal of autocrine growth factors through daily medium change, which otherwise caused maximal stimulation of the cells (see below).

The stimulatory effect of the conditioned medium is probably mediated through several substances, since melanoma cells constitutively express multiple growth factors (Rodeck et al. 1991). Several of these defined substances have been etiologically associated with melanoma growth. In the following, the most important of these factors are summarized.

Basic Fibroblast Growth Factor

bFGF, a 17.5-kDa polypeptide, is a prototype of autocrine growth factors for melanoma cells. It is a natural mitogen for melanocytes, found in extracts from keratinocytes (Halaban et al. 1988a), and it is produced by melanoma cells but not by melanocytes (Halaban et al. 1988b). Evidence for the existence of an autocrine loop for melanoma cells is given by the fact

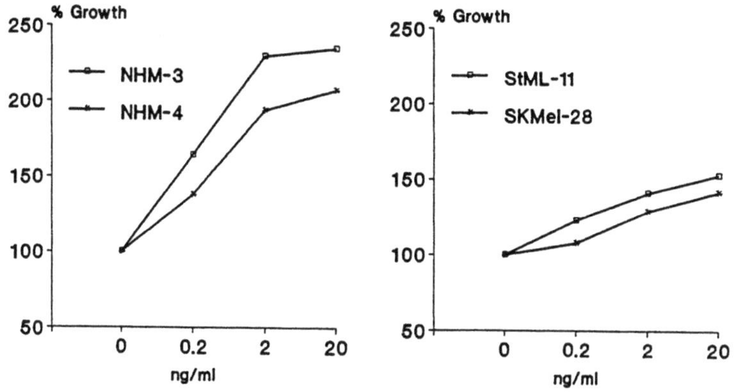

Fig. 3. Effect of basic fibroblast growth factor (bFGF) on proliferation of human melanocytes (NHM-3 and -4; *left*) and of melanoma cell lines (SKMel-28 and StML-11; *right*). Cells were seeded at 10^4 cells/ml in microtiter plates. Melanocytes were maintained in reduced melanocyte medium (RMM) and melanoma cells in normal medium (NM) + 1 mg/ml bovine serum albumin (BSA). Change of media containing 0.2–20 ng/ml bFGF was performed every 2 days in melanocytes and daily in melanoma cell cultures. Cell proliferation was evaluated on day 8 by the MUH method

that their proliferation is inhibited by antisense oligonucleotides targeted against bFGF and its receptor (Becker et al. 1989, 1992). In addition, transformation of murine melanocytes with bFGF gene resulted in autonomous growth of the cells in culture (Dotto et al. 1989).

In order to investigate the growth regulation of melanoma cells and melanocytes by bFGF, we cultivated melanocytes in a serum-free growth factor-reduced melanocyte medium (RMM). This medium consisted of MCDB 153 supplemented with amino acids, 2 m*M* Ca^{2+}, 5 μg/ml insulin, 10 μg/ml transferrin, 1 n*M* cholera toxin, and 50 μM hydrocortisone. Melanoma cells were maintained in serum-free DMEM/Ham's F12 medium supplemented with 1 mg/ml bovine serum albumin (BSA). Figure 3 illustrates comparatively the effect of bFGF on the proliferation of melanocytes and of melanoma cells. Both cell types were stimulated by this growth factor, but the growth stimulation of melanoma cells was less prominent than that of the melanocytes, possibly through the autocrine production of bFGF by these cells (NHM-3 235% and StML-11 153% of the controls at 2 ng/ml, $p < 0.001$). This is supported by the finding that bFGF had no effect on logarithmically growing dense monolayers of melanoma cell lines.

Melanoma Growth Stimulatory Activity/Interleukin 8

Melanoma growth stimulatory activity (MGSA) has been shown to have 50% homology to interleukin (IL)-8 and has been regarded as an autocrine growth factor for melanoma cells (Richmond et al. 1988). It is produced by nevus cells and by melanoma cells and stimulates the proliferation of melanoma cells and of melanocytes (Richmond and Thomas 1988; Bordoni et al. 1990). Evidence for the autocrine loop for MGSA is provided by the experiments by Lawson et al. (1987), which showed that antibodies against MGSA inhibited the autonomous growth of melanoma cells in vitro. Recently, IL-8 was identified as an essential autocrine growth factor for human malignant melanoma cells (Schadendorf et al. 1993). In this study, blockade of autocrine-produced IL-8 either at the mRNA level by antisense oligonucletides or at the protein level by monoclonal antibodies resulted in inhibition of cell proliferation and colony formation.

Epidermal Growth Factor/Transforming Growth Factor Alpha

Several lines of evidence suggest that the EGF/TGF-α system is important in the growth regulation of melanoma cells. Both substances possess similar properties and bind to the same cellular receptor which is designated the EGF-receptor (Carpenter and Cohen 1979). TGF-α is produced by melanoma cells but not by melanocytes (Herlyn et al. 1991; Albino et al. 1991).

Melanoma cells express EGF-receptor either in its normal form or in a truncated form, which is the protein product of the c-*erb-B2* oncogene (Chenevix-Trench et al. 1990). It has been reported that metastatic melanoma cells, but not primary melanoma cells or normal melanocytes, respond to EGF (Rodeck et al. 1987).

We investigated the effect of EGF on cultures of metastatic melanoma cells and normal human melanocytes. Melanocyte cultures were maintained in complete melanocyte medium (CMM, i.e., RMM supplemented with 2 ng/ml bFGF and 0.4% bovine pituitary extract) and the two metastatic melanoma cell lines maintained in NM. The proliferation of the melanocytes is not influenced by EGF at doses from 1–100 ng/ml ($p > 0.05$; Fig. 4). In contrast, dose-dependent stimulation of melanoma cell proliferation was seen after addition of EGF in sparse monolayers (SKMel-28; maximum 202% of the controls; $p < 0.01$). When EGF was added in dense monolayers of logarithmically growing cultures, no stimulation of proliferation in any of the cell lines was observed.

Interestingly, blockade of EGF-receptor by monoclonal antibodies (MAb) did not influence melanoma cell growth (Rodeck et al. 1991). It cannot be excluded however, that an intracrine loop exists allowing intracellular binding of EGF/TGF-α to the EGF-receptor.

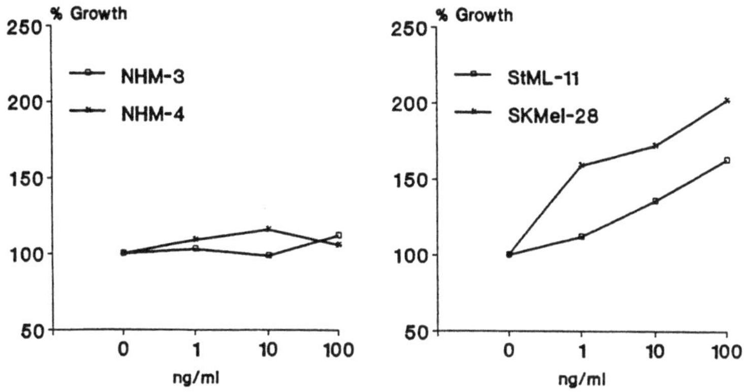

Fig. 4. Comparison of the effect of epidermal growth factor (EGF) on proliferation of melanocytes (*left*) and of melanoma cells (*right*). Cells were seeded at 10^4 cells/ml in microtiter plates. Melanocytes were maintained in complete melanocyte medium (CMM) and melanoma cells in normal medium (NM). Change of media containing 1–100 ng/ml EGF were performed every 2 days in melanocytes and daily in melanoma cell cultures. Cell proliferation was evaluated on day 8 by the 4-methylumbelliferyl heptanoate (MUH) method

Transforming Growth Factor Beta

TGF-β exists in mammalian cells in three forms (TGF-β_1, -β_2, -β_3), which have similar functions and bind to the same class of receptors (Cheifetz et al. 1987). mRNA for all three forms is produced by melanocytes and by melanoma cells, and TGF-β protein is secreted into the culture supernatant of melanoma cells (Albino et al. 1991).

We compared the effect of TGF-β in a series of experiments and found considerable differences in the response of normal melanocytes and malignant melanoma cells to TGF-β_1. Human melanocytes are strongly inhibited by exogenous TGF-β_1 (Fig. 5; NHM-4, 61% inhibition at 5 ng/ml; $p < 0.001$). In contrast, melanoma cells escape growth inhibition by this cytokine. In dense monolayers of logarithmically growing melanoma cell cultures, TGF-β_1 caused either no effect or slight inhibition of cell proliferation (SKMel-28; 16% growth inhibition at 5 ng/ml, $p < 0.05$; StML-11, no effect). When TGF-β_1 was added in sparse monolayers of slowly dividing melanoma cells and daily medium change was performed, it stimulated their proliferation (Fig. 5; SKMel-28, 199% of the controls at 5 ng/ml; $p < 0.001$). Similar findings describing altered sensitivity of minimally and highly metastatic melanoma cells to TGF-β_1 have been reported in the murine system (Mooradian et al. 1990). All these data suggest that alterations in the response of melanocytic cells to TGF-β_1 may play a role in melanoma pathogenesis.

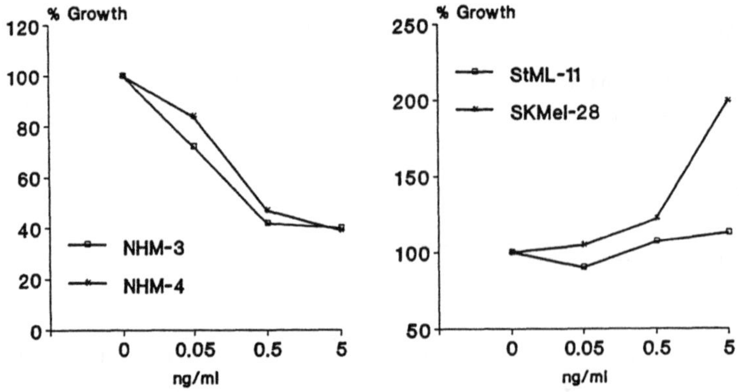

Fig. 5. Differential effect of transforming growth factor (TGF)-β1 on the proliferation of normal melanocytes (*left*) and of melanoma cells (*right*). Cultures were incubated with 0.05–5 ng TGF-β_1/ml as described in Fig. 4 and cell proliferation was evaluated on day 8 by the 4-methylumbelliferyl heptanoate (MUH) method

Other Growth Factors

The role of several other growth factors in human melanoma is less well understood. Nerve growth factor important for differentiation and survival of sympathic and sensory neurons, gained attention when it was found that metastatic melanoma cells express high levels of NGF-receptors (Fabricant et al. 1977; Herlyn et al. 1985). Low receptor levels have been detected in primary melanoma cells and melanocytes. Upregulation of NGF-receptor was induced after exposure of the cells to the tumor promoter 12-O-tetradecanoylphorbolacetate or to ultraviolet (UV) radiation (Peacocke et al. 1988; Krasagakis et al. 1993). Although NGF mainly increases melanoma cell survival, under certain conditions it may increase melanoma cell numbers in vitro (Mather and Sato 1979).

In our own experiments, we investigated the effect of NGF on proliferation of melanoma cells and normal melanocytes. These findings are illustrated in Fig. 6, showing a dose-dependent increase of melanoma cell growth by NGF (up to 240% of the controls at 100 ng/ml for StML-11). In contrast, melanocyte growth remained unaffected by 1–100 ng/ml NGF.

Insulin and insulin-like growth factor 1 (IGF-1) stimulate the proliferation of melanoma cells in vitro after binding to IGF-1-receptor (Rodeck et al. 1987). Up to now there have been no reports on production of these factors by melanoma cells. Melanoma cells may express the mast cell growth factor (MGF), as well as its ligand for the c-*kit* proto-oncogene (Turner et al. 1992). Although normal melanocytes respond to mast cell growth factor, MGF did not alter proliferation rates of most melanoma cell lines in vitro (Funasaka et al. 1992). Recently, Halaban et al. (1992a) reported that

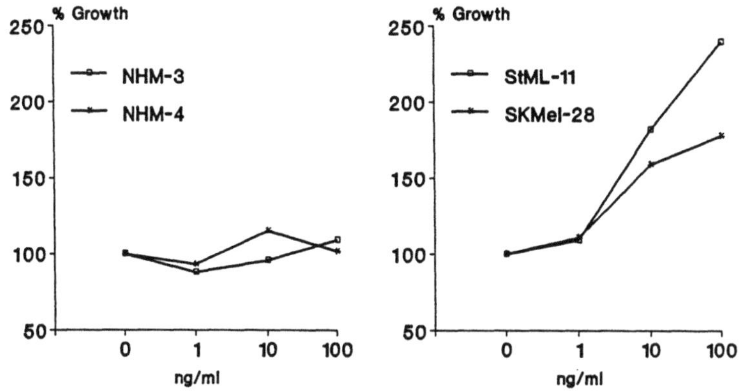

Fig. 6. Stimulation of melanoma cell (*right*) but not of melanocyte growth (*left*) by nerve growth factor (NGF). Cultures were incubated with 1–100 ng NGF/ml as described in Fig. 4 and cell proliferation was evaluated on day 8 by the 4-methylumbelliferyl heptanoate (MUH) method

hepatocyte growth factor/scatter growth factor (HGF/SF) is mitogenic for melanocytes in the presence of bFGF or MGF. c-Met and c-Kit, the receptors for HGF/SF and MGF are, in contrast to the bFGF receptor, not constitutively activated in melanoma cells (Halaban et al. 1992b).

Interleukins

Interleukins are cytokines which have been described as being produced by hemopoietic cells and as regulating their growth and differentiation. An analysis of the cytokine pattern expressed in melanocytic cells has been included in this volume. Production of several interleukins occurs in melanocytic cells, including IL-1_β, IL-6, IL-8, and IL-10 (Krüger-Krasagakes et al., this volume). IL-1 has been shown to inhibit the growth of both melanoma cells and melanocytes (Nakai et al. 1988; Mortarini et al. 1990; Swope et al. 1991). In contrast, it has been reported that IL-6 inhibits melanocyte growth (Swope et al. 1991), but its effects on melanoma cells depend on the stage of melanoma progression. Melanoma cells derived from radial growth phase or from early vertical growth phase are inhibited by IL-6 (Lu et al. 1992). In contrast, melanoma cells from advanced vertical growth phase lesions or metastasis are completely resistant to the IL-6-mediated growth inhibition. Recent work from the same group showed that endogenously produced IL-6 in metastatic melanoma cells may serve as an autocrine stimulator (Lu and Kerbel 1993). The contribution of other cytokines of the interleukin family on the growth control of melanoma needs further investigations. The role of TNF-α has not yet been completely elucidated. This cytokine is produced by melanocytes and melanoma cells

(Krüger-Krasagakes et al., this volume). Although melanocytes are strongly inhibited by TNF-α (Swope et al. 1991), only some of the melanoma cell lines respond to it (Mortarini et al. 1990). Due to its cytostatic and cytotoxic properties in vitro, TNF-α may result in selection of melanoma cells with enhanced malignancy (Zouboulis et al. 1990b).

Interferons

Interferons are substances which have been widely used in the systemic treatment of melanoma patients (Wadler and Schwartz 1990; Garbe et al. 1992). This has been attributed in part to the immunomodulating properties of the compounds and in part to the direct antiproliferative effect of IFN on melanoma cells. Although some investigators reported IFN-γ to be the most potent antiproliferative agent (Tyring et al. 1984), we and others demonstrated IFN-β to be more efficient than IFN-α or IFN-γ in inhibiting melanoma cell proliferation (Fisher et al. 1986; Garbe et al. 1990; Zouboulis et al. 1990a; Krasagakis et al. 1991).

We examined whether melanocytic cells develop an altered sensitivity to IFN in the course of malignancy. We cultured melanoma cells maintained in NM and melanocytes maintained in CMM in the presence of various IFN for 3 and 6 days respectively and observed an increased sensitivity of melanoma cells to IFN-α and IFN-γ, but similar sensitivity as melanocytes to IFN-β. These findings are presented comparatively in Fig. 7, showing 24% and 23% growth inhibition of melanocytes by 10^4 IU/ml IFN-α or IFN-γ, respectively,

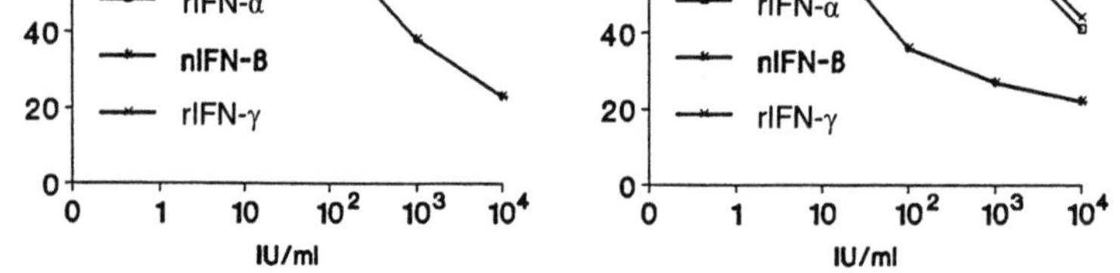

Fig. 7. Comparison of the inhibitory effect of recombinant (*r*) interferon (*IFN*)-α, natural (*n*) IFN-β, and recombinant IFN-γ on the proliferation of normal melanocytes (*left*) and of melanoma cell lines (*right*). Cultures were incubated with $1-10^4$ IU/ml of the various IFN. Medium change was performed every 2 days and cell proliferation was evaluated on day 4 for melanoma cells and day 7 for melanocytes by the 4-methylumbelliferyl heptanoate (MUH) method

compared to 59% and 56% of melanoma cells. Lower concentrations of IFN-α or IFN-γ had no effect on melanocyte proliferation. In contrast, even 1–10 IU IFN-β/ml significantly inhibited the proliferation of melanocytes and melanoma cells, and incubation with 10^4 U IFN-β/ml results in an 80% inhibition of cell growth in both cases.

Conclusion

Data from in vitro experiments revealed several alterations in growth control mechanisms of pigment cells by cytokines in the course of malignant transformation and progression. Few cytokines have been proven to be very important for direct regulation of melanomas. During the malignant transformation of pigment cells there is increased production of the stimulatory cytokines bFGF and MGSA. An altered sensitivity to some cytokines develops. Melanoma cells become sensitive to TGF-α, and IL-6 undergoes transition from paracrine growth inhibitor to autocrine growth stimulator, especially in late stages of tumor progression. Similar effects have been reported for TGF-β_1. In addition, the decreased sensitivity to the inhibitory cytokine TNF-α may further contribute to the escape of melanoma cells from negative growth control mechanisms. On the other hand, melanoma cells acquire an increased sensitivity to the growth-inhibitory effect of IFN-α and IFN-γ. The role of several other cytokines on the growth control of melanocytic cells is still unclear, and further investigations are needed to understand the complexity of the cytokine network in the pathogenesis of human melanoma.

References

Albino P, Davis BM, Nanus DM (1991) Induction of growth factor RNA expression in human malignant melanoma: markers of transformation. Cancer Res 51:4815–4820

Arita Y, O'Driscoll KR, Weinstein BI (1992) Growth of human melanocyte cultures supported by 12-O-tetradecanoylphorbol-13-acetate is mediated through protein kinase C activation. Cancer Res 52:4514–4521

Becker D, Meier CB, Herlyn M (1989) Proliferation of human malignant melanomas is inhibited by antisense oligonucleotides targeted against basic fibroblast growth factor. EMBO J 8:3685–3691

Becker D, Lee PL, Rodeck U, Herlyn M (1992) Inhibition of the fibroblast growth factor receptor 1 (FGFR-1) gene in human melanocytes and malignant melanomas leads to inhibition of proliferation and signs indicative of differentiation. Oncogene 7:2303–2313

Bordoni R, Fine R, Murray D, Richmond A (1990) Characterization of the role of melanoma growth stimulatory activity (MGSA) in the growth of normal melanocytes, nevocytes, and malignant melanocytes. J Cell Biochem 44:207–219

Carpenter G, Cohen S (1979) Epidermal growth factor. Annu Rev Biochem 48: 193–216

Cheifetz S, Weatherbee JA, Tsang ML, Anderson JK, Mole JE, Lucas R, Massague J (1987) The transforming growth factor-beta system, a complex pattern of cross-reactive ligands and receptors. Cell 48:409–415

Chenevix-Trench G, Martin NG, Ellem KAO (1990) Gene expression in melanoma cell lines and cultured melanocytes: correlation between levels of c-src-1, c-myc and p53. Oncogene 5:1187–1193

Dotto GP, Moelmann G, Ghosh S, Edwards M, Halaban R (1989) Transformation of murine melanocytes by basic fibroblast growth factor cDNA and oncogenes and selective suppression of the transformed phenotype in a reconstituted cutaneous enviroment. J Cell Biol 109:3115–3128

Eisinger M, Marco O (1982) Selective proliferation of normal human melanocytes in vitro in the presence of phorbol ester and cholera toxin. Proc Natl Acad Sci USA 79:2018–2022

Fabricant RN, DeLarco JE, Todaro GJ (1977) Nerve growth factor receptors on human melanoma cells in culture. Proc Natl Acad Sci USA 74:565–569

Fisher PB, Miranda AF, Babiss LE (1986) Measurement of the effect of interferons on cellular differentiation in murine and human melanoma cells. Methods Enzymol 119:611–618

Funasaka Y, Boulton T, Cobb M, Yarden Y, Fan B, Lyman SD, Williams DE, Anderson DM, Zakut R, Mishima Y, Halaban R (1992) c-Kit-kinase induces a cascade of protein tyrosine phosphorylation in normal human melanocytes in response to mast cell growth factor and stimulates mitogen-activated protein kinase but is down-regulated in melanomas. Mol Biol Cell 3:197–209

Garbe C, Krasagakis K, Zouboulis CC, Schröder K, Krüger S, Stadler R, Orfanos CE (1990) Antitumor activities of interferon alpha, beta and gamma and their combinations on human melanoma cells in vitro: changes of proliferation, melanin synthesis and immunophenotype. J Invest Dermatol 95:231S–237S

Garbe C, Kreuser ED, Zouboulis CC, Stadler R, Orfanos CE (1992) Combined treatment of metastatic melanoma with interferons and cytotoxic drugs. Semin Oncol 19 [Suppl 4]:63–69

Halaban R, Kwon BS, Ghosh S, Delli Bovi P, Baird A (1988a) bFGF as an autocrine growth factor for human melanomas. Oncogene Res 3:177–186

Halaban R, Langdon R, Birchall N, Cuono C, Baird A, Scott G, Moellmann G, McGuire J (1988b) Basic fibroblast growth factor from human keratinocytes is a natural mitogen for melanocytes. J Cell Biol 107:1611–1619

Halaban R, Rubin JS, Funasaka Y, Cobb M, Boulton T, Faletto D, Rosen E, Chan A, Yoko K, White W et al (1992a) Met and hepatocyte growth factor/scatter factor signal transduction in normal melanocytes and melanoma cells. Oncogene 7:2195–2206

Halaban R, Fan B, Ahn J, Funasaka Y, Gitay Goren H, Neufeld G (1992b) Growth factors, receptor kinases, and protein tyrosine phosphatases in normal and malignant melanocytes. J Immunother 12:154–161

Herlyn M, Thurin J, Balaban G, Benicelli JL, Herlyn D, Elder DE, Bondi E, Guerry D, Nowell P, Clark WH, Koprowski H (1985) Characteristics of cultured human melanocytes isolated from different stages of tumor progression. Cancer Res 45:5670–5676

Herlyn M, Kath R, Williams N, Valyi-Nagy I, Rodeck U (1990) Growth-regulatory factors for normal, premalignant and malignant human cells in vitro. Adv Cancer Res 54:213–234

Kim MK, Warren TC, Kimball ES (1985) Purification and characterization of a low molecular weight transforming growth factor from the urine of melanoma patients. J Biol Chem 260:9237–9243

Krasagakis K, Garbe C, Krüger S, Orfanos CE (1991) Effects of interferons on cultured human melanocytes in vitro: interferon-beta but not -alpha or -gamma inhibit proliferation and all interferons significantly modulate the cell phenotype. J Invest Dermatol 97:364–372

Krasagakis K, Garbe C, Krüger-Krasagakes S, Orfanos CE (1993) 12-O tetradecanoylphorbol-13-acetate not only modulates proliferation rates but also alters antigen expression and LAK-cell susceptibility of normal human melanocytes in vitro. J Invest Dermatol 100:653–659

Lawson DH, Thomas HG, Roy RGB, Gordon DS, Chawla RK, Nixon DW, Richmond A (1987) Preparation of a monoclonal antibody to melanoma growth stimulatory activity released into serum-free culture medium by Hs0294 malignant melanoma cells. J Cell Biochem 34:169–185

Lu C, Kerbel RS (1993) Interleukin 6 undergoes transition from paracrine growth inhibitor to autocrine stimulator during human melanoma progression. J Cell Biol 120:1281–1288

Lu C, Vickers MF, Kerbel RS (1992) Interleukin 6: a fibroblast derived growth inhibitor of human melanoma cells from early but not advanced stages of tumor progression. Proc Natl Acad Sci USA 89:9215–9219

Mather JP, Sato GH (1979) The growth of mouse melanoma cells in hormone-supplemented, serum-free medium. Exp Cell Res 120:191–200

Mooradian DL, Purchio AF, Furcht LT (1990) Differential effects of transforming growth factor β1 on the growth of poorly and highly metastatic murine melanoma cells. Cancer Res 50:273–277

Mortarini R, Belli F, Parmiani G, Anichini A (1990) Cytokine-mediated modulation of HLA-class II, ICAM-1, LFA-3 and tumor-associated antigen profile of melanoma cells. Comparison with anti-proliferative activity by rIL1-beta, rTNF-alpha, rIFN-gamma, rIL4 and their combinations. Int J Cancer 45:334–341

Nakai S, Mizuno K, Kaneta M, Hirai Y (1988) A simple, sensitive bioassay for the detection of interleukin-1 using human melanoma A375 cell line. Biochem Biophys Res Commun 154:1189–1196

Peacocke M, Yaar M, Mansur CP, Chao MV, Gilchrest BA (1988) Induction of nerve growth factor receptors on cultured human melanocytes. Proc Natl Acad Sci USA 85:5282–5286

Richmond A, Thomas HG (1988) Melanoma growth stimulatory activity: isolation from human melanoma tumors and characterization of tissue distribution. J Cell Biochem 36:185–198

Richmond A, Balentien E, Thomas HG, Flaggs G, Barton DE, Spiess J, Bordoni R, Francke R, Derynck R (1988) Molecular characterisation and chromosomal mapping of melanoma growth stimulatory activity, a growth factor structurally related to β-thromboglobulin. EMBO J 7:2025–2033

Rodeck U, Herlyn, M, Menssen HD, Furlanetto RW, Koprowski H (1987) Metastatic but not primary melanoma cell lines grow in vitro independently of exogenous growth factors. Int J Cancer 40:687–690

Rodeck U, Melber K, Kath R, Menssen H-D, Varello M, Atkinson B, Herlyn M (1991) Constitutive expression of multiple growth factor genes by melanoma cells but not normal melanocytes. J Invest Dermatol 97:20–26

Sauvaigo S, Fretts RE, Riopelle RJ, Lagard AE (1986) Autonomous proliferation of MeWo human melanoma cell lines in serum-free medium: secretion of growth-stimulating activities. Int J Cancer 37:123–132

Schadendorf D, Möller A, Algermissen B, Worm M, Sticherling M, Czarniecki BM (1993) IL-8 produced by human malignant melanoma cells in vitro is an essential autocrine growth factor. J Immunol 151:2667–2675

Sun WH, Kreisle RA, Phillips AW, Ershler WB (1992) In vivo and in vitro characteristics of interleukin 6-transfected B16 melanoma cells. Cancer Res 52:5412–5415

Swope VB, Abdel-Malek Z, Kassem LM, Nordlund JJ (1991) Interleukins 1 alpha and 6 and tumor necrosis factor-alpha are paracrine inhibitors of human melanocyte proliferation and melanogenesis. J Invest Dermatol 96:180–185

Todaro GJ (1988) Oncogenes and growth factors. In: Orfanos CE, Stadler R, Gollnick H (eds) Dermatology in five continents. Springer, Berlin Heidelberg New York, pp 11–25

Turner AM, Zsebo KM, Martin F, Jacobsen FW, Bennett LG, Broudy VC (1992) Nonhematopoietic tumor cells express stem cell factor and display c-kit receptors. Blood 80:374–381

Tyring SK, Klimpel G, Brysk M (1984) Eradication of cultured human melanoma cells by immune interferon and leukocytes. J Natl Cancer Inst 73:1067–1073

Wadler S, Schwartz EL (1990) Antineoplastic activity of the combination of interferon and cytotoxic agents against experimental and human malignancies: a review. Cancer Res 50:3473–3486

Zouboulis CC, Garbe C, Krüger S, Orfanos CE (1990a) Interferons and melanoma: comparison of the cytostatic and cytotoxic effects of natural and recombinant interferons, tumor necrosis factor-alpha and their combinations on human melanoma cells in vitro. Skin Cancer 5:137–145

Zouboulis CC, Schröder K, Garbe C, Krasagakis K, Krüger S, Orfanos CE (1990b) Cytostatic and cytotoxic effects of recombinant tumor necrosis factor-alpha on sensitive human melanoma cells in vitro may result in selection of cells with enhanced markers of malignancy. J Invest Dermatol 95:223S–230S

Zouboulis CC, Garbe C, Krasagakis K, Krüger S, Orfanos CE (1991) A fluorometric rapid microassay to identify antiproliferative compounds for human melanoma cells in vitro. Melanoma Res 1:91–95

Effects of Various Synthetic Retinoids on Proliferation and Immunophenotype of Human Melanoma Cells In Vitro

D. Schadendorf[1], M. Worm[1], K. Jurgovsky[1], E. Dippel[1], U. Reichert[2], and B.M. Czarnetzki[1]

[1] University Hospital Rudolf Virchow, Department of Dermatology, The Free University of Berlin, Augustenburger Platz 1, 13353 Berlin, Germany
[2] CIRD Galderma, 06902 Valbonne, France

Abstract

Since response rates in human melanoma are low with currently available therapeutic modalities, we have reevaluated the potential usefulness of retinoids as new alternatives for therapy of metastatic melanoma. Nine synthetic retinoids with high affinity and/or selectivity for the retinoic acid receptors (RAR) α, β, and γ were studied in comparison to all-*trans* retinoic acid (RA) for their in vitro effects on melanoma cell proliferation and for their immunomodulating capacities using four human melanoma cell lines.

Eight out of ten retinoids tested had no effect on melanoma cell growth, whereas the remaining two compounds with high RAR-γ selectivity (CD437 and CD2325) showed a dose-dependent antiproliferative effect on all melanoma cell lines with IC_{50} (concentration inhibiting response by 50%) values between 10^{-6} and 10^{-7} *M*. Further analyses showed that paracrine-mediated tumor cell growth inhibition such as induction of transforming growth factor (TGF)-β described as one mechanism of retinoid action and enzyme systems such as tyrosinase and monoamine oxidase were not involved in mediating the antiproliferative effects exerted by the two retinoids. Four of nine retinoids modulated HLA-DR expression on human melanoma cells, and expression levels of intercellular adhesion molecule 1 (ICAM-1) was increased by another subset of compounds. These effects were, however, not correlated to the receptor selectivity of the retinoids.

The potent growth inhibitory effect of the RAR-γ-selective retinoids and the immunomodulating capacities of the retinoids open an interesting alternative for new antiproliferative and immunomodulatory strategies in the treatment of metastatic melanoma.

Recent Results in Cancer Research, Vol. 139

Introduction

Human malignant melanoma remains a devasting disease because of its increasing incidence and mortality (Stat Bite 1992). Dissemination and progression of the disease are the major cause of death in affected patients, since melanoma cells are highly resistant to chemotherapeutic agents, with response rates below 30% in vivo (Ho and Sober 1990; McClay and Mastrangelo 1988) and in vitro (Schadendorf et al. 1994a). Recently combinations of chemotherapy and immunotherapy have been used to increase response rates (Falkson et al. 1991; Richards 1991), but final answers regarding improved overall survival time await larger, randomized studies. Strategies using alternative approaches for the treatment of metastatic melanoma must therefore be pursued with more intensity.

In vitro experiments performed in the early 1980s demonstrated the high potential of retinoic acid (RA) as an immunomodulating agent that also affects growth of tumor cells including melanoma (reviewed by Lotan et al. 1991). The mechanisms by which retinoids exert their antitumor effects as well as the mechanisms that may be operative in resistance or lower sensitivity of some melanoma cell lines to RA are still unclear.

With the recent detection of nuclear retinoic acid receptors (RAR), new compounds could be synthesized tailored to interact with specific RAR subtypes. Using such agents, we hoped to identify retinoids that might modulate various biological characteristics of melanoma cells more selectively and that might in the end provide more effective and reliable therapeutic tools for clinical application.

Material and Methods

Cell Culture

All cell lines (SK-Mel-23, -37, -186, MeWo, all melanoma cell lines, and HT-3, a cervical cancer cell line) were maintained as described using RPMI 1640 medium containing 10% fetal calf serum (FCS; Schadendorf et al. 1989). All melanoma cell lines used have been characterized before regarding their differentiation characteristics (Worm et al. 1993a).

Antibodies

Antibodies against HLA-DR and desmin were purchased from Dianova (Hamburg, Germany). The monoclonal antibody detecting ICAM-1 (CL 207.14) was generously provided by Dr. S. Ferrone (Valhalla, USA).

Immunohistochemistry

For immunohistochemistry (IHC), 10^{-5} cells/25-cm^2 tissue culture flask were grown with the various retinoids (10^{-6} *M*) for a minimum of 10 days. Cytospins were prepared and stained by the alkaline phosphate and monoclonal anti-alkaline phosphatase (APAAP) technique as described previously (Schadendorf et al. 1991). Quantitative evaluation was done by counting all positively stained cells. Results are expressed as means of positive cells grouped into five categories, defined as follows: negative, –; 1%–25%, (+); 26%–50% +; 51%–75%, ++, and 76%–100%, +++. Microscopic evaluation was done by two independent observers, and each experiment was done twice. Up- and downregulation for each retinoid was defined as changes from one category to another, in comparison to the untreated control.

Retinoids

A panel of ten different retinoids (Table 1) with different receptor selectivities were used. Their structures are published elsewhere (Reichert et al. 1993; Schadendorf et al. 1994c). All-*trans* retinoic acid (RA) is equivalent to CD 14 and was used in comparison to the synthetic retinoids. A stock solution of each substance was prepared in dimethyl sulfoxide (DMSO), and each compound was added after attachment of the cells over a concentration range from 10^{-8} to 10^{-5} *M*. As control, DMSO 0.1% was used in all

Table 1. Receptor specificity and relative molecular masses of the retinoids used (Martin et al. 1992; Bernard et al. 1992)

Retinoid	Receptor specificity		Molecular mass (g/l)
	(*K*d)	(n*M*)	
CD14[a]	α, β, τ	19, 5, 6	300
CD367	α, β, τ	5, 3, 1	358
CD394	β, τ	192, 70	405
CD270	β, τ	17, 56	364
CD417	β	36	334
CD2019	β	26	375
CD437	τ	77	398
CD666	τ	68	364
CD2247	τ	34	356
CD2325	τ	53	388

[a] CD14 is all-*trans* retinoic acid (RA).

experiments. Cells were cultured in the presence of the retinoids over 4–10 days.

3-(4,5-Dimethylthiazol-2-yl)-2,5-Diphenyltetrazolium Bromide Test

The 3-(4,5-dimethylthiazol-2-yl)-2,5-diphenyltetrazolium bromide (MTT) test was used to measure indirectly the proliferating cells in a sample, as described previously (Worm et al. 1993a; Schadendorf et al. 1994b). On each plate, wells with untreated cells were measured as controls, and their absorption was defined as 100%. Experiments were done in quadruplicate and repeated at least twice. Standard deviation in all tests was below 10%.

Flow Cytometric Analysis

Cells were cultured in 75-cm^2 flasks in the presence of retinoids at a concentration of $10^{-6} M$ for 8 days. Subsequently, cells were trypsinized and used for flow cytometric analysis to quantify HLA-DR and intercellular adhesion molecule 1 (ICAM-1) expression as described (Schadendorf et al. 1994b).

Modulation of Retinoid-Mediated Growth-Inhibitory Effects by Transforming Growth Factor and Neutralizing Antibodies

In order to evaluate one possible mechanism by which retinoids exert growth inhibitory effects, the influence of human recombinant protein transforming growth factor (TGF)-β_1 and TGF-β_2 (Genzyme, Cambridge, USA) was studied over a concentration range of 0.001–10 ng/m on melanoma cell proliferation. Neutralizing mouse anti-TGF-β_1, -β_2, and -β_3 monoclonal antibodies (Genzyme) over a concentration range between 0 and 100 ng/ml were evaluated as well for their effects on the growth-inhibitory effects exerted by CD 437 and CD2325. Human recombinant TGF-β or TGF-β-neutralizing antibodies were tested with and without CD437 and CD2325 at a fixed concentration of $10^{-6} M$ in order to assess possible retinoid-triggered, paracrine-mediated modulation of melanoma cell proliferation. All experiments were performed twice in all four cell lines.

Results

Effects of Retinoids no the Growth of Melanoma Cells

Eight out of ten retinoids had no effect on growth of human melanoma cells in vitro. The remaining two retinoids (CD437, CD2325) profoundly inhibited the growth of all melanoma cell lines tested. The antiproliferative action of

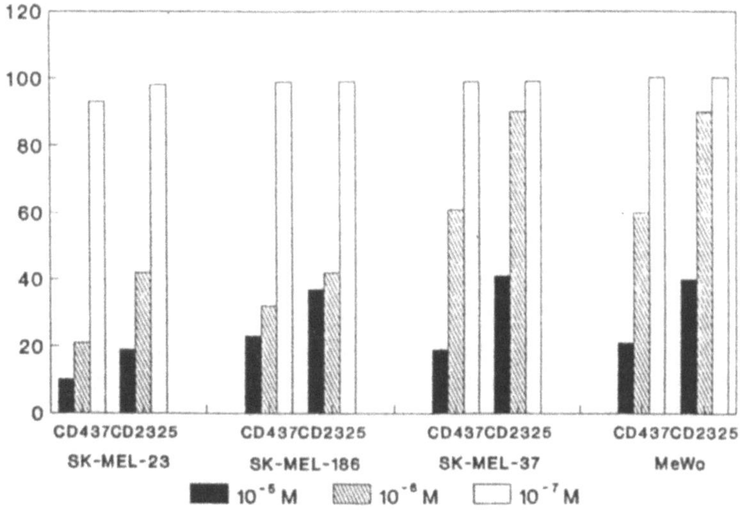

Fig. 1. Dose-dependent growth inhibition by retinoids CD437 and CD2325 on four human melanoma cell lines. The median of three independent experiments is given. Standard deviation for all experiments was below 10%

CD437 and CD2325 was dose dependent, with a reduction of viable cells down to 20% at a concentration of $10^{-5}\,M$ in all four cell lines (Fig. 1). For the majority of the retinoids, the IC_{50} was higher than $10^{-5}\,M$. The IC_{50} values for CD437 ranged between 2.5×10^{-7} to $1.2 \times 10^{-6}\,M$ and for CD2325 between 8×10^{-7} and $6.8 \times 10^{-6}\,M$ in the four melanoma cell lines tested. The differences in sensitivity did not correlate with degree of pigmentation or growth kinetics (data not shown).

In order to evaluate possible mechanisms by which retinoids exert their growth inhibitory effects, the influence of human recombinant protein TGF-β and TGF-β-neutralizing antibodies in combination with CD437 and CD2325 was tested. Antiproliferative effects mediated by both retinoids could not be changed or abolished by addition of human recombinant TGF-β antibodies (data not shown).

Other mechanisms of growth inhibition possibly involved in the action of CD437 and CD2325 were considered. Since melanogenesis generates a number of toxic intermediates including orthoquinones (reviewed by Riley 1991), we explored the possibility that enzyme systems such as tyrosinase or monoamine oxidase (MAO) are involved in the antiproliferative action. Inhibition of tyrosinase activity in melanoma cells by thiourea in the presence of the retinoids CD437 and CD2325 did not alter their dose-dependent antiproliferative effects (data not shown). This negative result is in agreement with the growth inhibition which can be observed in nonpigmented HT-3 cells upon incubation with CD437 or CD2325 (data not shown). Inhibition of MAO also had no effect on the antiproliferative action of the retinoids. These experiments suggest that enzyme systems involving tyrosinase and MAO are not involved in the growth-inhibitory action exerted by CD437 and CD2325.

Effects of Retinoids on HLA-DR and Intercellular Adhesion Molecule 1 Expression

The capacity of retinoids to modulate HLA-DR expression was divergent. Five out of nine retinoids (CD367, CD270, CD417, CD666, and CD2247) did not alter the HLA-DR expression on the surface of human melanoma cells (Table 2). CD394 and CD2019 increased HLA-DR levels on SK-Mel-37 cells, and CD437 and CD2325 the HLA-DR expression on SK-Mel-186 (Table 2). Furthermore, CD437 downregulated HLA-DR expression on SK-Mel-37, which was confirmed by fluorescence-activated cell sorter (FACS) analysis (Fig. 2).

ICAM-1 expression was already high on all human melanoma cell lines tested. On all of them only upregulation and no downregulation of ICAM-1 expression was observed (not shown). However, FACS analysis revealed a differential susceptability of the melanoma cell lines to the retinoid action. The two more intensely pigmented cell lines MeWo and SK-Mel-23 increased ICAM-1 expression in response to the retinoids CD367, CD394, CD270, CD417, CD437, CD2247, and CD2325 and CD367, CD394, CD2019, CD437, CD2247, and CD2325, respectively, whereas the less-pigmented cell lines SK-Mel-37 and SK-Mel-186 responded only to CD437, which was the

Table 2. Modulation of HLA-DR expression by synthetic retinoids (8 days, $10^{-6} M$) evaluated by immunohistology[a]

Retinoids	HLA-DR expression			
	SK-Mel-23[b]	SK-Mel-37[c]	SK-Mel-186[c]	MeWo[b]
CD367	•	•	•	•
CD394	•	↑	•	•
CD270	•	•	•	•
CD417	•	•	•	•
CD2019	•	↑	•	•
CD437	•	↓	↑	•
CD666	•	•	•	•
CD2247	•	•	•	•
CD2325	•	•	↑	•

↑, upregulation; ↓, downregulation.
[a] Alkaline phosphatase and monoclonal anti-alkaline phosphatase (APAAP) technique.
[b] Negative HLA-DR expression status of untreated cells.
[c] Positive HLA-DR expression status of untreated cells.

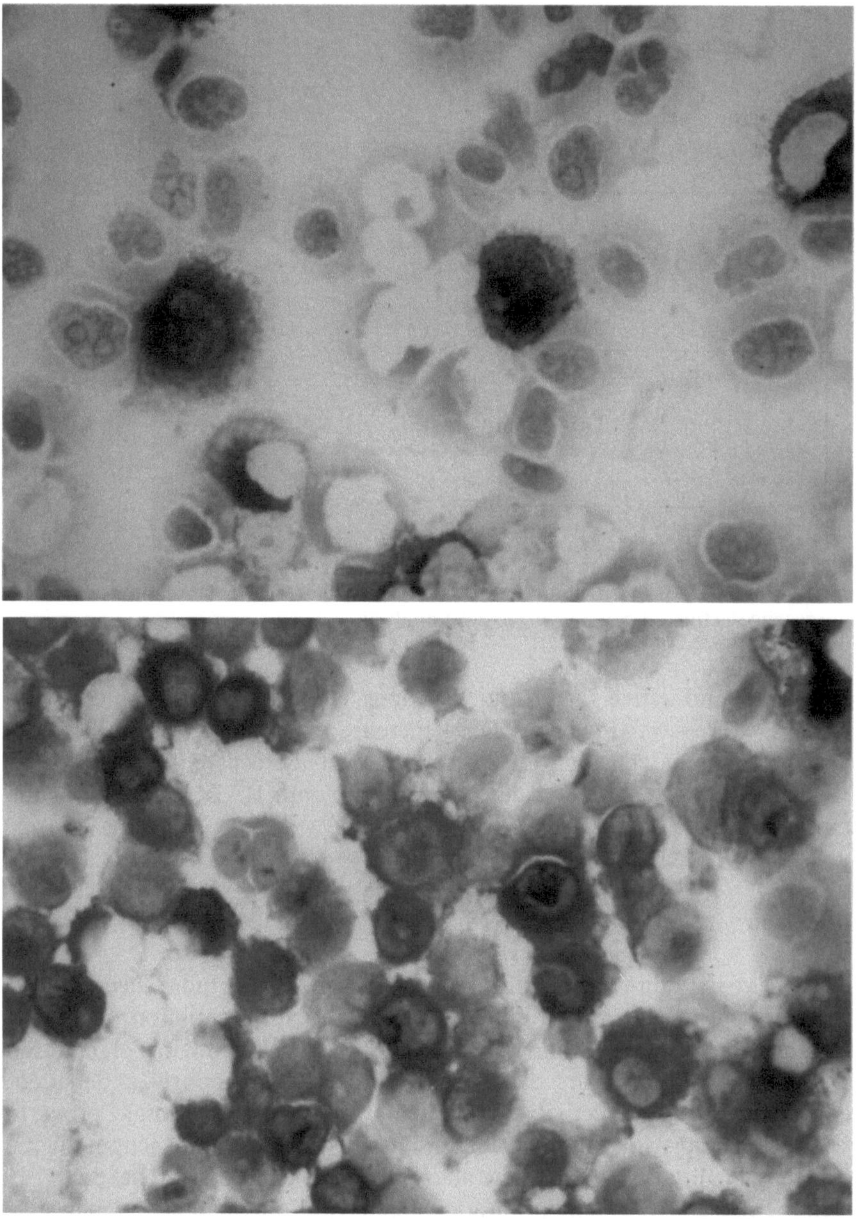

a

b

Fig. 2a,b. Cell surface expression of HLA-DR on SK-Mel-186 before (**a**) and after (**b**) treatment with CD437 (8 days, $10^{-6} M$). Cytospin preparations stained by the alkaline phosphatase and monoclonal anti-alkaline phosphate (APAAP) technique (×400)

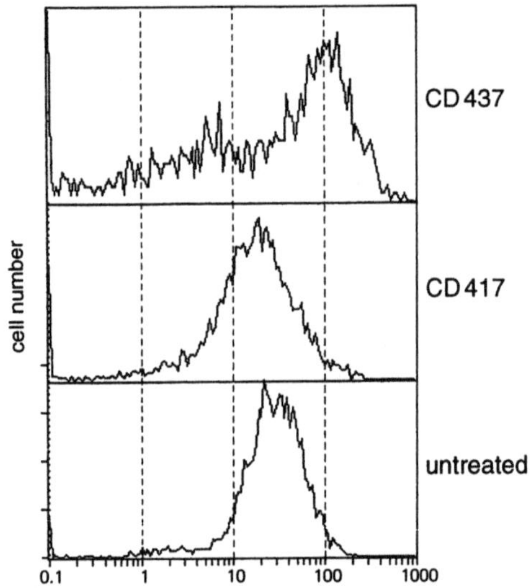

Fig. 3. Upregulation of intercellular adhesion molecule 1 (ICAM-1) expression on SK-Mel-37 by CD437, but not by CD417 (8 days, $10^{-6}\,M$), demonstrated by fluorescence-activated cell sorter (FACS) analysis

only compound active in all four cell lines, with a substantial increase in ICAM-1 expression (Fig. 3). CD394 increased ICAM-1 expression in SK-Mel-37 melanoma cells and CD2325 in SK-Mel-186 cells. Effects on HLA-DR and ICAM-1 expression did not correlate with RAR selectivity of the compounds tested.

Discussion

In recent years, there has been an impressive increase in studies investigating the mechanisms whereby retinoids inhibit the differentiation, alter the transformed phenotype, and change the biological behavior of cultured tumor cells. Although the exact mechanisms are still poorly understood, retinoids with high selectivity for particular RAR subtypes might prove to be effective tools for obtaining better insights into retinoid action. In the end, they might also provide new alternatives for clinical approaches.

In the present study, the proliferative behavior of human melanoma cells, as well as changes in the expression of the cell surface markers HLA-DR and ICAM-1 were monitored as markers of the immunomodulating capacity of synthetic retinoids. All compounds had previously been characterized regarding their selectivity for particular RAR (Table 2; Martin et al. 1992) and regarding their potential to activate the receptor complex (Bernard et al. 1992). Only two of these synthetic retinoids, both of which had high RARγ specificity, exhibited a dose-dependent, strong antiproliferative effect on all human melanoma cell lines tested, with an IC_{50} between 10^{-6} and $10^{-7} M$.

Whether the observed effect of both retinoids is truely RAR-γ mediated remains to be determined; more detailed studies at the structure–activity level as well as at the receptor level are needed and are currently in progress. Alternative explanations for the observed phenomena include a more rapid degradation or impaired cellular uptake of RARγ-specific retinoids other than CD437 and CD2325 in human melanoma cells. Differential binding and metabolism might be additional reasons for the differential effects observed. As pointed out by Lotan et al. (1991), our ability to accurately interpret the structure–activity results is limited because we do not know enough about factors such as the half-life of retinoids in growth medium, the rate of cellular retinoid uptake, or metabolic activation or inactivation reactions. Furthermore, although some progress has been made, the role of cellular retinoic-binding proteins in controlling the concentration of free retinoids and in directing protein-bound retinoids to key enzymes responsible for their metabolism is still not entirely clear (reviewed in Ross 1993).

Other mechanisms considered which have be shown to be involved in growth inhibitory effects of retinoids, such as paracrine-mediated growth inhibition by upregulation of TGF-β (DeBenedetti et al. 1991; Danielpour et al. 1993; Jakowlew et al. 1993), were not found to be involved in the antiproliferative effects of CD437 and CD2325 on melanoma cells. Furthermore, growth inhibition was independent of enzyme systems such as tyrosinase and MAO, in contrast to cytotoxic compounds such as cysteaminylphenols, which have recently been described as exerting melanocytotoxicity by generating toxic intermediates (Parsons et al. 1991).

Retinoids have been shown to modulate cell adhesion (Edward et al. 1992) and the expression of proteolytic enzymes (Hendrix et al. 1990). In contrast, the potential of synthetic retinoids to alter the expression of cell surface markers in the present experiments varied considerably. Additional data from our own laboratory and the literature describe the capacity of retinoids to profoundly regulate the expression of growth factor receptors (Worm et al. 1993b) as well as the regulation of ICAM-1 expression, independently of any growth inhibitory effects (Wang et al. 1992; Bouillon et al. 1991; Bouillon and Audette 1993), in line with the present observations. Similar to the modulation of the cell surface expression of ICAM-1 on melanoma cells, we demonstrate for the first time that retinoids are capable of modulating HLA-DR expression on human melanoma cells directly, reminiscent of immunoregulatory capacities of interferons. Recently, modulation of HLA-DR expression by RA was reported on human breast cancer cells (Gardner and Walker 1993).

In conclusion, apart from the direct antiproliferative effect of retinoids, their regulatory capacity on cell surface expression is of potential importance for malignant melanoma in vivo in terms of metastatic and immunocognative processes. Because of the potent antiproliferative capacity of two of the retinoids tested as well as the cell surface modulatory activity of several additional compounds, particularly regarding HLA-DR and ICAM-1 expression, a certain subset of aromatic retinoids might be a valuable addition to the therapeutic armamentarium targeted against malignant melanoma.

Acknowledgements. This work was supported in part by grants from the Trude Görke Stiftung, Berlin, and the Deutsche Krebshilfe (W 69/92/Scha 3).

References

Bernard BA, Bernadon JM, Delescluse C, Martin B, Lenoir MC, Maignan J, Charpentier B, Pilgrim WR, Reichert U, Shroot B (1992) Identification of synthetic retinoids with selectivity for human nuclear retinoic acid receptor γ. Biochem Biophys Res Commun 186:977–983

Bouillon M, Audette M (1993) Transduction of retinoic acid and γ-interferon signal for intercellular adhesion molecule-1 expression on human tumor cell lines: evidence for the late-acting involvement of protein kinase C inactivation. Cancer Res 53:826–832

Bouillon M, Tessier P, Boulianne R, Destrempe R, Audette M (1991) Regulation by retinoic acid of ICAM-1 expression on human tumor cell lines. Biochem Biophys Acta 1097:95–102

Danielpour D, Yip FA, Anzano MA, Smith JM, Sporn MB (1993) Growth inhibition of NRP-152 rat prostatic cells by retinoic acid is mediated via the induction of TGF-βs 2 and 3. Proc Am Assoc Cancer Res 34:128 (abstract)

DeBenedetti F, Falk L, Ruscetti FW, Colburn HN, Faltynek CR, Oppenheim JJ (1991) Synergistic inhibition of phorbol ester induced transformation of JB6 cells by transforming growth factor -β and retinoic acid. Cancer Res 51:1158–1164

Edward M (1992) Effect of retinoids on tumour invasion and metastasis. Pathobiology 60:271–277

Falkson CI, Falkson G, Falkson HC (1991) Improved results with the addition of interferon alfa-2b to dacarbazine in the treatment of patients with metastatic malignant melanoma. J Clin Oncol 9:1403–1408

Gardner FJE, Walker RA (1993) Modulation of cell surface components of human breast cancer cells by retinioc acid: enhanced HLA-DR expression. J Pathol 170:23–29

Hendrix MJC, Wood R, Seftor EA, Lotan D, Nakajima M, Misiorowski RL, Seftor REB, Stetler-Stevenson WG, Bevacqua SJ, Liotta LA, Sobel ME, Raz A, Lotan R (1990) Retinoic acid inhibition of human melanoma cell invasion through a reconstituted basement membrane and its relation to decreases in the expression of proteolytic enzymes and motility factor receptor. Cancer Res 50:4121–4130

Ho VC, Sober AJ (1990) Therapy of cutaneous melanoma: an update. J Am Acad Dermatol 22:159–176

Lotan R, Hendrix MJC, Lippman SM (1991) Retinoids in the management of melanoma. In: Marks R (ed) Retinoids in cutaneous malignancy, pp 133–149

Jakowlew SB, Mathius A, Zia F, Mulshine JL, Moody TW (1993) Retinoic acid stimulates transforming growth factor-beta mRNAs in non-small cell lung cancer cell lines. Proc Am Assoc Cancer Res 34:21 (abstract)

Martin B, Bernadon JM, Cavey MT, Bernard BA, Carlavan I, Charpentier B, Pilgrim WR, Shroot B, Reichert U (1992) Selective synthetic ligands for human nuclear retinoic acid receptor. Skin Pharmacol 5:57–65
McClay EF, Mastrangelo MJ (1988) Systemic chemotherapy for metastatic melanoma. Semin Oncol 15:569–577
Parsons DG, Favier D, McEwan M, Takahashi H, Jimbow K, Ito S (1991) Action of cysteaminylphenols on human melanoma cells in vivo: 4-S-cysteaminylphenol binds protein disulphide isomerase. Melanoma Res 1:97–104
Reichert U, Bernardon JM, Charpentier B, Nedoncelle P, Martin B, Bernard BA, Asslineau D, Michel S, Lenoir MC, Delescuse C, Pilgrim WM, Darmon YM, Shroot B (1993) Synthetic retinoids: receptor selectivity and biological activity. In: Bernadon BA, Shroot B (eds) From molecular biology to therapeutics. Pharmacol Skin 5:117–127
Richards JM (1991) Sequential chemoimmunotherapy for metastatic melanoma. Semin Oncol 5 [Suppl 7]:91–95
Riley PA (1991) Melanogenesis: a realistic target for antimelanoma therapy? Eur J Cancer 9:1172–1177
Ross AC (1993) Cellular metabolism and activation of retinoids: roles of cellular retinoid-binding proteins. FASEB J 7:317–327
Schadendorf D, Yamaguchi H, Old LJ, Srivastava PK (1989) A novel heteromorphic human cell surface alloantigen, gp60, defined by a human monoclonal antibody. J Immunol 142:1621–1625
Schadendorf D, Tiedemann KH, Haas N, Czarnetzki BM (1991) Detection of human papillomaviruses in paraffin-embedded condylomata – a comparison between immunohistology, in situ hybridization, and polymerase chain reaction. J Invest Dermatol 97:549–554
Schadendorf D, Worm M, Algermissen B, Kohlmus CM, Czarnetzki BM (1994a) Chemosensitivity testing of human malignant melanoma – retrospective analysis of clinical response and in vitro drug sensitivity. Cancer 73:103–108
Schadendorf D, Böhm M, Möller P, Grünewald T, Czarnetzki BM (1994b) Interleukin-7 induces differential lymphokine-activated killer cell activity against human melanoma cells, keratinocytes and endothelial cells. J Invest Dermatol 102:838–842
Schadendorf D, Worm M, Jurgovsky K, Dippel E, Michel S, Charpentier B, Bernardon JM, Reichert U, Czarnetzki BM (1994c) Retinoic acid receptor-8-selective retinoids exert antiproliferative effects on human melanoma cell growth in vitro. Int J Oncol 5 (in press)
Stat Bite (1992) Cancer incidence and mortality trends, 1973–1989. J Natl Inst Cancer 84:1862
Wang Z, Cao Y, D'Urso CM, Ferrone S (1992) Differential suseptibility of human melanoma cell lines to enhancement by retinoic acid of intracellular adhesion molecule 1 expression. Cancer Res 52:4766–4772
Worm M, Schadendorf D, Czarnetzki BM (1993a) Responsiveness to treatment of human melanoma cells correlates to immunophenotype. Melanoma Res 3:29–33
Worm M, Czarnetzki BM, Schadendorf D (1993b) Expression of growth factor receptors on human melanoma cells – comparison of modulating effects of interferons and retinoids. Exp Dermatol 2:217–223

Prognostic Significance of DNA Cytometry in Comparison with Histologic Measurements in Malignant Melanomas

T. Vogt, W. Stolz, U. Hohenleutner, R. Schiffner, and M. Landthaler

Department of Dermatology, University of Regensburg, Franz-Josef-Strauß-Allee 11, 93042 Regensburg, Germany

Abstract

In the present study we evaluated the prognostic impact of both DNA cytometry and quantitative histology in patients with malignant melanoma (MM). In contrast to previous investigations on sections, rapid image analysis (IA) of imprint specimens was performed to measure DNA cytometric features; 34 cases of stage I MM with low (<1.5 mm, $n = 20$) and higher tumor thickness (TTH) (>1.5 mm, $n = 14$) were analyzed.

We found significant correlations between cytometric features and TTH, which is accepted as the most important prognostic criterion in MM. Higher TTH was closely correlated with the rate of markedly aneuploid nuclei, which is indicated by the 5c exceeding rate (5cER; r, 0.89; $p < 0.001$). The gain of chromatin in thicker tumors was accompanied by higher mean nuclear area (MAREA; r, 0.60; $p < 0.001$) and mean DNA content (MDNA; r, 0.58; $p < 0.001$).

Additional evidence for prognostic significance of cytometry was obtained by preliminary survival analysis of 16 cases (four patients died within 2½ years and 12 patients survived for at least 4½ years). Applying multivariate stepwise discriminant analysis, a combination of TTH, level of invasion (LEV), 2c deviation index (2cDI), and modified standard deviation of the DNA values (SDNAM) proved to be most effective. One hundred percent of the cases were correctly classified as survivors or nonsurvivors. TTH and the 5cER were found to be the best univariate criteria for prognosis. In the U test according to Mann and Whitney, a significant discrimination of survivors and nonsurvivors was possible using either TTH or the 5cER, respectively ($p < 0.02$).

Thus, we would like to conclude that IA of imprint specimens can be recommended as a rapid and simple additional method for grading.

Recent Results in Cancer Research, Vol. 139

Introduction

It is generally accepted that histology is of paramount importance for the assessment of prognosis in malignant melanoma (MM). For histologic grading, quantitative features such as tumor thickness (TTH), level of invasion (LEV), mitotic counts (MC), and prognostic index (PI) are considered as well as qualitative criteria, i.e., ulceration, vertical growth pattern, inflammatory response of the host, and signs of regression (Ruiter 1992). Applying univariate and multivariate analysis, TTH proved to be the most consistent prognostic feature in several studies (Ronan et al. 1988). However, the individual clinical outcome of patients presenting with stage I MM remains variable, and for a significant subset of patients TTH fails to predict the outcome (Rowley and Cockerell 1991). An accuracy of only 76% in predicting 10-year survival was recently reported for a multimodal prognostic model (Soong et al. 1992).

To obtain more precise and objective prognostic information, several laboratory techniques were applied, i.e., morphometry (Leitinger et al. 1990), stereology (Binder et al. 1992), and DNA cytometry (Lindholm et al. 1990; Heenan et al. 1989; Zeng et al. 1990; Schmiegelow et al. 1987; Björnhagen et al. 1991; Bines et al. 1988; Bartkowiak et al. 1991; Zaloudik et al. 1988; Rode et al. 1991; Gattuso et al. 1990; Onishi and Ishikawa 1991). The latter can be performed either by flow cytometric analysis (FC; Bines et al. 1988; Bartkowiak et al. 1991; Zaloudik et al. 1988; Rode et al. 1991; Gattuso et al. 1990; Onishi and Ishikawa 1991) or by single cell rapid image analysis (IA; Lindholm et al. 1990; Heenan et al. 1989; Zeng et al. 1990; Schmiegelow et al. 1987; Björnhagen et al. 1991). Both methods are now applicable for fresh and paraffin-embedded tissue (Wied et al. 1989). In this study DNA measurements were performed by IA on Feulgen-stained imprint specimens, which can easily be prepared from fresh tissue and stored for several years.

In previous studies on ploidy characteristics the investigations often focused on the appearance of aneuploid stem lines, which is a rare event in stage I MM and might be more common in advanced stages and metastases of MM (Hansson et al. 1982). In our study we applied more sensitive algorithms for analysis of minor changes of DNA distribution, e.g., the 5c exceeding rate (5cER), the 2c deviation index (2cDI), and different percentiles (PERC) of the DNA histogram, respectively. In addition, morphometric criteria such as mean and standard deviation of nuclear surface area (MAREA/SAREA) were analyzed. Subsequently, univariate and multivariate dicriminant analysis was applied to evaluate the prognostic impact of the features.

Materials and Methods

In the 34 cases of MM analyzed here, the diagnosis was established by two independent dermatopathologists prior to DNA analysis; 19 cases were classified as superficial spreading MM and 14 as nodular MM. One MM could not be further classified. TTH was less than or equal to 1.5 mm in 20 cases, whereas thickness exceeded 1.5 mm in 14 cases. For a limited number of patients survival data were available: four patients died within 2½ years of follow-up, 12 patients survived for at least 4½ years. These cases were used for testing the real predictive power of the features analyzed.

Histologic Analysis

TTH was measured from the surface of the granular cell layer to the deepest location of neoplastic cells in mm using an ocular micrometer (Breslow 1970). LEV were defined according to Clark et al. (1969). MC was determined by counting the mitoses within ten high-power fields at ×400 magnification. Subsequently, the rate of mitoses per square millimeter was calculated. By multiplying the rate of mitoses per square millimeter and TTH, the PI was obtained according to Schmoeckel and Braun-Falco (1978).

Preparation of Imprint Specimens

Imprints were prepared on clean glass slides by touching with the freshly cut surface of a skin biopsy. The imprints were fixed in methanol (100%), formaldehyde (37%), and glacial acetic acid (96%) 85:10:5 (v/v/v). Feulgen staining was performed according to Böhm (1968) with hydrolysis in 5 N HCL for 50 min at 28°C and staining in Schiff's reagent for 60 min.

DNA Measurements

DNA analysis was performed by interactive IA using the IBAS system (Interaktives Bildanalysesystem; Kontron, Eching, Germany). The imprint specimens were digitized with a density of 16 pixels/μm using a TV Pasecon camera (Bosch, Stuttgart, Germany) connected with a 100-oil objective of an Axioplan microscope (Zeiss, Oberkochen, Germany). A total of 100 nuclei were randomly selected in each case. Fully automatic segmentation of the nuclei was achieved as follows: in a first step, the contrast within the original video image was increased by mapping the actual gray levels linearly into the full range between black (gray value, 0) and white (gray value, 255). The contour of the nuclei was then automatically found by use of the function EMPHASE, which performs an addition of the original image with the difference of the original image and the low-passed filtered version of it. Inaccurate segmentation could be rejected interactively, because the contour was given in the overlay of the original image at the end of the segmentation process.

Parameters Calculated

For each nucleus the optical density (OD) and the surface area were calculated. The integrated optical density (IOD) was obtained as the product of OD and nuclear area. In Feulgen-stained nuclei, the IOD is linearly correlated with the DNA content (Böhm 1968). In each slide 20 chicken erythrocytes were used as an internal reference. In a previous pilot study a comparison of chicken erythrocytes and normal human lymphocytes revealed the following relationship: $OD_{ery} \times 3.26 = 2cDNA$, where 2c is the normal DNA content of a human cell. An euploid cell in G_2 phase contains 4cDNA. In this study the relative DNA content in each of the 100 randomly selected cells was calculated as follows: relative DNA content = $IOD_{nucleus}/IOD_{1cDNA}$.

Algorithms for Evaluation of DNA Values

Beside morphometric variables of the nuclei (mean and standard deviation of the nuclear area, MAREA/SAREA), mean and standard deviation of nuclear DNA values (MDNA/SDNA) as well as percentiles of the DNA histograms (80th/90th/95th) were calculated as rough DNA distribution criteria. For a more detailed analysis of DNA distributions, the 5cER and the 2cDI were determined in each case. The 5cER is defined as the percentage of cells with a DNA content equal to or higher than 5c. Since euploid–polyploid cells should not contribute to the 5cER, cells with DNA values which are integer-valued exponents of 2c ± 12.5% are not taken into account. The 2cDI is defined as the ratio between the sum of the squares of the differences between the DNA values of individual cells and the 2c value and the number of cells measured. In contrast to simple standard deviation, the 2cDI reflects the variation of the nuclear DNA content around the 2c value within one case. In addition, modified variables were calculated from 2cDI and DNA values omitting all nuclei with values that were integer-valued exponents of 2c ± 12.5%; thus euploid–polyploid cells were not taken into account (2cDIM, MDNAM, SDNAM).

Statistical evaluation of the features analyzed was performed by the SPSS statistical program (SPSS, Munich). SPSS routines for U testing and univariate as well as multivariate discriminant analysis were applied.

The reproducibility of DNA measurements was tested by demonstration of the different ploidy peaks in rat liver imprints.

Results

The most interesting result was the finding of significant correlations between TTH, which is considered as the most effective histologic criterion for prognosis, and both DNA cytometric and morphometric features (see Table 1). The close linear correlation between the rate of aneuploid nuclei exceeding a DNA value of 5c (normal value, 2c), the so-called 5cER, and TTH reflects a tendency of thicker tumors to produce cell subsets with a considerable gain of chromatin (r, 0.89; $p < 0.001$). This is also demonstrated by the significant association of higher TTH with higher values of MAREA and MDNA ($p < 0.001$). In accordance with these findings, close correlations were detected between MDNA and MAREA (r, 0.77; $p < 0.001$). On a lower level of signficance it was shown that higher TTH and increasing MDNA are accompanied by higher variability of the DNA values indicated by the 2cDI values ($p < 0.01$). Significant correlations were also obtained between TTH, LEV, and MC ($p < 0.001$). Furthermore, MC correlated with the 5cER ($p < 0.001$), but not with nuclear area or other DNA cytometric features. Similar results were obtained for the histologic LEV according to Clark (see Table 1).

To examine the real prognostic impact of the features analyzed, we performed a preliminary survival analysis of 16 cases. The predictive power of the features was tested by univariate and multivariate analysis. Univariate analysis (step 0 of stepwise discriminant analysis) revealed significant F

Table 1. Correlations between DNA cytometry and histologic measurements

Histolocic feature	Cytometric feature	Coefficient of correlation (Pearson)	Level of significance
Tumor thickness	5cER	0.89	$p < 0.001$
	MAREA	0.60	$p < 0.001$
	MDNA	0.58	$p < 0.001$
	2cDI	0.50	$p < 0.01$
	PERC95	0.44	$p < 0.01$
Level of invasion	5cER	0.72	$p < 0.001$
	MAREA	0.58	$p < 0.001$
	MDNA	–	n.s.
	2CDI	–	n.s.
	PERC95	–	n.s.
Mitoses/mm^2	5cER	0.63	$p < 0.001$
	MAREA	–	n.s.
	MDNA	–	n.s.
	2cDI	–	n.s.
	PERC95	–	n.s.

5cER, 5c exceeding rate; MAREA, mean nuclear area; MDNA, mean DNA content; 2cDI, 2c deviation index; PERC95, 95th percentile; n.s., not significant.

values only for TTH and the 5cER values (F = 13 and 11, respectively; for $p < 0.001$ a F value higher than 10 is required). If one of these criteria was used to discriminate between survivors and nonsurvivors in a non-parametric test (U test according to Mann and Whitney), a significant discrimination was obtained for both on a low level of significance ($p < 0.02$) showing an overlap between the groups (Fig. 1a,b).

To further improve on this differentiation, the most effective combination of features was selected by multivariate analysis. By cytometric criteria alone (5cER, MAREA, MDNA, 2cDI), prediction of the outcome was possible in 88% of the cases ($n = 14$), whereas histometric criteria (TTH, LEV, MC, PI) allowed correct classification of 94% ($n = 15$). Further improvement of the classification rate up to 100% correct prediction of

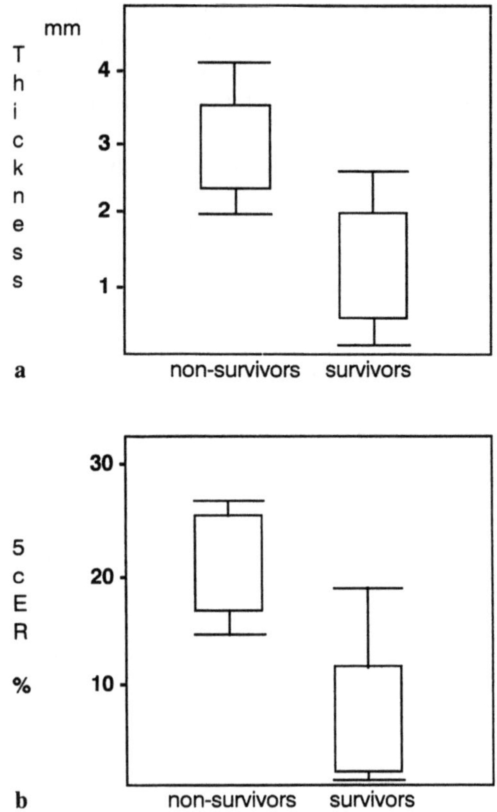

Fig. 1a,b. Applying the U test a significant discrimination between survivors (4½ years' survival or more; $n = 12$) and nonsurvivors (death within 2½ years after excision of primary tumor; $n = 4$) was possible with the best univariate prognostic criteria: tumor thickness TTH (**a**) and 5cER (5c exceeding rate; **b**). $p < 0.01$ and $p < 0.02$, respectively

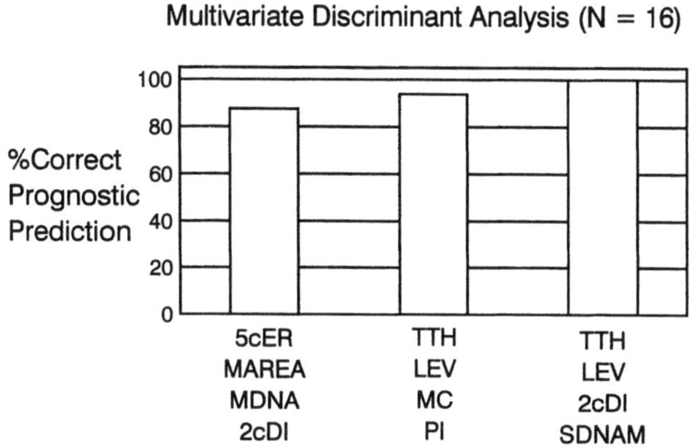

Fig. 2. Results of multivariate analysis. A combination of tumor thickness (*TTH*) level of invasion (LEV), and 2c deviation index (*2cDI*), and modified standard deviation of DNA values (*SDNAM*) proved to be most valuable for prediction of 5-year survival. *MAREA*, mean nuclear area; *MDNA*, mean DNA content; *5cER*, 5c exceeding rate; *MC*, mitotic count; *PI*, prognostic index. For explanations see methods

survival was only possible by combining cytometric and histometric features (TTH, LEV, 2cDI, SDNAM; Fig. 2).

Discussion

There is increasing evidence of an additional prognostic impact of morphometry and DNA cytometry in stage I MM (Heenan et al. 1989; Zeng et al. 1990; Schmiegelow et al. 1987; Björnhagen et al. 1991). This study stresses the fact that DNA cytometric and morphometric features extracted from imprint specimens of MM by image analysis are closely correlated to TTH, which is considered a very important prognostic factor in MM. This was demonstrated by highly significant correlations between TTH and both 5cER and MAREA (r, 0.89 and 0.60; $p < 0.001$). In addition, we found a significant association between the 5cER values and both LEV (r, 0.72; $p < 0.001$) and MC (r, 0.63; $p < 0.001$), respectively (see Table 1). Thus our study provides further evidence that a poor prognosis in MM correlates not only with higher TTH, but also with features indicating the gain of nuclear chromatin (5cER, MDNA, MAREA). In addition, as has already been shown for cutaneous lymphomas (Vogt et al. 1991), a higher variability of the DNA values indicated by higher 2cDI and SDNAM values can be considered as bad prognostic sign. Close associations between TTH and most cytometric features on the one hand, and missing correlations between most cytometric features and both LEV and MC on the other, show that MC and LEV do not describe the malignant potential of MM as accurately. Another explanation for this observation might be a lower reproducibility of LEV and MC, as has also been shown in literature (Rowley and Cockerell 1991).

The potential benefit of combining quantitative histology and DNA cytometry was additionally documented by a preliminary survival analysis. Multivariate stepwise analysis in 16 cases showed that a combination of TTH, LEV, 2cDI, and SDNAM allowed a prediction of the outcome of the patients with an accuracy of 100%. The best univariate criteria in our analysis were TTH and 5cER. Using these criteria alone, a significant discrimination ($p < 0.02$, U test) of survivors and nonsurvivors was also possible (see Fig. 1a,b). Due to its close correlation to TTH, the 5cER dropped out of multivariate analysis when the most appropriate combination of features was selected.

Our data are in accordance with some previous studies (Heenan et al. 1989; Zeng et al. 1990; Schmiegelow et al. 1987; Björnhagen et al. 1991), which were, however, exclusively performed on paraffin sections. Similar to the 2cDI, which was used in our study, the variation of the DNA values around the diploid peak was found to influence survival independently of TTH and age (Heenan et al. 1989). In addition, Zeng et al. (1990) analyzed 22 metastases by IA and found significant correlations between low survival time and increased variation of DNA values and the presence of multiple clonality. Bartkowiak et al. (1991) and Hansson et al. (1982) measured the rate of S phase cells by flow cytometry (FC), showing lower survival probability for increasing rates of cells cycling through S phase. A significant correlation between the appearence of aneuploid peaks in FC (defined as differing by more than 10% from the diploid value) and disease-free survival was also demonstrated (Gattuso et al. 1990). Bines et al. (1988) investigated 177 cases of MM. Aneuploidy turned out to be the most significant prognostic factor after thickness adjustment. There are, however, studies which do not fully agree with the hypothesis that aneuploidy and specific changes of nuclear morphology really indicate a worse prognosis (Lindholm et al. 1990; Zaloudik et al. 1988; Rode et al. 1991; Mukonen et al. 1991). However, most of these studies used FC (Zaloudik et al. 1988; Rode et al. 1991; Mukonen et al. 1991). In contrast to single-cell IA, FC only allows us to study ploidy in large amounts of nuclei, and the probability of detecting small numbers of aneuploid cells and S phase cells is limited (Ploem-Zaajer et al. 1987). For example, in gynecologic cancer it was recently shown that single-cell measurements of cellular and DNA features can provide more prognostic information than FC, even if the number of cells analyzed by IA is 1000-fold lower than that in FC (Kaern et al. 1992). In contrast to time-consuming single-cell analysis on paraffin sections, this study introduces a practical and feasible approach due to the developmet of simple and time-saving semiautomatic routines using imprint specimens. The time for analyzing one specimen could be reduced to 30 min. This was possible because of fully automatic segmentation of nuclei, which cannot be done in sections. Retrospective studies can also be done with this technique by microdissection of tumor tissue and preparation of single-cell specimens from paraffin material (Wied et al. 1989).

Nevertheless, it should be kept in mind that exceptions to the rules of quantitative pathology always exist and prognosis should not be based on such laboratory results alone, but should also include the whole spectrum of clinical features, for instance, the sex of the patients and their immunologic status (Balch 1992).

Acknowledgements. This work was supported by the Deutsche Forschungsgemeinschaft (Grant Sto 189/1-1 and 189/1-2). The skillful technical assistance of Mrs. M. Deutscher is gratefully acknowledged.

References

Balch CM (1992) Cutaneous melanoma: prognosis and treatment results worldwide. Semin Surg Oncol 8:400–414

Bartkowiak D, Otto F, Schuman J, Lippold A, Drepper H (1991) Sequential DNA flow cytometry in metastatic malignant melanoma. Oncology 48:154–157

Binder M, Dolezal I, Wolff K, Pehamberger H (1992) Stereologic estimation of volume-weighted mean nuclear volume as a predictor of prognosis in "thin" malignant melanoma. J Invest Dermatol 99:180–183

Bines SD, von Roenn JH, Kheir SM, Coon JS (1988) Flow cytometry in melanoma. In: Nathanson L (ed) Malignant melanoma: biology, diagnosis, and therapy. Kluwer Academic, Boston, pp 155–169

Björnhagen V, Auer G, Lagerlöf B, Erhardt K, Mansson-Brahme E (1991) Nuclear DNA analyses in archival material from primary malignant melanoma. A pilot study. Anal Quant Cytol Histol 13:335–342

Böhm N (1968) Einfluß der Fixierung und der Säurekonzentration auf die Feulgen Hydrolyse bei 28°C. Histochemie 14:201–211

Breslow A (1970) Thickness, cross-sectional areas and depth of invasion in the prognosis of cutaneous melanoma. Ann Surg 172:902–908

Clark WH Jr, From L, Bernardino EA (1969) The histogenesis and biologic behavior of primary human malignant melanomas of the skin. Cancer Res 29:705–726

Gattuso P, Reddy V, Solans E, Kathuria S, Araha GV, Jacobs HK, Walloch J (1990) Is DNA ploidy of prognostic significance in stage I cutaneous melanoma? Surgery 108:702–709

Hansson J, Tribukait B, Lewensohn R, Ringborg U (1982) Flow cytofluorometric DNA analyses of metastases of human malignant melanomas. Anal Quant Cytol 4:99–104

Heenan PJ, Jarvis LR, Armstrong BK (1989) Nuclear indices and survival in cutaneous melanoma. Am J Dermatopathol 11:308–312

Kaern J, Wetteland J, Trope CG, Farrants GW, Juhn SW, Pettersen EO, Reith A, Danielsen HE (1992) Comparison between flow cytometry and image cytometry in ploidy distribution assessments in gynecologic cancer. Cytometry 13:314–321

Leitinger G, Cerroni L, Soyer HP, Smolle J, Kerl H (1990) Morphometric diagnosis of melanocytic skin tumors. Am J Dermatopathol 12:441–445

Lindholm C, Hofer PA, Jonsson H (1990) Single cell DNA cytophotometry in clinical stage I malignant melanoma. Relationship to prognosis. Acta Oncol 29:147–150

Mukonen T, Pyrkonen S, Laasonen A, Asko-Seljavaara S, Franssila K (1991) DNA aneuploidy and low S-phase fraction as favourable signs in metastatic melanoma. Br J Cancer 64:749–752

Onishi K, Ishikawa H (1991) Flow cytometric DNA analysis of primary cutaneous malignant melanoma. Acta Derm Venereol (Stockh) 71:525–528

Ploem-Zaajer JJ, van Driel-Kulker AM, Mesker WE, Cornelisse CJ (1987) Advantages and limitations of retrospective DNA cytometry by flow and image analysis. In: Burger G, Ploem JS, Goerttler K (eds) Clinical cytometry and histometry. Academic, London, pp 176–179

Rode J, Williams RA, Dhillon AP, Moss E (1991) Nuclear DNA profiles in primary melanomas and their metastases. Cancer 67:2333–2336

Ronan SG, Han MC, Das Gupta TK (1988) Histologic prognostic indicators in cutaneous melanoma. Semin Oncol 15:558–565

Rowley MJ, Cockerell CJ (1991) Reliability of prognostic models in malignant melanoma. Am J Dermatopathol 13:431–437

Ruiter DJ (1992) Clinical and pathologic diagnosis, staging and prognostic factors of melanoma and management of primary disease. Curr Opin Oncol 4:357–367

Schmiegelow P, Oppermann T, Nüßgen A, Schroiff R, Jänner M (1987) Melanoma in situ adjacent to an invasive nodular melanoma and metastases – DNA-cytophotometry, mitotic index, and anisokaryosis. Vichows Archiv [A] 411:871–2873

Schmoeckel C, Braun-Falco O (1978) Prognostic index in malignant melanoma. Arch Dermatol 114:871–873

Soong SJ, Shaw HM, Balch CM, McCarthy WH, Urist MM, Lee JY (1992) Predicting survival and recurrence in localized melanoma: a multivariate approach. World J Surg 16:191–195

Vogt T, Stolz W, Braun-Falco O, Kaudewitz P, Eckert F, Abmayr W, Dummer R, Burg G (1991) Prognostic significance of DNA cytometry in cutaneous malignant lymphomas. Cancer 68:1095–1100

Wied GL, Bartels PH, Bibbo M, Dytch HE (1989) Image analysis in quantitative cyto- and histopathology. Hum Pathol 20:549–71

Zaloudik J, Moore M, Ghosh AK, Mechl Z, Rejthar A (1988) DNA content and MHC class II antigen expression in malignant melanoma: clinical course. J Clin Pathol 41:1078–1084

Zeng QS, Fu YS, Alistair A, Cochran J (1990) Nuclear DNA measurements of metastatic melanoma by a computerized digital imaging system. Hum Pathol 21:1112–1116

Lymphocyte–Melanoma Interaction: Role of Surface Molecules

J.C. Becker and E.B. Bröcker

Department of Dermatology, University of Würzburg, Josef-Schneider-Straße 2, 97080 Würzburg, Germany

Abstract

The coexistence of tumor-specific immunity with a progressing tumor is observed in most experimental systems and remains one of the major paradoxes of tumor immunology. Expression of several surface molecules on melanoma cells, e.g., intercellular adhesion molecule 1 (ICAM-1) or major histocompatibility complex (MHC) class II, has been associated with an aggressive tumor growth and an reduced host antitumor response.

HLA class I expression is also frequently altered in melanoma compared to melanocytes. Given the central role of these molecules in the restriction of T cell recognition, regulation of tumor HLA class I expression might also be a strategy for the evasion of immune surveillance by the malignant cells.

The fact that it is now possible to clone antigen-specific T cells from tumor patients, as well as the relevant autologous tumor cell lines, enabled us to establish a model system to investigate possible tumor escape mechanisms from immunosurveillance.

Using this system, we were able to demonstrate that purified soluble ICAM-1 or 12-fold-concentrated cell-free melanoma supernatants, containing shed ICAM-1, were able to inhibit conjugate formation between T cell clones and the autologous melanoma cells as efficiently as monoclonal antibodies against CD11a, Soluble ICAM-1 also abrogated the MHC-restricted killing of the melanoma by T cell clones.

We further observed that a number of $CD4^+$ T cell clones and melanoma cell lines established from the same tumors form conjugates with each other, leading to an increase of $[Ca^{2+}]_i$ in the T cell clone; however, this interaction failed to induce interleukin-2 production or proliferation of the T cell clone. Furthermore, this interaction rendered the T cell clone unresponsive to subsequent stimulation. All these effects were MHC class II restricted. Therefore, the melanoma was capable of delivering antigen-specific signals to the T cell clone, but did not deliver the costimulatory signals, e.g., a

Recent Results in Cancer Research, Vol. 139

B7/CD28 interaction, necessary for full T cell activation. Transfection of the melanoma with an expression vector containing a B7 cDNA with subsequent B7 expression on its cell surface renders the melanoma a fully competent antigen-presenting cell which is able to induce a nuclear factor binding to the interleukin-2 promoter in the specific T cell clone, followed by enhanced interleukin-2 transcription, synthesis, and T cell proliferation.

Introduction

The phenomenon of spontaneous regression and also the late onset of metastatic spread in a number of patients explain the early interest of tumor immunologists in investigating human melanoma and the eagerness of clinicians to influence the course of disease by immunotherapy (Carrel and Johnson 1993; Lejeune et al. 1993; Lanzaveechia 1993). There is now a large consensus that melanoma cells are antigenic in the sense that they express tumor-associated antigens (TAA) that can be recognized by T cells in a syngeneic host (Topalian et al. 1989; Van den Eynde et al. 1989; Van der Bruggen et al. 1991; Becker et al. 1993a). Indeed, as demonstrated by immunohistology and cell extractions, the cellular components which should be able to reject the tumor, i.e., T lymphocytes and macrophages, infiltrate primary as well as metastatic melanomas (Becker et al. 1993a,b; Bröcker et al. 1988). Furthermore, in contrast to other malignancies melanoma patients seem to be fully immunocompetent. However, the prognosis of melanoma which cannot be cured by surgical resection is one of the most unfavorable in medicine. The coexistence of tumor-specific immunity with a progressing tumor remains one of the major paradoxes of tumor immunology. In this contribution we demonstrate some mechanisms by which human melanoma may escape immune surveillance.

Loss of Major Histocompatibility Complex Class I Expression

In the course of local and systemic progression of melanoma, an increasing proportion of tumor cells lack detectable major histocompatibility complex (MHC) class I (HLA-A, -B, -C) molecules on the cell surface. This was demonstrated in vivo by immunohistology using monoclonal antibodies against epitopes on the constant, invariant part of these molecules (van Duinen et al. 1988; Ruiter et al. 1991; Carrido et al. 1993). The loss of MHC class I antigens on metastatic melanoma is associated with poor prognosis, probably because these tumor cells cannot be recognized by specific cytotoxic T cells. A number of different changes in melanoma cell biology might account for this effect:

1. High constitutive expression of the c-*myc* oncogene in human melanoma leads to down-regulation of expression of HLA class I genes (Versteeg et

al. 1989; Schrier and Peltenberg 1993). The genes at the HLA-B locus are preferentially affected. Recent studies have confirmed the regulatory role of the c-*myc* oncogene on MHC class I expression at the level of transcription. However, the main enhancer of the MHC class I genes (enhancer A) is not involved in this process (Peltenberg et al. 1993).

2. Intracellular antigens must be processed before presentation to $CD8^+$ T cells by MHC class I molecules (Townsend 1992). Recent studies have shown that a number of tumor cell lines fail to process endogenously synthesized proteins for presentation. Pulse-chase experiments showed that MHC class I molecules were not transported from the endoplasmatic reticulum to the cell surface in these cell lines (Restifo et al. 1993). This suggested that peptides were not available for binding to nascent MHC molecules in the endoplasmatic reticulum. Further characterization of these cell lines revealed that they lack expression of the MHC-encoded proteasome as well as the putative peptide transporter. Treatment of these cells with interferon (IFN) alpha or gamma enhanced expression of these molecules and reversed the observed functional and biochemical deficits (Restifo et al. 1992). Treatment of melanoma cells with interferon can restore MHC class I expression in vitro and in vivo; treatment of melanoma patients with IFN-α increased MHC class I expression on metastases (von Stamm et al. 1993).
3. The loss of MHC class I expression might also be due to an inability to synthesize β_2-microglobulin. This has been shown for the melanoma cell line SK-MEL 33 (Wang et al. 1993). The lack of HLA class I expression by this cell line is caused by a unique lesion in the synthesize β_2-microglobulin gene. Sequencing of β_2-microglobulin mRNA detected a guanosine deletion on position 323 in codon 76 that causes a frameshift with a subsequent introduction of a stop codon at a position 54 base upstream of the normal position of the stop codon in the message. The loss of 18 amino acids and the change of six amino acids are likely to cause marked changes in the structure of the polypeptide, which may account for the inability of β_2-microglobulin to associate with MHC class I heavy chains. A similar defect has been shown for another melanoma cell line, FO-1, which showed a gross deletion of the 5′ region and a portion of the coding region of the β_2-microglobulin gene, preventing its transcription and subsequently MHC class I expression (D'urso et al. 1991).

Role of Intercellular Adhesion Molecule 1

Cell surface adhesion molecules are thought to play an important role in establishing the intercellular contacts that are essential for immunological reactions (Springer 1990; Larson and Springer 1990). One of these adhesion pathways in man involves the β_2-leukocyte integrin LFA-1 (CD11a/CD18) and its ligand, the intercellular adhesion molecule 1 (ICAM-1; CD54). This interaction appears critical for immunosurveillance during inflammation or neoplastic transformation.

The ICAM-1 molecule has a molecular weight of 90000 and is composed of five immunoglobulin-like extracellular domains, a hydrophobic transmembrane domain, and a short cytoplasmic domain (Springer 1990). ICAM-1 is constitutively expressed or can be induced on a wide range of cells of hematopoietic and nonhematopoietic origin, such as keratinocytes, fibroblasts, endothelial cells, and tumor cells, including melanoma (Hogg et al. 1991). ICAM-1 may be induced or upregulated by proinflammatory cytokines such as IFN-γ and tumor necrosis factor (TNF)-α in vitro. In vivo, it is not expressed in benign melanocytic nevi, but occurs in proportion to local and systemic melanoma progression, thus being regarded as a progression marker (Holzmann et al. 1987; Natali et al. 1990). Its prognostic relevance has been shown in a clinical study of acral melanoma (Kageshita et al. 1991). We found a correlation of ICAM-1 expression on tumor cells with intratumoral infiltrates only in primary melanoma, but not in metastases (Bröcker et al. 1988). Treatment of patients with low doses of IFN-α led to increased ICAM-1 expression in cutaneous metastases independent from the amount of T cell infiltrates (von Stamm et al. 1993). The cytolytic conjugate between cytotoxic T cells and tumor cells is stabilized by interactions between the LFA-1 integrin on the lymphocytes and the ICAM-1 ligand expressed by the target cell. Lack of expression of ICAM-1 appear to permit circulating tumor cells to avoid establishing stable cytolytic conjugates and provide a means of evading T cell-mediated killing (Hart and Saini 1992). Paradoxically, progression towards metastasis in melanoma is accompanied by upregulated expression of ICAM-1, and this might be expected to facilitate the formation of cytolytic conjugates, leading to reduced tumor cell survival rather than to increased tumor burden (Johnson et al. 1989). However, the finding of soluble ICAM-1 in the serum of melanoma patients suggests that release of this molecule by high-producing tumor cells could block the receptor on cytotoxic T cells (Becker et al. 1992; Altomonte et al. 1992). It has been shown that some soluble forms of cell surface macromolecules seem to compete with membrane-bound forms in binding to their ligands. For example, the soluble TNF receptor is able to neutralize the cytopathic activity of TNF-α. The soluble ligand of the lymphocyte-homing receptor inhibits binding of lymphocytes to high endothelial venules. Soluble forms of ICAM-1 inhibit: (a) rhinovirus infection, (b) binding of *Plasmodium falciparum*-infected erythrocytes to membrane-bound ICAM-1, (c) adherence of the lymphocytic cell line MOLT-4 to endothelial cells, (d) aggregation of Epstein-Barr virus-transformed cell lines, and (e) non-MHC-restricted cytotoxicity exerted by NK and LAK cells (Gearing and Newman 1993; Greve et al. 1989; Ockenhouse et al. 1992; Becker et al. 1991).

The fact that it is now possible to clone and maintain in culture antigen-specific T cells from tumor patients, as well as the relevant autologous tumor cell lines, enabled us to establish a model system to investigate the effect of soluble tumor-derived ICAM-1 on MHC-restricted T cell–melanoma interaction (Becker et al. 1993a,b). In this system, purified soluble ICAM-1 produced in Chinese hamster ovary (CHO) cells as well as concentrated cell-free supernatants containing ICAM-1 shed from a human melanoma cell line inhibited: (a) T cell–melanoma conjugate formation, (b) MHC-restricted cytotoxicity, and (c) antigen-triggered induction of cytokine production in T cells (Becker et al. 1993c). Since it has been shown that several forms of soluble ICAM-1 are able to bind either LFA-1 or erythrocytes infected with *Plasmodium falciparum*, it seems likely that this inhibition is mediated by competition between membrane-bound and soluble ICAM-1. The inhibition achieved with approximately 1000 ng/ml was as efficient as that mediated by monoclonal antibodies against ICAM-1.

In our model system not all forms of soluble ICAM-1 seem to be functionally active, since concentrated culture supernatants from keratinocytes containing soluble ICAM-1 were not able to inhibit MHC-restricted T cell–melanoma interaction (own unpublished observations). This might be due to diversity of soluble ICAM-1 derived from different sources (Hogg et al. 1991). ICAM-1 demonstrates a cell type-dependent variability in the molecular weight: the molecule expressed by melanoma cells is larger than that expressed by B cells from the same individual. These differences reflect primarily changes in asparagine-linked carbohydrates. Tissue-specific changes in glycosylation are common features of adhesion molecules and have been shown to influence the affinity of mediated adhesion. Recently, a gene regulating cell adhesion by altering the affinity of different adhesion molecules to their ligands has been cloned and it is differently expressed in malignant and nonmalignant cells (Pullman and Bodmer 1992).

The mechanism of shedding of ICAM-1 remains to be characterized. Soluble ICAM-1 could be the result of an alternatively spliced mRNA which deletes the transmembrane and cytoplasmatic domains, but to our knowledge no such mRNA has been detected yet. Alternatively, soluble ICAM-1 may be the result of proteolytic cleavage close to the cell membrane. Precedence for other adhesion molecules being cleaved at the cell surface exists as evidence by the discovery of a shed form of LECAM-1 in neutrophil culture supernatants in conjunction with a simultaneous loss of cell surface expression. This mechanism seems to be unlikely, at least for melanoma, since increasing concentrations of soluble ICAM-1 after adequate stimulation in melanoma supernatants are associated with an increasing ICAM-1 cell surface expression (Becker et al. 1991). Finally, soluble ICAM-1 might simply be the consequence of cell death, nonspecific proteolysis, and soluble membrane debris. In the case of melanoma cells, the observation that soluble ICAM-1 is induced most efficiently by the combination of IFN-γ and TNF-α, cytokines which not only induce ICAM-1 expression, but also can be cytotoxic, corroborates with the latter hypothesis.

Although the concentrations of soluble ICAM-1 detected in the serum of melanoma patients would not be sufficient to block non-MHC-restricted cell–cell interactions, nothing is known about the concentrations of soluble ICAM-1 in the microenviroment of the tumor.

An in vivo experiment which may be relevant to the role of ICAM-1 in melanoma metastasis has recently been carried out in humans (Meyskens et al. 1990). In a clinical trial, patients with stage I and II melanoma were injected with IFN-γ. This trial was stopped after 2 years because of occurrence of increased death and relapse rates as well as decreased disease-free intervals in the treated patients. Injection of IFN-γ has been shown to induce ICAM-1 expression in vivo. Furthermore, the induction of circulating ICAM-1 in serum of melanoma patients receiving interleukin-2 (IL-2) therapy has been described. This induction correlated with the induction of IFN-γ in those patients. The results of this trial together with these observations provide some evidence that one or more IFN-γ regulated functions do indeed foster the development of metastasis in melanoma patients.

The natural ligand for the CD28 molecule was reported to be the B cell activation antigen B7 (Norton et al. 1992). It is a 44- to 54-kDa glycoprotein and also a member of the immunoglobulin superfamily. While B7 is constitutively expressed on dendritic cells, it is only present in substantial levels after activation of B cells and monocytes. Recently, B7 has also been detected on activated human peripheral blood T cells, T cell clones, NK cell clones, HTLV-1-transformed T cells, and PMA-activated keratinocytes (Chen et al. 1993).

Induction of unresponsiveness in T_H1 cells to a specific antigen by MHC class II-expressing tumor cells might have major implications for tumor immunology. We recently reported that a human melanoma cell line expressing MHC class II was able to induce clonal anergy in a specific, MHC-restricted $CD4^+$ T cell clone (Becker et al. 1993d). The $CD4^+$ T cell clone and an autologous melanoma cell line form conjugates with each other, leading to an increase of $[Ca^{2+}]_i$ in the T cell clone; however, this interaction failed to induce interleukin-2 production or proliferation of the T cell clone. Furthermore, the interaction rendered this T cell clone unresponsive to subsequent stimulation. All these effects were MHC class II restricted. Therefore, the human melanoma cell line SMC was capable of delivering antigen-specific signals to the T cell clone, but did not deliver the costimulatory signals, e.g., a B7/CD28 interaction, necessary for full T cell activation. Transfection of the melanoma cells with an expression vector containing a B7 cDNA, which resulted in subsequent expression of B7 on its cell surface, rendered it a fully competent antigen-presenting cell which is able to induce a nuclear factor binding to the IL-2 promoter in the specific T cell clone, resulting in enhanced IL-2 transcription, synthesis, and T cell proliferation.

These findings suggest that manipulation of costimulation may offer new strategies for future tumor immunotherapy. In this regard Townsend and Allison recently demonstrated that transfection of murine melanoma cells bearing MHC class II molecules with a B7 cDNA expression vector induces the rejection of these tumor cells in vivo (Townsend and Allison 1993). This treatment also primed for a response against subsequent challenge by the wild-type melanoma.

It has been shown that anergic T cells have a defect in antigen-induced transcription of the IL-2 gene. This defect may be due to an inhibition of the transcription factor AP-1 and its corresponding *cis* element (Kang et al. 1992). Exposure of anergic T cells to IL-2 restores the activity of the AP-1 element and therefore antigen responsiveness. In our system the full restoration of antigen responsiveness was achieved after a 14- to 21-day culture in IL-2-supplemented medium (data not shown). This observation provides further insight into the mechanisms of IL-2-based immunotherapy of melanoma.

Consequences of Major Histocompatibility Complex Class II Expression

For several years now it has been known that in vivo expression of HLA-DR on melanoma cells is not a favorable prognostic sign, but rather the contrary (Bröcker et al. 1984; van Duinen et al. 1988; Ruiter et al. 1991; Carrido et al. 1993). This holds true for primary melanoma as well as for locoregional metastases. Benign melanocytic nevi with the exception of Halo nevi do not express MHC class II molecules. As was found with ICAM-1, a positive correlation of HLA-DR with the amount of intratumoral T lymphocytes was found in primary melanoma but not in metastases. To our surprise we observed an inverse relation between CD25-positive T cells and HLA-DR expression on tumor cells in primary melanoma, suggesting a suppression of autologous immune response by HLA-DR antigen-positive melanoma cells in vivo (Bröcker et al. 1988).

A possible explanation for this observation might be that occupancy of the antigen-specific T cell receptor by antigen presented by nonprofessional antigen-presenting cells in the absence of a costimulatory signal is not a neutral event for the T cell (Schwartz 1990; Müller 1989; Chen et al. 1993). In general, recognition of antigen presented by antigen-presenting cells to T_H1 lymphocytes leads to T cell activation manifested by IL-2 production and proliferation; however, occupancy of the antigen-specific T cell receptor in the absence of a costimulatory signal results in a state of profound unresponsiveness. This long-lasting tolerant or anergic state is characterized by an inability to produce IL-2 when cells are subsequently exposed to both antigen-receptor occupancy and a costimulatory signal. The induction of tolerance has primarily been observed after coculture of T cell clones either with specific peptides presented by artificial planar membranes impregnated with MHC class II molecules or class II MHC-bearing nonprofessional antigen-presenting cells such as T cells, keratinocytes, or pancreatic beta cells.

The conditions that lead to T cell anergy appear to be caused by receipt of signals transduced through the TCR/CD3 complex in the absence of vital second signals. CD28 was reported to mediate one of these signals (Ghosh et al. 1993). This 44-kDa homodimeric T cell surface protein is a member of the immunoglobulin (Ig) superfamily and was shown to gain an accessory function during T cell activation. Following suboptimal activation of T cells via the TCR in the absence of costimulatory signals, cross-linking of CD28 results in enhanced T cell IL-2 production and proliferation and prevents induction of anergy. IL-2 gene transcription is regulated by a 300-bp enhancer in the 5′ flanking region of the IL-2 gene. This enhancer mediates signals from the T cell receptor and also CD28. Cross-linking of CD28 with antibodies leads to the formation of a protein complex binding the so-called CD28-responsive element (CD28 RE) of the IL-2 enhancer and subsequently increases gene transcription up to fivefold. In addition, stimulation of CD28 alters IL-2 gene expression by inducing specific changes in the mRNA degradation. Therefore, the observed increase in IL-2 production via CD28 stimulation results from an increase in transcription and stabilization of IL-2 mRNA.

References

Altomonte M, Colizzi F, Esposito G, Maio M (1992) Circulating ICAM-1 as a marker of disease progression in cutaneous melanoma. N Engl J Med 327:959

Becker JC, Dummer R, Hartmann AA, Burg G, Schmidt RE (1991) Shedding of ICAM-1 from human melanoma cell lines induced by IFNγ and TNFα: functional consequences on cell mediated cytotoxicity. J Immunol 147:4398–4001

Becker JC, Dummer R, Schwinn A, Hartmann AA, Burg G (1992) Circulating ICAM-1 in melanoma patients: induction by interleukin-2 therapy. J Immunotherapy 12:147–151

Becker JC, Schwinn A, Dummer R, Burg G, Bröcker EB (1993a) Lesion-specific activation of cloned tumor infiltrating lymphocytes by autologous tumor cells: induction of proliferation and cytokine production. J Invest Dermatol 101:15–21

Becker JC, Schwinn A, Dummer R, Burg G, Bröcker EB (1993b) Tumor infiltrating lymphocytes in primary melanoma: functional consequnces of differential IL-2 receptor expression. Clin Exp Immunol 91:121–125

Becker JC, Termeer C, Schmidt RE, Bröcker EB (1993c) Soluble intercellular adhesion molecule 1 inhibits MHC-restricted T cell/tumor interaction. J Immunol 151:7224–7232

Becker JC, Brabletz T, Czerny C, Termeer C, Bröcker EB (1993d) Tumor escape mechanisms from immunosurveillance: induction of unresponsiveness in a specific MHC-restricted $CD4^+$ human T cell clone by the autologous MHC class II^+ melanoma. Int Immunol 5:1501–1508

Bröcker EB, Suter L, Sorg C (1984) HLA-DR antigen expression in primary melanomas of the skin. J Invest Dermatol 82:244–247

Bröcker EB, Zwadlo G, Holzmann B, Macher E, Sorg C (1988) Inflammatory cell infiltrates in human melanoma at different stages of tumor progression. Int J Cancer 41:562–567

Carrel S, Johnson JP (1993) Immunologic recognition of malignant melanoma by autologous T lymphocytes. Curr Opin Oncol 5:383–389

Carrido F, Cabrera T, Concha A, Glew S, Ruiz-Cabello F, Stern PL (1993) Natural history of HLA expression during tumor development. Immunol Today 14: 491-499
Chen L, Linsley PS, Hellström KE (1993) Costimulation of T cells for tumor immunity. Immunol Today 14:483-486
D'Urso CM, Wang Z, Cao Y, Tatake R, Zeff RA, Ferrone S (1991) Lack of HLA class I expression by cultured melanoma cells FO-1 due to a defect in beta2-mircoglobulin gene expression. J Invest Dermatol 87:284-292
Gearing AJH, Newman W (1993) Circulating adhesion molecules in disease. Immunol Today 14:506-512
Ghosh P, Tan TH, Rice NR, Sica A, Young HA (1993) The interleukin 2 CD28-responsive complex contains at least three members of the NF kB family: c-Rel, p50, and p65. Proc Nate Acad Sci USA 90:1696-1700
Greve JM, Davis G, Meyer AM, Forte CM, Yost SC, Marlor CW, Kamarck ME, McClelland A (1989) The major human rhinovirus receptor is ICAM-1. Cell 56:839
Hart IR, Saini A (1992) Biology of tumor metastasis. Lancet 339:1453-1457
Hogg N, Bates PA, Harvey J (1991) Structure and function of intercellular adhesion molecule 1. In: Hogg N (ed) Integrins and ICAM-1 in immune responses. Chem Immunol 50:98-121
Holzmann B, Bröcker EB, Lehmann JM, Ruiter DJ, Sorg C, Riethmüller G, Johnson JP (1987) Tumor progression in human malignant melanoma: five stages defined by their antigenic phenotypes. Int J Cancer 39:466-471
Johnson JP, Stade BG, Holzmann B, Schwäble R, Riethmüller G (1989) De novo expression of ICAM-1 in melanoma correlates with increased risk of metastasis. Proc Natl Acad Sci USA 86:641-644
Kageshita T, Nakamura T, Yamada M, Kuriya N, Arao T (1991) Differential expression of melanoma asscociated antigens in acral lentiginous melanoma and in nodular melanoma lesions. Cancer Res 51:1726-1732
Kang SM, Beverly B, Tran SC, Brorson K, Schwartz RH, Lenardo M (1992) Transactivation by AP-1 is a molecular target of T cell clonal anergy. Science 257:1134-1138
Lanzavecchia A (1993) Identifying strategies for immune intervention. Science 260:937-944
Larson RS, Springer TA (1990) Structure and function of leukocytes integrins. Immunol Rev 114:181-204
Lejeune F, Bauer J, Leyvraz S, Lienard D (1993) Disseminated melanoma, pre-clinical therapeutic studies, clinical trials, and patient treatment. Curr Opin Oncol 5:390-396
Meyskens FL, Kopecky K, Samson M, Hersch E, McDonald J, Jaffe H, Crowley J, Coltman C (1990) Recombinant human interferon gamma: adverse effect in high risk stage I and II cutaneous melanoma. J Natl Cancer Inst 82: 1071
Müller DL (1989) Do tolerant T cells exist? Nature 339:513-514
Natali P, Nicotra MR, Cavaliere R, Bigotti A, Romano G, Temponi M, Ferrone S (1990) Differential expression of ICAM-1 in primary and metastatic lesions. Cancer Res 50:1271-1278
Norton SD, Zuckerman L, Urdahl KB, Shefner L, Miller J, Jenkins MK (1992) The CD28 ligand, B7, enhances IL-2 production by providing a costimulatory signal to T cells. J Immunol 149:1556-1561
Ockenhouse CF, Betageri R, Springer TA, Staunton DE (1992) Plasmodium falciparum-infected erythorcytes bind ICAM-1 at a site distinct from LFA-1 Mac-1 and human rhinovirus. Cell 68:63

Peltenburg LCT, Dee R, Schrier PI (1993) Downregulation of HLA class I expression by c-myc in human melanoma is independent of enhancer A. Nucleic Acid res 21:1179–1185
Pullman WE, Bodmer WF (1992) Cloning and characterization of a gene that regulates cell adhesion. Nature 356:529
Restifo NP, Spiess PJ, Karp SE, Mule JJ, Rosenberg SA (1992) A non immunogenic sarcoma treatment with the cDNA for interferon gamma elicts CD8+ T cells against the wildtype tumor: correlation with antigen presentation capability. J Exp Med 175:1423–1430
Restifo NP, Esquivel F, Kawakami Y, Yewdell JW, Mule JJ, Rosenberg SA, Bennink JR (1993) Identification of human cancers deficient in antigen processing. J Exp Med 177:265–272
Ruiter DJ, Mattijissen V, Bröcker EB, Ferrone S (1991) MHC antigens in human melanoma. Semin Cancer Biol 2:25–45
Schrier PI, Peltenberg LTC (1993) Relationship between myc oncogene activation and MHC class I expression. Adv Res 60:181–245
Schwartz RH (1990) A cell culture modell for T lymphocyte clonal anergy. Science 248:1349–1356
Springer TA (1990) Adhesion receptors of the immune system. Nature 346:425–434
Topalian S, Solomon D, Rosenberg SA (1989) Tumor specific cytolysis by lymphocytes infiltrating human melanomas. J Immunol 142:3714–3724
Townsend A (1992) A new presentation pathway? Nature 356:386–387
Townsend SE Allison JP (1993) Tumor rejection after direct constimulation of CD8+ T cells by B7-transfected melanoma cells. Science 259:368–370
Van den Eynde B, Hainaut P, Herin M, Knuth A, Lemoine C, Weynants P, van der Bruggen P, Fauchet R, Boon T (1989) Presence on a human melanoma of multiple antigens recognized by autologous CTL. Int J Cancer 44:634–640
Van der Bruggen P, Traversari C, Chomez P, Lurquin C, de Plaen E, van der Eynde B, Boon T (1991) A gene encoding an antigen recognized by CTL on a human melanoma. Science 254:1643–1647
van Duinen SG, Ruiter DJ, Broecker EB, van der Velde EA, Sorg C, Welvaart K, Ferrone S (1988) Level of HLA antigen in locoreginal metastases in clinical course of the disease in patients with melanoma. Cancer Res 48:1019–1025
Versteeg R, Krüse-Wolters K, Plomp AC, van Leuwen A, Stam NJ, Ploegh HL, Ruiter DJ, Schrier PI (1989) Suppression of class I human histocompatibility leukocyte antigen by c-myc is locus specific. J Exp Med 170:621–635
von Stamm U, Bröcker EB, von Depka Prondzinski M, Ruiter DJ, Rümke P, Broding C, Carrel S, Lejeune FJ (1993) Effects of systemic IFN alpha on the antigenic phenotype of melanoma metastases. EORTC melanoma cooperative study 18852. Melanoma Res 3:173–180
Wang Z, Cao Y, Albino AP, Zeff RA, Houghton A, Ferrone S (1993) Lack of HLA class I antigen expression by melanoma cells SK-MEL-33 caused by a reading frameshift in beta2-microglobulin messenger RNA. J Clin Invest 91:684–692

Melanoma Control in the United States: Current Status

H.K. Koh[1-3] and A.C. Geller[1,3]

[1] Departments of Dermatology and Medicine, Boston University School of Medicine, 80 East Concord Street, C-3, Boston, MA 02118, USA
[2] Department of Epidemiology and Biostatistics, Boston University School of Public Health, Boston, USA
[3] The Cancer Prevention and Control Center, Boston University Medical Center, Boston, USA

Abstract

Screening and education for melanoma/skin cancer are receiving increasing worldwide attention. In an attempt to improve melanoma control in the United States, where incidence and mortality rates continue to increase, the American Academy of Dermatology (AAD) has provided free skin cancer screenings to more than 600 000 Americans and prevention messages to millions more. This chapter reviews and summarizes ongoing melanoma control activities in the United States, including prevention, education, and early detection/screening. We also address outcome measures in melanoma control and suggest that the unique external and visible nature of skin cancer blurs the distinction between screening and education. Measuring and evaluating the benefits of international melanoma control activities presents many challenging tasks. Future collaborative work must include complementary strategies in melanoma/skin cancer prevention, education, and screening to combat the worldwide increase in melanoma incidence and mortality.

Introduction

Cutaneous melanoma has become an increasingly common cancer in the United States, constituting a growing public health problem (Koh 1991). Rising incidence and death rates now contribute to an estimated 32 000 cases and 7000 deaths for 1993 (Boring et al. 1993). In theory, prevention, education, and early detection should decrease melanoma morbidity and mortality, since sunlight is considered a major contributing factor for melanoma, the cancer is external and visible, risk factors are known, and early detection of melanoma is associated with a high 5-year survival rate (Koh 1991).

Recent Results in Cancer Research, Vol. 139

In an attempt to improve melanoma control, the American Academy of Dermatology (AAD) has provided skin cancer education and prevention messages to millions of Americans and free skin screenings for more than 600000 Americans since 1985 (AAD 1993). However, measuring and rigorously evaluating the benefits of any melanoma control program present many challenges. This chapter will address some of the major questions of melanoma/skin cancer control in the United States and summarize its current status.

Outcome Measures

The ideal measure of the success of a melanoma control program should come from a randomized trial demonstrating a sustained reduction in the mortality rates of melanoma in a defined population (compared to a control population). Because such trials have formidable logistical challenges (involving randomizing and following hundreds of thousands of subjects for years), no such randomized trial currently exists anywhere in the world (Koh et al. 1993). Alternatively, tracking intermediate or short-term outcome measures in interventions outside of a randomized trial could serve as an indicator of future progress (Marks and Hill 1992). Such intermediate outcome measures in prevention may include:

1. Increase in sales of sunscreens and protective clothing
2. Decreased rates of sunbathing in hot, sunny climates over time
3. Decreased rates of sunburns over time
4. Increased self-reported rates of use of sunscreens, hats, and protective clothing
5. Increased knowledge, attitudes, and beliefs about sun protection

Intermediate measures of the success of skin cancer education may include:

1. Increased information reaching the proper target audience
2. Greater societal awareness of significant risk factors and susceptibility of risk
3. Improved skin awareness and self-examination rates by individuals at risk
4. Increased requests for skin cancer examinations

Intermediate measures of the success of screening programs may include:

1. Lower rates of thick melanomas in screened populations
2. Overall reduction in tumor thickness of screenees compared with comparison groups (unscreened population)
3. Greater proportion of high-risk persons attending screenings
4. Increased self-screening by participants (compared to practice prior to screening)

Data available on these end points are just beginning to emerge, as noted below.

Prevention

Since case-control studies identify sunlight as a probable "cause" of melanoma (and childhood sunburns have been associated with increased risk of melanoma in later years), primary prevention efforts have tried to limit overexposure to sunlight using educational messages aimed to different audiences (Marks and Hill 1992). Intensive educational approaches in Australia have reached children, using creative, visually striking, and nonthreatening messages and requiring collaboration between schools, peers, and family (Marks and Hill 1992). Some studies have stressed the importance of parental influences in delivering this message (Cockburn et al. 1989; Maducdoc et al. 1992; Banks et al. 1992).

Similar efforts have begun in the United States; for example, two simple educational teaching tools to boost sun protection in youth include the ABCS of sun protection (Away from sun, Block, Coverup, Speak out) promoted by the American Cancer Society and the American Academy of Dermatology. Both hold promise as easy-to-remember teaching methods. Secondly, the "shadow rule" teaches children that when a child's shadow is shorter than he or she is, it is time to use sunscreens, hats, and shades. This learning device, developed by an astronomer and published in the medical literature, may be useful for children who are not aware of the time of day and do not wear a watch (Holloway 1992). Future studies of younger children and adolescents should test their knowledge, awareness, and practice of these two important messages.

Successful sun protection approaches for adults must first identify and target population subgroups least likely to practice adequate sun protection measures. A recent random digit dial survey of 2458 US white adults (>16 years of age) found that less than 50% of all sunbathers use sunscreen, with compliance lowest in men and persons with lower education levels. Furthermore, among sunscreen users, less than 50% reported using the widely recommended sun protection factor (SPF) 15^{+} (Koh et al. 1992a). Other studies also note a range of 26% to 70% compliance, with generally higher sun protection practice among women (Cockburn et al. 1989; Banks et al. 1992; Johnson and Lookingbill 1984; Hill and Rassaby 1984). Special outreach may need to target men (who have higher melanoma mortality rates than women) and persons with lower educational status (Geller et al. 1992a).

Education

Presently in the United States, skin cancer education primarily occurs during the spring of each year when national and local media publicize the availability of free skin cancer screening programs and at the same time disseminate education messages (through newspaper, radio, and television) alerting the public to the warning signs of skin cancer risk factors and the importance of early detection and sun protection. For example, in May 1992, 238 TV stations in more than 150 U.S. cities (with populations greater than 50 000) carried skin cancer broadcasts during prime-time news coverage. These messages penetrated all 30 of the top TV markets in the United States, reaching an estimated 50 million Americans (AAD 1993).

As Morrison has noted, "publicity efforts for cancer control have now given large numbers of well people advice as to when and how they should be examined for various diseases during their early, asymptomatic phases." (Morrison 1985) In this vein, AAD educational efforts complement screening as part of an overall cancer control effort. Such publicity can have a variety of public health effects, improving knowledge and changing attitudes and behavior through both primary prevention (such as the modification of sun exposure behavior) and early detection outside of screening (such as increased self-examination of the skin or a direct visit to their physician for a skin examination). However, documentation of these changes is sparse. In a recent nationally representative sample of 502 white Americans (50 years of age and above,) awareness of skin cancer was relatively high (74% had heard of melanoma) and the major risk factors were widely known. However, skin cancer knowledge and prevention practices were significantly worse among men and people with no education beyond high school (Miller et al. 1993).

Professional education of medical providers should also be an essential component of a melanoma control strategy, as visual screening by a qualified health provider should enhance early detection and patients at risk appear to be integrated into the health care system (Koh 1991; Geller et al. 1992b). One survey of melanoma patients in Massachusetts indicated that patients had extensive contact with physicians in the year prior to diagnosis (Geller et al. 1992b). Specifically, of 216 patients, 87% had regular physicians and 63% had seen those physicians in the year prior to diagnosis, but only 24% had examined their own skin prior to diagnosis and 20% reported physician skin examinations (Geller et al. 1992b). However, there is little data on the performance of the skin cancer examination during the routine medical visit or the teaching of skin cancer education in American medical schools.

The Australian Cancer Society has recommended that education about diagnosis and management of skin cancers and their precursors begin in medical schools. Further, they urge that major components of professional education programs include the ability to detect individuals at high risk within day to day medical practice, the role of opportunistic screening, and the ability to develop selective screening for high risk individuals (Marks and Hill 1992).

Early Detection/Screening

Annual free AAD skin cancer screening programs have provided skin examinations by dermatologists to more than 600 000 Americans (1985–1993) (AAD 1993; Koh et al. 1993). As noted above, the media help publicize the times of these clinics and invite the public to attend. At screening, participants first complete a standardized form which asks about risk factors, changing moles, and family and personal history of skin cancer and melanoma. Then, AAD physicians perform visual examinations for skin cancer; persons with possible skin cancer found at screening are asked to visit their own doctor for diagnosis and treatment. Hence, the AAD activity qualifies as what Miller terms "mass screening," i.e., screening activities of a large segment of the public.

In analyzing the impact of this program, one must start with the recognition that the AAD screening programs also uniquely delivers education through three means:

1. Prescreening publicity not only disseminates the availability of screening sessions, but also publicizes melanoma risk factors and warning signs of skin cancer.
2. At the screenings, physicians and staff first provide attendees with visually striking brochures and videos on sun protection, excessive sun exposures, tanning parlors, guides to self-examination, and the importance of early detection. Moreover, during the actual screening examination, the participant's questions about particular skin lesions or risk factors can prompt the screening dermatologist to deliver personalized education about skin cancer while visually reviewing skin lesions together with the attendee. We suggest that in this way, screening programs represent a teachable moment to counsel patients at a time when a learner is ready to accept new information for use conceptually or in practice.
3. After the screening, for all persons with suspected melanoma, the AAD provides essential information on the importance of follow-up care, increased attention to skin self-examination, avoidance of the sun during peak times, and on screening family members of confirmed cases. In 1992 and 1993, AAD staff contacted more than 3000 people with suspected melanoma by letter or telephone call (AAD 1993).

Initial attempts to evaluate these efforts are just beginning. Leffell et al. (1993) found that screening participants who received education literature were less likely to be anxious about a full body examination than those who did not receive any information. Brandberg et al. (1993) found an increase in attention to nevi in 190 persons after attendance at a skin cancer screening clinic in Sweden. Using surveys at the day of screening and seven months later, they concluded that those who were concerned about their nevi were reassured, while those not so interested learned to pay more attention to their nevi (Brandberg et al. 1993). Preliminary studies in Massachusetts found populations at risk attending the AAD screening programs; more than 86% of attendees had at least one risk factor and 78% had at least two risk factors (Koh et al. 1991). Future studies should clarify what publicity messages arouse concern among those at highest risk and what intensity of concern convinces them to be screened.

How Do Cancer Screening Principles Apply to Skin Cancer?

The above discussion begins to show how closely education and screening are intertwined in a cancer uniquely visible as skin cancer. Further examination of the textbook definitions of cancer screening also demonstrates the blurred distinction between education and screening for skin cancer. The object of skin cancer screening (as for all cancer screening) is "testing of apparently healthy volunteers from the general population for the purpose of separating them into groups with high and low probabilities for a given disorder" and ". . . the early detection of those diseases whose treatment is either easier or more effective when undertaken at an earlier point in time" or "a process which allows detection of disease at an early or preinvasive stage before symptoms prompt the diagnosis" (Sackett and Holland 1975). Moreover, though, Sackett defines screening as an "organized attempt to detect among apparently healthy people in the country, disease or risk factors of which they are *unaware*" (Sackett et al. 1985). Miller defines screening as "the presumptive identification of *unrecognized* disease by the application of tests, examinations or other procedures that can be applied rapidly" (Miller 1985). The International Union Against Cancer (UICC) defined screening as an "organized program in which *unsuspected* lesions in asymptomatic subjects in a defined population are found" (Miller et al. 1990). Morrison defined screening as a "purposeful extension of the process by which people *perceive symptoms* of their own illnesses and then consult physicians for diagnosis and treatment" (Morrison 1985).

In the light of these definitions, some would not consider the AAD programs as screening, since many participants have some level of awareness or suspicions about certain skin lesions. However, as skin cancer usually does not exhibit symptoms (defined as any subjective evidence of disease or of a patient's condition, i.e., such evidence as perceived by the patient), these traditional textbook definitions may not readily apply to skin cancer (Koh et al. 1994a). One could either argue that most patients with skin cancer are asymptomatic (since skin cancer uncommonly causes itching, discomfort, or pain) or that they are symptomatic (since they may be able to see, and therefore perceive, their own skin cancer). It is probably more reasonable to consider skin cancer not as a symptom but a sign, i.e., "an indication of the existence of something; any objective evidence of disease" (Anderson et al. 1988; Koh et al. 1994c).

As there have been few discussions about the nuances of the definitions of skin cancer screening, these issues were presented to scientists attending the Second Epidemiology of Melanoma Conference in Vancouver, Canada (1991) (Koh et al. 1994a). These experts generally agreed that the unique external and visible nature of skin cancer blurred the distinction between screening and education and in fact made them inseparable. They gave less importance to what constitutes skin cancer screening using such definitions of awareness and suspicion and more weight to whether the program resulted in more early detection and decreased mortality (Koh et al. 1994a).

Screening Results and Access to Screening

AAD skin cancer screenings appear to detect early melanoma (almost 99% of all screen-detected melanomas are stages 1 and 2), with stage and thickness comparing favorably with those of the United States Surveillance, Epidemiology, and End Results (SEER) registry. Specifically, of those subjects with a screening diagnosis of melanoma attending the 1992–1993 AAD national programs, we have so far confirmed 261 melanomas in 257 individuals (Koh et al. 1994b). All but four persons had localized disease. In comparison with SEER population-based data, screen-detected persons (1992–1993) with confirmed melanoma were less likely to have regional and metastatic disease and more likely to have thinner lesions. However, we caution that these results are preliminary, and without a formal control group we cannot make any projections about improved mortality. Also, self-selection bias and other screening biases exist (Koh et al. 1994b).

Cole and Morrison noted that "another objective proposed for screening programs is to provide a mechanism whereby persons, especially the poor, can gain access to medical care" (Cole and Morrison 1980). AAD screening programs for melanoma/skin cancer in the United States may serve as the sole opportunity for skin cancer examinations for some participants. In an analysis of insurance status and prior dermatologic care among participants (1992 and 1993), more than 75% of screenees reported not having a regular dermatologist, 47% would not have seen their physician without the screen, and 9% had no health insurance. Eighty percent of persons were attending their first program, suggesting screenings also offer an opportunity for many to receive their first "expert" complete skin examination (AAD 1993).

The AAD screening and education programs are just one part of melanoma control. Professional education could improve melanoma case-finding in the United States population (defined as the "testing of patients who have sought health care for disorders which may be unrelated to their chief complaints. The encounter is initiated by the patient and the purpose here is a comprehensive assessment of health") (Sackett et al. 1975). Studies of melanoma case-finding note that an estimated 14%–25% of melanoma is discovered by the doctor (at a time when the patient had not noticed anything wrong) (Green 1982; Elwood and Gallagher 1988; Koh et al. 1992b).

Current Skin Cancer Screening Recommendations and the Prospect of Targeting High-Risk Populations

Because there is so little data, making public health skin cancer recommendations today is a difficult process. Currently, recommendations about skin cancer screening are diverse. Some groups, such as the UICC, recommend no skin cancer screening. Others, including the American Cancer Society, the American Academy of Dermatology, and the 1992 National Institutes of Health Consensus Conference on Early Melanoma, do recommend screening. The 1989 report of the United States Preventive Services Task Force recommends screening only for high-risk populations. These recommendations will change and evolve over time (Koh et al. 1993).

Screening and education programs must be able to reach persons with risk factors and especially population subgroups with the highest risk for late-stage disease and death. New data from the United States, Australia, and New Zealand indicate that melanoma mortality is rising fastest in white men over age 50, for reasons that are unclear (Marks and Hill 1992; Geller et al. 1992a; Cooke and McNoe 1990). Until further data accrue, it may be reasonable to focus future screening and educational efforts particularly on this group as a strategy to prevent death. As part of this strategy, the AAD launched a national public service announcement entitled "You May be a Marked Man" targeting older men. Public response is currently being evaluated.

Targeted screening may also need to concentrate on persons with atypical moles/dysplastic nevi. Surveillance of such high-risk patients coupled with patient education has resulted in early discovery of melanoma (Masri et al. 1990; Vasen et al. 1989).

Conclusion

Over the next few decades, screening and education for melanoma/skin cancer will receive increasing worldwide attention. Multiple strategies will be required to combat increasing incidence and mortality rates. AAD screening and educational programs have begun, but data on their effects are only just beginning to become available. Future collaborative work in melanoma/skin cancer prevention, education, and screening holds promise as a way to improve early detection and save lives.

Acknowledgments. We would like to thank the American Academy of Dermatology Committee on Melanoma/Skin Cancer Screening Program, Ms. Ruth Sikes, Dr. Donald Miller, and Dr. R. Lew.

References

AAD (American Academy of Dermatology) Committee on Melanoma (1993) Skin cancer screening summary report. American Academy of Dermatology, Schaumburg

Anderson DM, Patwell JM, Plaut K, McCullough K (1988) Dorland's illustrated medical dictionary, 27th edn. Saunders, Philadelphia

Banks BA, Silverman RA, Schwartz RH et al (1992) Attitudes of teenagers toward sun exposure and sunscreen use. Pediatrics 89:40–42

Boring CC, Squires TS, Tong T (1993) Cancer statistics. CA Cancer J Clin 43:7–26

Brandberg Y, Bolund C, Michelson H et al (1993) Psychological reactions in public melanoma screening. Eur J Cancer 29A:860–863

Cockburn J, Hennrikus D, Scott R et al (1989) Adolescent use of sun-protection measures. Med J Aust 151:136–140

Cole P, Morrison AS (1980) Basic issues in population screening for skin cancer. JNCI 64:1263–1272

Cooke KR, McNoe BM (1990) Targeting early detection of malignant melanoma of the skin. NZ Med J 103:551–553

Elwood JM, Gallagher RP (1988) The first signs and symptoms of melanoma: a population based study. In: Elwood JM (ed) Nevi and melanoma: incidence, interrelationships and implications. Karger, Basel, pp 140–152 (Pigment cell, no 9)

Geller AC, Koh HK, Miller DR et al (1992a) Death rates of malignant melanoma among white men in the United States, 1973–1988. MMWR 41:20–21, 27

Geller AC, Koh HK, Miller DR et al (1992b) Use of health services before the diagnosis of melanoma. Implications for early detection and screening. J Gen Intern Med 7:154–157

Green A (1982) Incidence and reporting of cutaneous melanoma in Queensland. Aust J Dermatol 23:105–109

Hill D, Rassaby J (1984) Determinants of intentions to take precautions against skin cancer. Comm Health Stud 8:33–44

Holloway L (1992) Atmospheric sun protection factor on clear days: its observed dependence on solar zenith angle and its relevance to the shadow rule for sun protection. Photochem Photobiol 56:229–234

Johnson EY, Lookingbill DP (1984) Sunscreen use and sun exposure. Arch Dermatol 120:727–731

Koh HK (1991) Cutaneous melanoma. N Engl J Med 325:171–182

Koh HK, Geller AC, Miller DR et al (1991) Who is being screened for melanoma/skin cancer? Characteristics of persons screened in Massachusetts. J Am Acad Dermatol 24:271–277

Koh HK, Bak SM, Geller AC et al (1992a) Sunbathing habits and sunscreen use in 2458 Caucasian adults: results of a national survey. Abstract presented at American Public Health Association, Washington DC

Koh HK, Miller DR, Geller AC et al (1992b) Who discovers melanoma? Patterns from a population-based survey. J Am Acad Dermatol 26:914–919

Koh HK, Geller AC, Miller DR et al (1993) Early detection of melanoma: an ounce of prevention may be a ton of work. J Am Acad Dermatol 28:645–647

Koh HK, Miller DR, Geller AC et al (1994a) Skin cancer screening in Massachusetts: the program and methodologic questions. In: Gallagher RP, Elwood JM (eds) Epidemiology of malignant melanoma. Kluwer Academic Publishers, Boston

Koh HK, Norton LA, Geller AC et al (1994b) Evaluation of national skin cancer screening. Cancer (submitted)

Leffell DJ, Berwick M, Bolognia J (1993) The effect of pre-education on patient compliance with full-body examination in a public skin cancer screening. J Dermatol Surg Oncol 19:660–663

Maducdoc LR, Wagner RF, Wagner KW (1992) Parents' use of sunscreen on beach-going children. The burnt child dreads the fire. Arch Dermatol 128:628–629

Marks R, Hill D (eds) (1992) The public health approach to melanoma control: prevention and early detection. International Union Against Cancer

Masri GD, Clark WH Jr, Guerry D IV et al (1990) Screening and surveillance of patients at high risk for malignant melanoma result in detection of earlier disease. J Am Acad Dermatol 22:1042–1048

Miller AB (ed) (1985) Screening for cancer. Academic Press, Orlando

Miller AB, Chamberlain J, Day NE et al (1990) Report on a workshop of the UICC project on evaluation of screening for cancer. Int J Cancer 46:761–769

Miller DR, Koh HK, Geller AC et al (1993) National survey of skin cancer awareness and prevention in older Americans. Abstract, presented at the American Public Health Association, San Francisco, CA

Morrison AS (1985) Screening in chronic disease. Oxford University Press, New York

Sackett DL, Holland WW (1975) Controversy in the detection of disease. Lancet 2:357–359

Sackett DL, Haynes RB, Tugwell P (1985) Clinical epidemiology Little Brown, Boston; pp 139–155

Vasen HFA, Bergman W, VanHaeringen A et al (1989) The familial dysplastic nevus syndrome: natural history and the impact of screening on prognosis. A study of nine families in the Netherlands. Eur J Cancer Clin Oncol 25:337–341

III. Cutaneous Lymphoma

New Perspectives in Experimental and Clinical Research for Cutaneous T Cell Lymphomas

G. Burg[1], A. Häffner[2], R. Böni[1], S. Dommann[1], and R. Dummer[1]

[1] Department of Dermatology, University of Zurich Medical School, Gloriastr. 31, CH-8091 Zurich, Switzerland
[2] Department of Dermatology, Case Western Reserve University, Cleveland, Ohio, USA

Abstract

Cutaneous T cell lymphomas (CTCL) are lymphoproliferative disorders, which can be classified by an adaptation of the Kiel classification. The most common CTCL, Mycosis fungoides (MF) and Sézary syndrome (SS), are monoclonal T helper memory lymphomas. They belong to the group of peripheral T cell lymphomas. However, CTCL includes other disease entities such as granulomatous slack skin, pagetoid reticulosis, and lipotropic CTCL. Polymerase chain reaction of the T cell receptor (TCR)-γ and screening of the PCR products for sequence-specific mobility in acrylamide gels has increased the detection limit for clonal T cells in the skin. This method will help to define the relationship of CTCL to other lymphoproliferative disorders and may contribute to the early diagnosis of CTCL. In SS, the malignant CTCL clone secretes a T helper-2 cytokine pattern, which might be responsible for the systemic immunosuppression in CTCL patients. New treatment modalities (IL-12) might correct these immunologic abnormalities. Cutaneous B cell lymphomas mostly are follicular center cell derived and usually have a good prognosis. Therapy of cutaneous lymphomas should take into account prognostic factors, the most reliable of which in CTCL is the tumor mass expressed by the tumor burden index.

Introduction and Classification

Our understanding of cutaneous lymphomas has continuously been expanded by the application of newer methods such as labeled antibody studies, electron microscopy, and molecular biology, which have led to new inter-

Recent Results in Cancer Research, Vol. 139

pretations of clinical and histologic features of these heterogeneous diseases. The enormous increase in knowledge in these scientific fields still continues to model the pathophysiologic concepts and clinical and histologic classifications of lymphoproliferative disorders. This review can only address some of the issues based on the current scientific background.

Classification of Cutaneous Lymphomas

Extranodal sites including the skin provide distinct microenvironments for the proliferation of lymphoid cells; nevertheless we are dealing with the same pathogenetic process as found in lymph node-based lymphomas. Therefore, the classification given for cutaneous lymphomas in the following table (Table 1) is adapted to the Kiel classification (Kerl et al. 1991; Lennert and Feller 1992) and the Working Formulation (1982), respectively. This classification is clinically useful due to its simple application, although approximately 15%–20% of cases do not fit into this scheme (Kerl et al. 1991).

Table 1. Non-Hodgkin Lymphomas

Lymphoma	Working formulation
T-cell lymphomas	
Lymphomas of T precursor cells	
T lymphoblastic lymphoma/leukemia[a]	ML, lymphoblastic(I)
Lymphomas of peripheral T cells	
T chronic lymphocytic leukemia[a]	ML, small lymphocytic, consistent with CLL (A)
Mycosis fungoides (MF)	Mycosis fungoides (A)
Sézary syndrome	Sézary syndrome (A)
Pagetoid reticulosis, circumscribed, desseminated	–
Pleomorphic T cell lymphoma, HTL V-I± (small, medium, large)	ML, polymorphous (H)
Immunoblastic lymphoma, T cell type (Ki-1+)	ML, large cell, immunoblastic (H)
Large cell anaplastic lymphoma, T cell type (Ki-1+)	
B cell lymphomas	
B chronic lymphocytic leukemia[a]	ML, small lymphocytic, consistent with CLL (A)
Lymphoplasmocytoid immunocytoma	ML, small lymphocytic plasmacytoid (A)
Plasmacytoma	Extramedullary plasmacytoma
Centroblastic/centrocytic lymphoma	ML, mixed small cleaved and larger (B-G)

Table 1. (*Contd.*)

Lymphoma	Working formulation
Centroblastic lymphoma	ML, large cell noncleaved (G)
Centrocytic (mantle cell) lymphoma	ML, small cleaved (E, G)
Immunoblastic lymphoma	ML, large cell, immunoblastic (H)
Burkitt's lymphoma	ML, small noncleaved, Burkitt (J)
Skin-associated lymphoid tissue (SALT) lymphoma (?)	–
Rare and distinct forms of lymphoproliferative and related disorders	
Granulomatous slack skin/MF	
Lymphoepitheloid lymphoma (Lennert)[a]	
Midline granuloma[a]	
Lymphomatoid papulosis	
Systemic angioendotheliomatosis (angiotropic lymphoma)(B > T)	
Lymphomatoid granulomatosis (Liebow)[a], angiocentric, angiodestructive	
Angiolymphoid hyperplasia with eosinophilia (Kimura)	
Syringolymphoid hyperplasia with alopecia	
Subcutaneous (lipotropic) T cell lymphomas	
Sinus histiocytosis with massive lymphadenopathie (Rosai-Dorfman)[a]	
Peripheral T cell lymphoma of the AILD type[a]	
T cell-rich large B cell lymphoma	
B cell-rich T cell lymphoma	
Large cell lymphoma of the multilobated cell type (B or T)	
T cell lymphoma expressing delta TCR	

AILD, angioimmunoblastic lymphadenopathy with dysproteinemia; CLL, chronic lymphocytic leukemia; TCR, T cell receptor; ML, malignant lymphoma.
[a] Usually secondary skin involvement.

Cutaneous T cell lymphomas (CTCL) represent the largest part (65%) of all primary cutaneous lymphomas (CL). Besides classical mycosis fungoides (MF) and its erythrodermic form, Sézary's syndrome, there are many unusual variants.

Cutaneous B cell lymphomas (CBCL; Burg et al. 1985) comprise about 25% of CL, whereas in the lymph node they are much more frequent than T cell lymphomas. The head and neck area for some unknown reasons seem to be preferentially involved by infiltrates and tumors, which in the face may lead to the special feature of facies leonina. Almost 50% of CBCL are follicular center cell (FCC)-derived lymphomas.

The physiological development of T lymphocytes occurs first in an antigen-independent phase, which is morphologically characterized by the blastic appearance of the T lymphocytes. This first phase is followed by a second antigen-dependent phase. T lymphocytes in the second antigen-dependent phase are designated peripheral T lymphocytes. They appear cytologically as small, cerebriform, pleomorphic, T immunoblastic or large anaplastic cells, depending on their state of activation. Since pathophysiological classification of T cell lymphomas is not possible, the Kiel classification based on the normal counterpart of T cell development was introduced (Stansfeld et al. 1988). Figure 1 gives an overview on the ontogeny of B lymphocytes and the respective malignant B cell lymphomas arising from the various stages of differentiation. B lymphocytes are produced in the bone marrow. Following stimulation by an antigen in secondary lymphoid tissue, only a small proportion of these cells survive and differentiate to become part of the relatively stable pools of peripheral B cells (Burg et al. 1994), which need to receive regular signals in order to become long-lived cells.

In addition to CTCL and CBCL, the skin may be primarily or secondary involved in rare and distinct forms of lymphoproliferative and related disorders of various lineage derivation: granulomatous forms of CTCL, unusual morphologic features due to strong tropism of neoplastic T or B cells to distinct morphologic structures such as blood vessels (malignant angioendo-

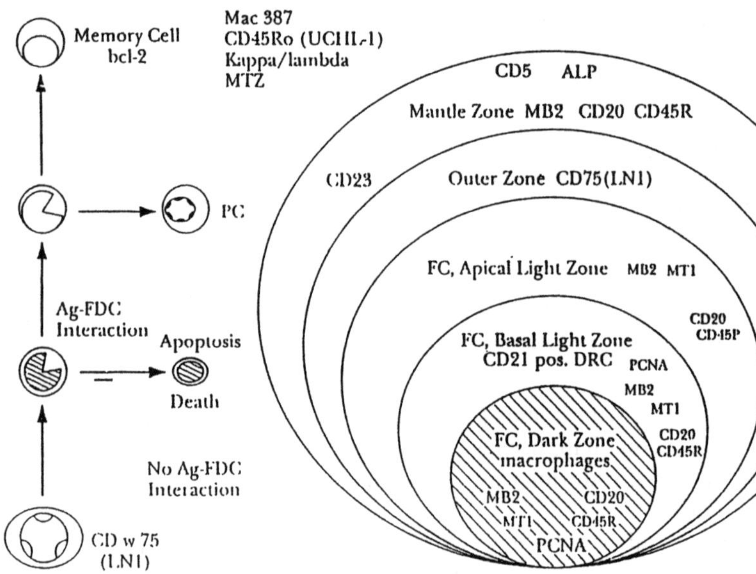

Fig. 1. Cellular and compartmental composition of secondary lymph follicle after antigen stimulation (according to Liu et al. 1992). *FDC*, follicular dendrite cell; *MTZ*, mantle zone; *FC*, follicular center; *DRC*, dendritic reticulum cell; *PCNA*, proliferating cell nuclear antigen

theliomatosis; angiocentric lymphoma), adnexal structures (syringolymphoid hyperplasia) (Burg and Schmöckel 1992), or subcutaneous lymphoma (Burg et al. 1991; Gonzalez et al. 1991), or B cell-rich T cell lymphoma and T cell-rich large B cell lymphoma (Dommann et al.; Ramsay et al. 1988) with scarce neoplastic T and B cell populations, respectively, effaced by the reactive T or B cells, rendering diagnosis difficult even if genotyping is performed.

Diagnosis of Cutaneous Lymphomas

For routine diagnostic purposes, morphology always has been and will be in the future the gold standard for the classification of lymphoproliferative disorders. Based on clinical and histo- and cytomorphological features, almost 75% of cutaneous lymphomas can be properly diagnosed and classified as B cell or T cell with low-grade or high-grade malignancy. Immunophenotyping using a panel of appropriate monoclonal antibodies for paraffin-fixed or cryo tissue samples and additional genotyping by Southern blot analysis to detect clonal rearrangement of T cell receptor or immunoglobulin genes increase diagnostic reliability up to 85%–90% (Fig. 2).

Unusual Nosologic Entities of Cutaneous Lymphomas

Advances in immunophenotyping and molecular biology have led to the identification of several clinical conditions as CTCL. One of them is the granulomatous slack skin (LeBoit 1991). The clinical appearance presents pendulous skin folds in the intertriginous body regions due to elastolysis.

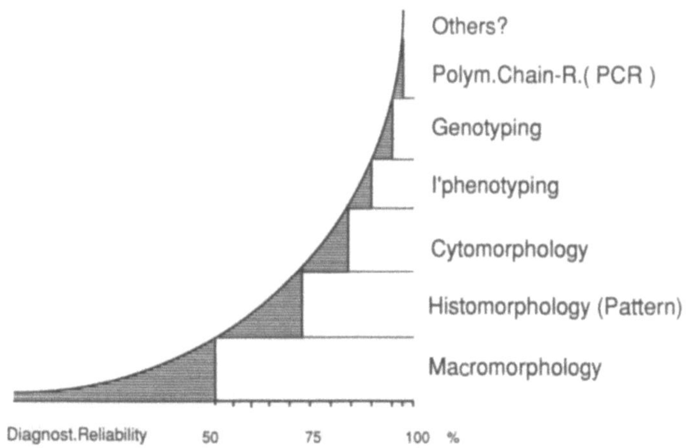

Fig. 2. Reliability of methods used for the diagnosis of cutaneous lymphomas

Another entity is pagetoid reticulosis. The localized type (Woringer-Kolopp) presents with long-standing hyperkeratotic plaques. In some cases, the epidermal lymphocytes have been shown to express the T cell receptor γ/δ on their surface (Alaibac and Chu 1992; Heald et al. 1992; Ralfkiaer et al. 1992). In the murine system, in contrast to humans, this subtype of T lymphocytes shows preferential homing into the epithelium of skin and gut (Carter et al. 1988). The relationship between the γ/δ cells physiologically confined to the epidermis and the malignant cell clones in pagetoid reticulosis remains unclear.

A small proportion of CTCL show a T suppressor/cytotoxic phenotype. These lymphomas consist of CD4-negative, CD8-positive lymphocytes. In a series of nine CD8-positive CTCL patients, rapidly progressive disease was associated with a CD2-positive and CD7-negative phenotype. A slowly progressing clinical course was predicted by a CD2-negative and CD7-positive phenotype (Agnarsson et al. 1990). We have observed a young female patient with a CD8-positive CTCL presenting with extensive erosions of the skin due to an "epidermolytic" infiltrate as well as tumors, with an aggressive course of the disease.

Recently we reported a patient with subcutaneous "lipotropic" CTCL (Burg et al. 1991). Immunophenotyping and rearrangement analysis demonstrated large blastic tumor cells with rearrangement of the δ chain of the T cell receptor (TCR) and expression the TCR γ/δ. Cloning of the infiltrating cells detected high interferon-γ production by γ/δ lymphocytes, which could explain the enormous serum levels of this cytokine and the elevated natural killer cell activity in the peripheral blood of this patient (Burg et al. 1991).

Different from primary nodal B cell lymphomas leading to extranodal involvement during the course of the disease, most follicular center cell-derived CBCL primarily occurring in the skin remain confined to the skin, have a excellent prognosis, and therefore are referred to as "semimalignant" CBCL. They differ from pseudolymphomas by kappa or lambda light chain restriction and tendency of the skin lesions to relapse (Burg et al. 1985).

T cell-rich B cell lymphoma is a distinct entity described in the lymph node (Ramsay et al. 1988), but occasionally also occurring in the skin (Dommann et al.). Since in these cases the reactive lymphoid cell component exceeds the number of tumor cells, the nature of the neoplastic cell type has to be confirmed by polymerase chain reaction (PCR)-assisted demonstration of clonality.

Etiology and Pathogenesis of Cutaneous Lymphomas

The role of HTLV-I in the pathogenesis of CTCL has been extensively studied. After a latent period of about 20–30 years, adult T cell lymphoma/leukemia develops in about 1% of individuals infected with HTLV-I retrovirus due to monoclonal integration of the HTLV-I provirus into the host T cell. Mycosis fungoides and Sezary syndrome patients are HTLV-I seronegative with conventional screening methods. Nevertheless, retroviral genomic information could be integrated into tumor cells without induction of antibodies. Screening skin biopsies from patients with CTCL with primers for the pol region and for the px region of the retrovirus, genomic integration was demonstrated only in a minority of patients, indicating that HTLV-I might be a cofactor in the malignant transformation of the host cell in some of the patients.

During the thymic development, T lymphocytes are generated by several molecular genomic events of T cell development as well as positive and negative selection. The present model of thymic T cell development suggests that hematopoetic stem cells enter the thymus via the cortex with a TCR in germline configuration. In addition to the acquirement of T cell epitopes on their surface, most, if not all, lymphocytes undergo rearrangement of the TCR γ and δ chain. During the following steps, TCR δ rearrangement is deleted and substituted by TCR α rearrangement (Wood et al. 1994). TCR β rearrangement also occurs, which is the target for detection of clonality by conventional Southern blot technique. The sensitivity limit of this method is approximately 2%. In nonlymphatic tissues such as the skin, where a considerable amount of DNA is contributed by various cell types, this limitation can be particularly problematic (Wood et al. 1994). Unlike the deletion of the δ rearrangements, the TCR γ gene remains in the genome. its expression is suppressed by yet undefined silencer mechanisms. Although there are only a limited number of TCR γ-variable and -constant regions, the insertion of a few nucleotides forming the N-region creates a unique fingerprint for the specific T cell clone on a DNA level. Using appropriate primers for the $V\gamma$ and $J\gamma$ gene segments, PCR can selectively amplify T cell DNA. The γ PCR products can be screened by their sequence rather than their size with denaturing gradient gel electrophoresis, temperature gradient electrophoresis (Staib et al. 1993), or cRNA electrophoresis (Volkenandt et al. 1993). These methods allow the analysis of these clone-specific properties and are used in the early diagnosis of CTCL (Wood 1992). A T cell clone can be detected if its DNA contributes at least 0.1% to the total specimen DNA (Wood et al. 1994).

The pathophysiology of CTCL relies on interactive immunological events involving lymphocytes and accessory cells, which functionally also include keratinocytes. Clinical as well as histologic features suggest that CTCL clones in most cases need the presence of epidermal cells to survive and thus depend on the epidermal cytokine network. Epidermal keratinocytes and Langerhans cells have been identified as a potent source of a broad range of immunoregulatory factors, which include several T cell growth factors as well as T cell growth inhibitors. These cytokines might act alone or in combination with other proliferation-inducing agents such as superantigen (Tokura et al. 1992). Paracrine loops between epidermal cells and lymphocytes seem to be involved in the pathogenesis. In addition, keratinocyte-derived factors might contribute to creating a microenvironment which allows the growth of malignant T cell clones, but suppresses reactive cells such as macrophages, natural killer cells, or cytotoxic T cells. If the conditions are changed and lymphocytes isolated from a skin biopsy are cultured in the presence of interleukin (IL)-2 and IL-4, only the reactive, not tumor-clone derived cells expand (Reinhold et al. 1991).

The tumor cells in cutaneous T cell lymphomas commonly show a T helper memory phenotype. These lymphocytes play a central role in the regulation of immune defense (Sanders 1988). It is tempting to speculate that the malignant cell clones in these lymphoproliferative disorders have systemic immunoregulatory capacities, even if the disease is clinically restricted to the skin.

In the majority of mycosis fungoides patients, very few of the circulating peripheral blood mononuclear cells (PBMC) belong to the malignant T cell clone (Bakels et al. 1992). Nevertheless, the PBMC of these patients demonstrate immunologic deficiencies. They exhibit a reduced capacity to lyse tumor cells, referred to as natural killer cell activity (Dummer et al. 1991; Laroche and Kaiserling 1983); however, phenotypic analysis of the PBMC did not show decreased numbers of natural killer cells (our own unpublished observations). The extent of the reduced cytotoxic potential correlates with soluble IL-2 receptor serum levels. These soluble receptor molecules are able to neutralize IL-2 activity in vitro (Dummer et al. 1992).

A decreased potential to generate lymphokine-activated killer cell activity (Wood et al. 1990) has been reported. Another phenomenon in these patients are alterations in immunoglobulin production (van der Putte et al. 1988; Venencie et al. 1984).

Recently, we have analyzed IL-4, IL-6, interferon-γ, and soluble IL-2 receptor release of phytohemagglutinin (PHA)-stimulated PBMC of CTCL patients and compared it to the release of these cytokines from age-matched control patients' PBMC. IL-6 is produced by macrophages and B and T cells (Hirano et al. 1990). No difference in the IL-6 production was noted, but there was a significant decrease in the interferon-γ release and an increase in the IL-4 and soluble IL-2 receptor release in the PHA-stimulated PBMC from CTCL patients (Dummer et al. 1993a,b). Regarding the cytokine production profile, two major subdivisions of the murine T helper system were proposed: T helper-1 clones, which synthesize and secrete mainly IL-2 and interferon-γ, and T helper-2 clones, which produce IL-4, IL-5 and IL-10 (Mosmann et al. 1986; Romagnani 1991).

Although there are only a few circulating malignant cells in the peripheral blood of nonleukemic patients, a change in the T helper phenotype with a selective decrease of naive lymphocytes has been documented (Gilmore et al. 1991). We suggest that the cytokine secretion pattern in CTCL patients reflects the functional counterpart of these phenotypic changes of the PBMC. Due to the low number of circulating morphologically malignant cells, it seems unlikely that the malignant cell clones are responsible for the phenomenon that we observed. We favor the hypothesis that during tumor development a switch from T helper-1 to T helper-2 in the T cell compartment takes place. It remains to be seen whether this switch is specific for malignant lymphoproliferative disorders and which cytokines are involved in this process. It is tempting to speculate that it weakens T cell-based immunosurveillance. Several clinical features such as increased risk of second malignancy (Kantor et al. 1989), elevated immunoglobulin E and A serum levels, hypereosinophilia, and reduced cellular response after antigen challenge may be explained by this hypothesis (Dummer et al. 1993b).

In CBCL, pathophysiologic considerations have been addressed to the expression of the *bcl-2* suppressor gene: t 14/18 translocation leads to juxtapositioning of the immunoglobulin heavy chain gene to the *bcl-2* gene, resulting in increased expression of the bcl-2 protein and thus preventing apoptosis. Whereas in follicilar center cell-derived nodal lymphomas *bcl-2* translocation plays an important pathogenetic role, the t 14/18 translocation is involved only in a minority of CBCL.

The presence of CD21-positive dendritic reticulum cells in most of the follicular center cell-derived B cell lymphomas indicates that cellular or cytokine-mediated interactions between lymphoid tumor cells and accessory cells are mandatory for the development and progression of the proliferative neoplastic process.

Therapy of Cutaneous Lymphomas

The treatment of cutaneous lymphomas remains a challenging problem. Their highly variable natural history, with episodes of spontaneous remissions and exacerbations, raises the question about optimal management.

Because in a recent randomized study aggressive combination therapy with high-dose chemotherapy and radiotherapy failed to improve survival of patients with MF (Kaye et al. 1989), a nonaggressive stage-adapted, sequential application of topical therapies is the preferred first-line treatment for peripheral CTCL without transformation. In addition, the advanced mean age of these patients requires a nonaggressive therapy. Choice of the treatment should consider extent and aggressiveness of the disease as well.

A reliable parameter for the evaluation of appropriate therapeutic measurements is the determination of the tumor burden index (TBI) and the shift of TBI during lymphoma progression. The calculation of the TBI is based on the rough estimation of lymphoma mass as the product of the percentage of body surface covered by patches or plaques or the numbers of tumors multiplied by a constant factor for the category of tumor "thickness." The procedure for calculating the TBI is given in Table 2 (Burg et al. 1994; Burg and Bojahr, unpublished data). For example, a patient with patches covering 15% of his body surface (BS), plaques covering 10%, and three

Table 2. Tumor burden index (TBI) for cutaneous T cell lymphomas (CTCL)

	Skin involvement (%)		Tumors[c] (n)	TBI
	Patch[a]	Plaque[b]		
CF	×1	×10	×100	

CF, constant factor.
[a] Histologically eczemtous patchy infiltrate in the stratum papillare, compatible with early CTCL.
[b] Histologically dense subepidermal band-like infiltrate, filling the stratum papillare, typical for CTCL.
[c] Histologically diffuse infiltrate reaching into or covering the stratum reticulare or the subcutaneous tissue.

tumors has a TBI of (1 × 15) + (10 × 10) + (3 × 100) = 415; a patient showing erythroderma with plaque-like infiltrate has a TBI of 1000; if in addition he has three tumorous lesions, the TBI is 1300.

It has been clearly demonstrated that a change of the TBI strongly correlates with the level of soluble IL-2 receptor as a marker for disease activity and progression (Dummer et al. 1991, 1992).

There are only a limited number of nonaggressive therapeutic alternatives such as topical steroids and photochemotherapy (Roenigk and Caro 1981). Phospholipids might be another treatment option. In a clinical trial using topical hexadecylphosphocholine, we observed partial and complete responses in lesions of CTCL and CBCL (Dummer et al. 1993c). Additional trials will help to define the future role of phospholipids in the treatment of CTCL. More aggressive treatment options include radiotherapy or the topical application of cytotoxic drugs such as nitrogen mustard and carmustine. This treatment may be associated with local or systemic side effects such as thrombocytopenia (Zackheim et al. 1990). Other promising approaches include immunomodulation using interferon-α (Dreno et al. 1991). Regarding the discussed imbalance of the T helper-1/T helper-2 system in CTCL patients, it is interesting to speculate that interferon-α might be able to restore the T helper-1 part. This cytokine might decrease the proliferation of the malignant cell clones and render them more susceptible for lysis by major histocompatibility complex (MHC)-restricted cytotoxic lymphocytes through the induction of MHC class I expression (Balkwill 1989). Especially in combination with retinoids (Knobler et al. 1991; Zachariae and Thestrup 1990) or psoralens and ultraviolet A (PUVA) therapy (Roenigk et al. 1990;

Roenigk and Caro 1981; Staib et al. 1993), this cytokine is an important contribution to the systemic therapy of cutaneous lymphoma patients.

References

Agnarsson BA, Vonderheid EC, Kadin ME (1990) Cutaneous T cell lymphoma with suppressor/cytotoxic (CD8) phenotype: identification of rapidly progressive and chronic subtypes. J Am Acad Dermatol 22:569–577

Alaibac M, Chu AC (1992) Pagetoid reticulosis: a gamma/-delta T-cell lymphoma? Eur J Dermatol 2:109–111

Bakels V, van Oostveen J, Gordijn L, Walboomers J, Meijer C, Willemze R (1992) Frequency and prognostic significance of clonal T-cell receptor beta gene rearrangements in the peripheral blood of patients with mycosis fungoides. Arch Dermatol 128:1602–1607

Balkwill FR (1989) Interferons. Lancet 1:1060–1063

Burg G, Schmöckel CH (1992) Syringolymphoid hyperplasia with alopecia. A syringotropic cutaneous T-cell lymphoma? Dermatology 184:306–307

Burg G, Kaudewitz P, Klepzig K, Przybilla B, Braun-Falco O (1985) Cutaneous B-cell lymphoma. Dermatol Clin 3:689–704

Burg G, Dummer R, Wilhelm M, Nestle F, Ott MM, Feller A, Hefner H, Lanz U, Schwinn A, Wiede J (1991) A subcutaneous delta-positive T-cell lymphoma that produces interferon gamma. N Engl J Med 325:1078–1081

Burg G, Dummer R, Kerl H (1994) Classification of cutaneous lymphomas. Dermatol Clin 12:213–217

Carter L, DenHollander N, Ramaswamy K, Riley D, Befus D (1988) Expression of TCR types on gut intraepithelial lymphocytes. Immunol Today 9:368–369

Dommann S, Dommann-Scherrer CC, Burg G. Cutaneous T-cell rich large B-cell lymphoma. (submitted for publication)

Dreno B, Claudy A, Meynadier J, Verret JL, Souteyrand P, Ortonne JP, Kalis B, Godefroy WY, Beerblock K, Thill L (1991) The treatment of 45 patients with cutaneous T-cell lymphoma with low doses of interferon-alpha 2a and etretinate. Br J Dermatol 125:456–459

Dummer R, Nestle F, Wiede J, Schäfer E, Röger J, Erhard H, Hefner H, Burg G (1991) Coincidence of increased soluble interleukin-2 receptors, diminished natural killer cell activity and progressive disease in cutaneous T-cell lymphomas. Eur J Dermatol 1:135–138

Dummer R, Posseckert G, Nestle F, Witzgall R, Burger M, Becker JC, Schäfer E, Wiede J, Sebald W, Burg G (1992) Soluble interleukin-2 receptors inhibit interleukin-2 dependent proliferation and cytotoxicity: explanation for diminished natural killer cell activity in cutaneous T-cell lymphomas in vivo? J Invest Dermatol 98:50–54

Dummer R, Burg G, Nestle F, Kohl O (1993a) Soluble interleukin-2 receptor and cutaneous T-cell lymphoma. Cancer 71:3793–3794

Dummer R, Kohl O, Gillisson J, Kägi M, Burg G (1993b) Peripheral blood mononuclear cells in non-leukemic cutaneous T-cell lymphoma patients: reduced proliferation and preferential secretion of a T helper 2 like cytokine pattern upon stimulation Arch Dermatol 129:433–436

Dummer R, Krasovec M, Roger J, Sindermann H, Burg G (1993c) Topical application of hexadecylphosphocholine in patients with cutaneous lymphomas. J Am Acad Dermatol 29:963–970

Gilmore SG, Benson EM, Kelly JW (1991) T-cell subsets with a naive phenotype are selectively decreased in the peripheral blood of patients with mycosis fungoides. J Invest Dermatol 96:50–56

Gonzalez CL, Medeiros LJ, Braziel RM, Jaffe ES (1991) T-cell lymphoma involving subcutaneous tissue: a clinico-pathologic entity commonly associated with hemophagocytic syndrome. Am J Surg Pathol 15:17–27

Heald P, Buckley P, Gilliam A, Perez M, Knobler R, Kacinski B, Edelson R (1992) Correlations of unique clinical, immunotypic, and histologic findings in cutaneous gamma/delta T-cell lymphoma. J Am Acad Dermatol 26:865–870

Hirano T, Akira S, Taga T, Kishimoto T (1990) Biological and clinical aspects of interleukin-6. Immunol Today 11:443–449

Kantor AF, Curtis RE, Vonderheid EC, van Scott EJ, Fraumeni JF (1989) Risk of second malignancy after cutaneous T-cell lymphoma. Cancer 63:1612–1615

Kaye FJ, Bunn PJ, Steinberg SM, Stocker JL, Ihde DC, Fischmann AB, Glatstein EJ, Schechter GP, Phelps RM, Foss FM et al (1989) A randomized trial comparing combination electron-beam radiation and chemotherapy with topical therapy in the initial treatment of mycosis fungoides. N Engl J Med 321:1784–1790

Kerl H, Cerroni L, Burg G (1991) The morphologic spectrum of T-cell lymphomas of the skin: a proposal for a new classification. Semin Diagn Pathol 8:55–61

Knobler RM, Trautinger F, Radaszkiewicz T, Kokoschka EM, Micksche M (1991) Treatment of cutaneous T cell lymphoma with a combination of low-dose interferon alfa-2b and retinoids. J Am Acad Dermatol 24:247–252

Laroche L, Kaiserling D (1983) Decreased natural-killer cell activity in cutaneous T-cell lymphomas. N Engl J Med 308:101–102

LeBoit PE (1991) Variants of mycosis fungoides and related cutaneous T-cell lymphomas. Semin Diagn Pathol 8:73–81

Lennert K, Feller AC (1992) Histopathology of non-Hodgkin's lymphomas. Springer, Berlin Heidelberg New York

Liu YJ, Johnson GD, Gordon J, MacLennan ICM (1992) Germinal centers in T-cell-dependent antibody responses. Immunol Today 13:17–21

Mosmann TR, Cherwinski H, Bond MW, Giedlin MA, Coffman RL (1986) Two types of murine helper T cell clone. I. Definition according to profiles of lymphokine activities and secreted proteins. J Immunol 136:2348–2357

Ralfkiaer E, Wollf-Sneedorff A, Thomsen K, Geisler C, Vejlsgaard G (1992) T-cell receptor gamma/delta-positive peripheral T-cell lymphomas presenting in the skin: a clinical, histological and immunophenotypic study. Exp Dermatol 1:31–36

Ramsay AD, Smith WJ, Isaacson PG (1988) T-cell-rich B-cell lymphoma. Am J Surg Pathol 12:433–443

Reinhold U, Abken H, Kukel S, Goeden B, Uerlich M, Neumann U, Kreysel HW (1991) Tumor-infiltrating lymphocytes isolated from a Ki-1-positive large cell lymphoma of the skin. Phenotypic characterization and analysis of cytokine secretion. Cancer 68:2155–2160

Roenigk H, Kuzel TM, Skoutelis AP, Springer E, Yu G, Caro W, Gilyon K, Variakojis D, Kaul K, Bunn PJ et al (1990) Photochemotherapy alone or combined with interferon alpha-2a in the treatment of cutaneous T-cell lymphoma. J Invest Dermatol 95:198S–205S

Roenigk HJ, Caro WA (1981) Skin cancer in the PUVA-48 cooperative study. J Am Acad Dermatol 4:319–324

Romagnani S (1991) Human TH1 and TH2 subsets: doubt no more. Immunol Today 12:256–257

Sanders ME (1988) Human naive and memory T-cells: reinterpretation of helper-inducer and suppressor-inducer subsets. Immunol Today 9:195–198

Staib G, Mielke V, Griesser H, Menke M, Duller B, Sterry W (1993) PCR-analysis of T-cell receptor (TCR)-gamma genes to differentiate between malignant and reactive T-cell infiltrates of the skin. J Invest Dermatol 100:458 (abstr)
Stansfeld A, Diebold J, Kapanci Y (1988) Updated Kiel classification for lymphomas. Lancet 1i:292–293
Tokura Y, Heald PW, Yan SL, Edelson RL (1992) Stimulation of cutaneous T-cell lymphoma cells with superantigenic staphylococcal toxins. J Invest Dermatol 98:33–37
van der Putte SCJ, Toonstra J, van Wichen DF, van Unnik JAM, van Vloten W (1988) Abberant immunophenotype in mycosis fungoides. Arch Dermatol 124: 373–380
Venencie PY, Winkelmann RK, Friedman SJ, Kyle RA, Puissant A (1984) monoclonal gammopathy and mycosis fungoides. J Am Acad Dermatol 11:576–579
Volkenandt M, Wienecke R, Koch O, Buer J, Probst M, Atzpodien J, Horishi T, Danenberg K, Danenberg P, Bertino J (1993) Conformational polymorphisms of cRNA of T-cell receptor genes as a clone-specific marker for cutaneous lymphoma. J Invest Dermatol 101:514–516
Wood GS (1992) Cutaneous lymphoproliferative disorders: strategies for molecular biological analysis and their major findings. Springer Semin Immunopathol 13: 387–399
Wood GS, Haeffner AC, Dummer R, Crooks C (1994) Molecular biology techniques for the diagnosis of CTCL. Dermatol Clin (in press)
Wood NL, Kitces EN, Blaylock K (1990) Depressed lymphokine activated killer cell activity in mycosis fungoides. Arch Dermatol 126:907–913
Working Formulation (1982) The non-Hodgkin's lymphoma pathologic classification project. National Cancer Institute sponsored study of classification of non-Hodgkin's lymphoma. Summary and description of Working Formulation for clinical usage. Cancer 49:2112–2135
Zachariae H, Thestrup-Pedersen K (1990) Interferon alpha and etretinate combination treatment of cutaneous T-cell lymphoma. J Invest Dermatol 95:206S–208S
Zackheim HS, Epstein EJ, Crain WR (1990) Topical carmustine (BCNU) for cutaneous T cell lymphoma: a 15-year experience in 143 patients. J Am Acad Dermatol 22:802–810

Use of Polymerase Chain Reaction in the Detection of Clones in Lymphoproliferative Diseases of the Skin

G. Staib and W. Sterry

Department of Dermatology, University of Ulm, Oberer Eselsberg 40, 89070 Ulm, Germany

Abstract

Early-stage mycosis fungoides shows similar clinical symptoms and histological and immunophenotypical features to several benign lymphoproliferative skin disorders. We analyzed T cell receptor gamma gene rearrangementment by polymerase chain reaction in the search for monoclonal lymphoid subpopulations in skin infiltrates.

Totally, 283 skin biopsies (paraffin-embedded and frozen material) from patients with different malignant and reactive skin diseases were investigated. Using primers for the T cell receptor gamma chain gene, monoclonality was detected in 59 out of 66 (89%) cases of pleomorphic cutaneous lymphoma, in 60 out of 78 (77%) patients with mycosis fungoides, in 11 out of 22 (50%) cases of parapsoriasis en plaques, in five out of 35 (14%) cases of pseudolymphoma, in six out of 15 (40%) patients with lymphomatoid papulosis, and in none out of 64 patients with inflammatory skin diseases.

The results show that clonal T cell population can be detected in the majority of patients with cutaneous T cell lymphoma, but the findings have to be correlated with the histological and morphological features.

Introduction

Cutaneous malignant lymphomas comprise a group of rare and heterogeneous diseases. Their diagnosis depends on clinical appearance, histological and cytological characteristics, and the expression of cell surface molecules as detectable by the use of monoclonal antibodies (Sterry 1992; Verga and Braver man 1991). Using these criteria, it is possible to diagnose typical and more advanced cases of cutaneous lymphomas without any problem. However, it is only the availability of molecular biology techniques, particularly

Recent Results in Cancer Research, Vol. 139

the possibility of amplifying specific DNA sequences using polymerase chain reaction (PCR), that allows a reliable diagnosis of atypical or early cases.

In this review, we will describe the currently used methods for detection of T and B cell clones in lymphoproliferative malignancies by means of PCR, summarize our own data of more than 250 patients, and outline future uses of this powerful approach in the management of patients with malignant lymphomas of the skin.

Definition of Genes with Potential Use for Detection of T or B Cell Clones

The characteristics of a gene to be used for detection of a T or B cell clone should be as follows: (a) such a gene should have a unique sequence, making it a specific marker for the cell that carries this gene; (b) it should have regions flanking the unique sequence that ideally are constant, allowing the use of a single primer pair to amplify the region of interest; (c) this unique region should be present in every patient with a given lymphoma; (d) this sequence also should be present in the DNA of every tumor cell, from the initial stages of the disease to the final highly transformed lymphoblasts; (e) the unique sequence should not become lost or changed during tumor progression.

Such an ideal gene combining these characteristics has not yet been identified, thus making it necessary to use genes that have only two or three of these features. On the basis of theoretical considerations, three types of genes could be used to detect clone-specific gene sequences: (1) Genes coding for cell surface antigen receptors, i.e., heavy and light chain genes of the immunglobulin, or the genes of the α/β or γ/δ T cell antigen receptor (TCR) (Reis et al. 1990). The antigen recognition site of the antigen receptor with its virtually unlimited variability is localized at the junction of V and D or J segments, generated by random insertion or deletion of nucleotides, and referred to as complementarity determining region 3 (CDR3). The CDR3 region can be regarded as the genetic fingerprint of T or B cells (Quertermous et al. 1986, 1987). (2) Oncogenes relevant for the respective tumor carrying specific mutations in the clone deriving from the cell initially affected by the mutation. Examples are p53, *ras*, or *myc* oncogenes. (3) Fusion genes resulting from chromosomal translocations or deletions, particularly if they have been generated by illegimate action of recombinases generating unique DNA sequences.

However, these candidate genes for clone detection have specific disadvantages: antigen receptor genes do not exhibit constant areas flanking the unique DNA sequence, since hundreds of different V segments and several J and C segments are localized up- and downstream. Oncogenes may be mutated at different sites, which would require various primer sets to identify at least the most frequent mutation hot spots. Furthermore, such genes may become deleted during tumor progression, making their use as clonal marker less attractive. Fusion genes generated by translocation or deletion have the advantage of having constant flanking regions, allowing their easy detection; however, while such fusion genes occur very frequently in certain leukemias and can be used as clonal markers, they are rare and highly variable in cutaneous malignant lymphomas known so far. Of all the candidate genes, the antigen receptor genes are at present the only ones that are used for detection of clones in cutaneous lymphomas, since they are present in virtually every case, are not subject to further modification or gene loss, and are absolutely tumor specific (Sklar and Weiss 1988). The major problem, the highly variable flanking regions, has been overcome in recent years by either using consensus primers or primer mixes.

T Cell Receptor Gene Polymerase Chain Reaction for Detection of T Cell Clones

Since T cells may express receptors either of the α/β or γ/δ type, there are principally four genes available for diagnostic purposes. The vast majority of cutaneous T cell lymphomas express the α/β type TCR (Leftanc et al. 1986a). Since the δ chain, which is localized within the α chain locus, is eliminated during α chain rearrangement, it is not available for analysis. On the other hand, both the α and the β chain contain numerous V segments, making it difficult to amplify the unique CDR3. Although some authors have used TCR RNA for identifying the unique messenger RNA of the malignant clone, this requires frozen material and prevents this approach from being routinely used (Volkenandt et al. 1991).

At present, most groups take advantage of the fact that all α/β TCR-positive T cells also contain at least one rearranged allele of the γ chain gene. The relatively simple structure of this gene is illustrated in Fig. 1: in contrast to α and β TCR genes, the γ gene contains only a very limited number of V segments, some of them being pseudogenes that cannot be rearranged since they lack the recombinase recognition sites, and only two C regions (Griesser et al. 1990).

Two possible PCR techniques exist to amplify the CDR3 region of the TCR γ chain gene. One group of authors uses a pair of consensus primers, annealing to the V segment between nucleotides 272 and 290 and to the J segment between nucleotides 45 and 62 (Lefranc et al. 1986b). Other groups, including our own, use specific primers for all known V and J segments, which are combined intwo primer mixes (Trainor et al. 1991). Mix I contains TCR γ V 2, 3, 4, 8, and 9 primers; mix II contains TCR γ V 5, 10, 11, and 12 primers. The three J segment primers are included in each of the two mixes. The obtained PCR products are analyzed by use of temperature gradient gel electrophoresis (TGGE) as described by Rosenbaum and Riesner (1987). In Fig. 2 such a gel is shown; Table 1 summarizes our data generated by TCR γ chain PCR in cutaneous T cell-dominated skin diseases.

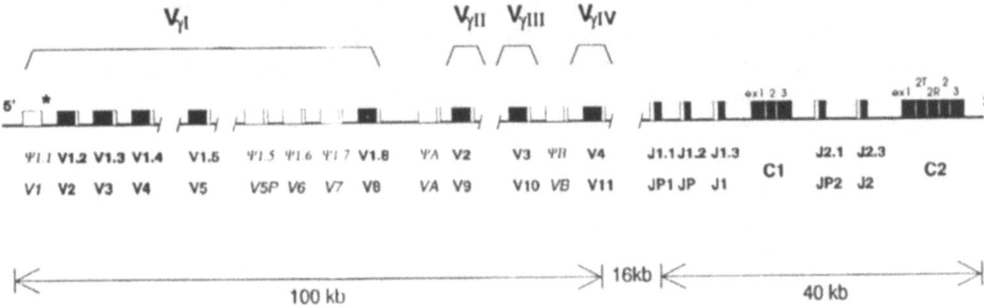

Fig. 1. Human T cell receptor (TCR) gamma locus. Two alternative nomenclatures are used: *upper* according to Quertermous et al. (1986), *lower* according to Lefranc et al. (1986a). V genes are clustered over about 100 kb and are divided into four subgroups (I–IV). *Asterisk* indicates the incomplete recombination signal sequences (RSS) 3′ of V1. V pseudogenes (*white*) are nonfunctional. J regions are divided into two arrays 5′ from C1 and C2, respectively. J1.2 has no analogue in the second J group and significantly differs from the others in its heptamer/nonamer sequences

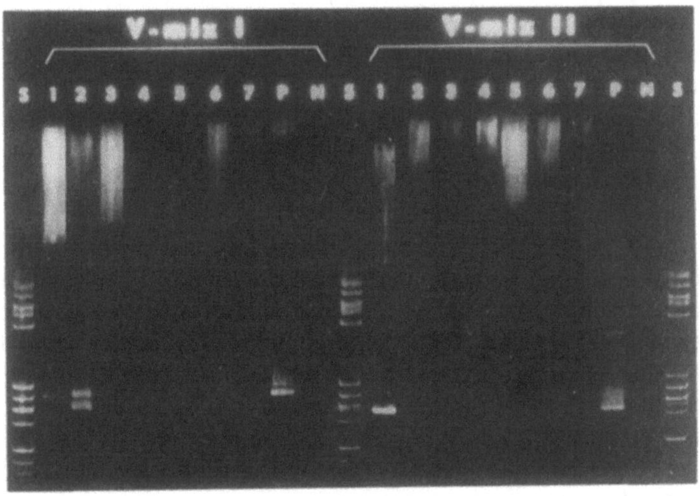

Fig. 2. Temperature gradient gel electrophoresis (TGGE) of seven skin infiltrates (*1–7*), positive (*P*) and negative (*N*) controls, and a low molecular weight DNA marker (*S*, pBR 322 HaeIII-digest.), performed after polymerase chain reaction (PCR) of T cell receptor (TCR) gamma chain genes. Both primer mixtures are shown separately. Gel slots *1* and *2*, monoclonal (positive) infiltrates of patients with pleomorphic T cell lymphoma; gel slots *3–7*, polyclonal (negative) skin infiltrates of parapsoriasis, pseudolymphoma, early stage of mycosis fungoides, patch test reaction, and psoriasis

Table 1. Clonality in cutaneous T cell infiltrates; polymerase chain reaction (PCR) of T cell receptor gamma chain genes

Diagnosis	Total	Monoclonal	
	(*n*)	(*n*)	(%)
Cutaneous T cell lymhomas	145	120	82
Pleomorphic T cell lymphomas	66	59	89
Mycosis fungoides	78	60	77
Patch stage	56	40	71
Plaque stage	17	15	88
Tumor stage	5	5	100
Sézary syndrome	1	1	100
T cell lymphoma-associated diseases	72	19	26
Parapsoriasis en plaques	22	11	50
Lymphomatoid papulosis	15	3	20
Pseudolymphomas	35	5	14
Inflammatory skin disorders	64	0	0
Psoriasis	14	0	0
Pityriasis lichenoides	10	0	0
Positive patch test reaction	10	0	0
Dermatitis (toxic, allergic contact)	20	0	0
Lichen planus	10	0	0
Total	281	139	49

Immunoglobulin Heavy Chain Polymerase Chain Reaction for Detection of B Cell Clones

With the same sensitivity as for cutaneous T cell lymphomas, in B cell-dominated infiltrates the detection of a clonal B cell population is possible using PCR for the immunoglobulin (Ig) heavy chain gene. The Ig heavy chain gene contains a sequence that is suitable for use of consensus primers in the PCR (Wan et al. 1990). For its amplification, we use a seminested PCR with three primers: a first round of 30 cycles with LJH and FR3A and then a second round of 20 cycles with primers VLJH and FR3A (Fig. 3). The amplification product is analyzed on an agarose gel with standard ethidium bromide staining (Fig. 4). Table 2 shows the results for different B and T cell-infiltrated skin biopsies using lg heavy chain gene PCR.

Fusion Gene Polymerase Chain Reaction for Detection of Tumor Cell Clones

The activation of the *bcl-2* gene by the (14;18) translocation in follicular lymphomas is well established, occurring in over 85% of cases. It seems that the translocation occurs at the same time as the lg gene rearrangement,

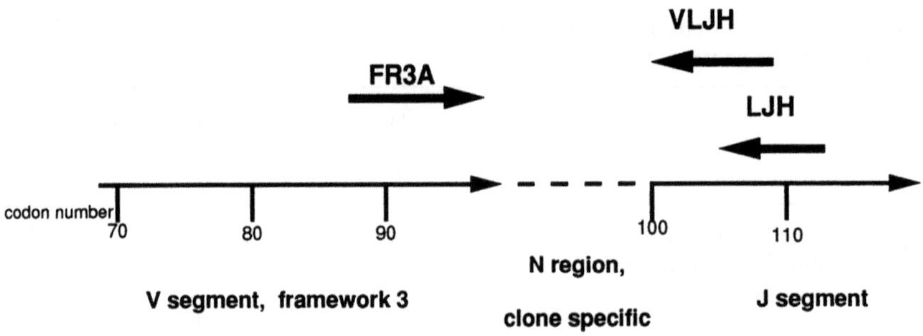

Fig. 3. Location of the primer sequences in the immunoglobulin heavy chain gene

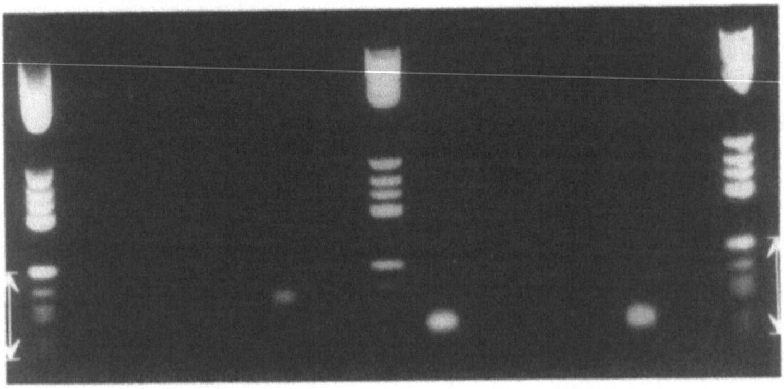

Fig. 4. Agarose gel electrophoresis of three probes, positive (*P*) and negative (*N*) controls and a low molecular weight DNA marker (*S*, pBR 322 HaeIII-digest.), performed after seminested polymerase chain reaction (PCR) of immunoglobulin heavy chain genes. The amplification products of the first 30 cycles are separated in the slots *left* of the middle DNA marker and the products of all 50 cycles are shown *right* of the marker. Gel slot *1*, monoclonal case of B cell lymphoma of the skin. Only the positive control (Ramos cell line) already shows a slight band after the first round

Table 2. Seminested polymerase chain reaction (PCR) of immunoglobulin heavy chain genes

Diagnosis	Analyzed (*n*)	Monoclonal (*n*)
Cutaneous B cell lymphoma	15	13
Pseudolymphoma	19	0
Cutaneous T cell lymphoma	19	4

since the breakpoint appears at a J segment adjacent to a heptamer–nonamer signal sequence. The consequence of the (14;18) translocation is a deregulation of the *bcl-2* gene, which has recently been shown to act as an inhibitor of apoptosis, thus prologing the life span of B cells. However, several groups that have investigated the occurrence of (14;18) translocations in follicular lymphomas of the skin have demonstrated that (14;18) translocations are extremely rare and may only occur if there is secondary skin involvement of nodular follicular lymphomas. Therefore, *bcl-2* breakpoint analyses as tumor-specific markers are not possible in primary cutaneous follicular B cell lymphomas (Jansen et al. 1993).

Another fusion gene which is relatively frequent in lymphatic leukemia of T cell type is the SIL/TAL translocation. This translocation also generates unique DNA sequences, which can be used as clone-specific markers. However, when we analyzed 16 cutaneous T cell lymphomas, we could not find a single case in which this SIL/TAL translocation was demonstrated, again excluding this fusion gene for use in the detection of clones in cutaneous malignant lymphomas.

Therefore, we summarize that in cutaneous malignant lymphomas there are no known translocations that occur with a frequency sufficently high for use as clone-specific markers.

Monitoring of Patients with Cutaneous Malignant Lymphomas

For a few weeks now we have been able to detect a clonal T cell population in the peripheral blood of patients with cutaneous malignant lymphomas. Therefore, the mononuclear cells are separated out of 20 ml heparinized blood (Ficoll gradient) and an average of 10×10^6 cells are used for the PCR. The amplification conditions are the same as described for the PCR of the T cell gamma chain gene in the skin infiltrate. Our first results for the detection of clonal cell population in the peripheral blood are summarized in Tabel 3.

The possibility of amplifying the CDR3 regions of the antigen receptors of both T and B cells also allows us to sequence these regions and thus to construct clone-specific primers that will only amplify the malignant clone of the patient. Having such primers in hand, one may then be able to monitor patients specifically during treatment as well as during remission. If these investigations are performed on a broader scale using patient-specific primers, we may be able to analyze how the tumor burden in the skin, the lymph nodes, and the peripheral blood of patients with cutaneous malignant lymphomas behaves during therapy. We may anticipate from similar studies in leukemias that not all patients that are in clinical remission will show a complete disappearance of the malignant cells in the physiological compartments of the respective lymphocyte subpopulation. We will have to discover how big the remaining tumor burden may be without leading to clinical

Table 3. Clonal T cell population in the peripheral blood of patients with cutaneous malignant lymphoma[a]

Diagnosis	Analyzed (*n*)	Clonality	
		Skin (*n*)	Blood (*n*)
Pleomorphic T cell lymphoma	7	7	7
Mycosis fungoides			
Patch stage	16	5	8
Plaque + tumor stage	6	5	6

[a] Average of 12×10^6 mononuclear cells; polymerase chain reaction (PCR) analyses of the T cell receptor (TCR) gamma chain before treatment

relapses and where the threshold concentrations requiring further treatment have to be defined. Investigations of this type will most likely lead to more specific and more clearly defined treatment protocols.

References

Griesser H, Feller A, Sterry W (1990) T-cell receptor and immunoglobulin gene rearrangement in cutaneous T-cell rich pseudolymphomas. J Invest Dermatol 95(3):292–295

Jansen J, Ludwig W, Sterry W (1993) SIL-TAL 1 deletion in T-cell acute lymphoblastic leukemia. Leukemia 7:1204–1210

Lefranc M, Forster A, Rabbits T (1986a) Rearrangement of two distinct T-cell gamma-chain variable-region genes in human DNA. Nature 319:420–422

Lefranc M, Forster A, Bear R (1986b) Diversity and rearrangement of the human T-cell rearranging gamma gene: nine derm-line variable genes belonging to two subgroups. Cell 45:237–246

Quertermous T, Strauss W et al. (1986) Human T-Cell gamma genes contain N segments and have marked junctional variability. Nature 322:184–187

Quertermous T, Strauss W, Dongen J (1987) Human T-cell gamma chain joining regions and T-cell development. J Immunol 138(8):2687–2690

Reis M, Griesser H, Mak T (1990) T-cell receptor and immunoglobin genes in hematologic malignancies. Tumor Biol 11(1):59–77

Rosenbaum V, Riesner D (1987) Temperature-gradient gel electrophoresis. Thermodynamic analysis of nuceic acids and proteins in purified form and in cellular extracts. Biophys Chem 26:235–246

Sklar J, Weiss L (1988) Applications of antigen receptor gene rearrangements to the diagnosis and characterization of lymphoid neoplasms. Annul Rev Med 39:315–334

Sterry W (1992) Mycosis fungoides and other T-cell lymphomas of the skin. Dermatology 4:1–22

Trainor KJ, Brisco M, Wan J (1991) Gene rearrangement in B- and T- lymphoproliferative disease detected by the polymerase chain reaction. Blood 78(1):192–196

Verga M, Braverman I (1991) The use of immunohistologic analysis in differentiating cutaneous T-cell lymphoma from psoriasis and dermatitis. Arch Dermatol 127: 1503–1510

Volkenandt M et al (1991) Development of a highly specific and sensitive molecular probe for detection of cutaneous lymphoma. J Invest Dermatol 97:137

Wan J, Trainor K, Brisco M (1990) Monoclonality in B-cell lymphoma detected in paraffin embedded sections by use of the polymerase chain reaction. J Clin Pathol 43:888–890

bcl-1, bcl-2, p53, c-myc, and lyt-10 Analysis in Cutaneous Lymphomas

S.A. Garatti[1,2], E. Roscetti[1,2], D. Trecca[1], N.S. Fracchiolla[1], A. Neri[1], and E. Berti[2]

[1] Laboratorio di Ematologia Sperimentale e Genetica molecolare, Servizio di Ematologia, Istituto di Scienze Mediche, Via Pace 9, 20122 Milan, Italy
[2] Istituto di Scienze Dermatologiche, Università degli Studi di Milano, Ospedale Maggiore IRCCS, 20122 Milan, Italy

Abstract

In the present study we investigated the pathogenetic role of c-*myc*, *bcl*-2, and *lyt*-10 oncogenes, *bcl*-1 locus, and p53 suppressor gene in a representative panel of cutaneous lymphomas, including 25 cases of cutaneous B cell lymphoma (CBCL) and 29 cases of cutaneous T cell lymphoma (CTCL). In our analysis four cases of CBCL were found rearranged for *bcl*-2 and two for the *bcl*-1 locus. Two cases of CTCL and one case of CBCL were found rearranged for *lyt*-10. No rearrangements of c-*myc* oncogene were found in CBCL. Analysis of p53 gene showed mutation only in one case of mycosis fungoides in tumoral stage, at codon 163 of p53 gene (TAC → CAC; Tyr → Asp). Our data suggest that in primary CBCL *bcl*-2 oncogenes and *bcl*-1 locus are rarely involved. Furthermore, in primary CTCL p53 gene is not affected at significant frequency. The occurrence of p53 mutation in a patient affected by mycosis fungoides in tumoral stage may represent an involvement of p53 gene in tumor progression of CTCL, a finding observed in several types of human cancer.

Introduction

Cutaneous lymphomas represent a heterogeneous group of lymphoid malignancies. Cutaneous T cell lymphomas (CTCL) have been extensively investigated over the last 10 years, allowing the definition of several pathological entities. The most frequent CTCL are represented by mycosis fungoides (MF), Sezary's Syndrome (SS), T pleomorphic lymphomas (PTL) HTLV-1 +/−, and anaplastic large cell lymphoma (ALCL; Kerl et al. 1991; Le Boit 1991). It is not universally agreed upon whether CBCL originate from germinal center cells, mantle cells, or marginal B cell. On the basis of cytotype, the majority of these cases were classified as germinal centre-

Recent Results in Cancer Research, Vol. 139

derived B lymphomas (Willemze et al. 1987; Berti et al. 1991). Another frequent type of CBCL is the immunocytoma. Very rare CBCL are lymphoblastic and immunoblastic primary ones.

Human cancers are generally associated with alterations of particular genes which normally appear to control cellular growth and differentiation. These genes, called "proto-oncogenes," may be activated in human cancer by several mechanisms, such as chromosome translocations, point mutations, insertions or deletions, and genic amplification; their activated forms are called "oncogenes." Up to now, more than 50 proto-oncogenes and loci frequently associated with cancers have been found. They have been subdivided into classes and families on the basis of various criteria (Dalla Favera and Ceserman 1986). In the context of lymphoid malignancies, four oncogenes have been extensively characterized: c-*myc*, *bcl*-2, *ras*, and c-*abl* (Krolewski and Dalla Favera 1989). In addition, the *bcl*-1 locus, involved in chromosomic translocation t(11;14)(q13;q32), was found in some lymphoid malignancies, in particular in about 30%–50% of lymphocytic lymphomas of intermediate differentiation/centrocytic lymphomas (IDL/Cc; Tsujimoto et al. 1984; Weisenburg et al. 1987; Rimokh et al. 1990; Medeiros et al. 1990; Raffeld and Jaffe 1991). The last two oncogenes, *ras* and c-*abl*, were not found to be involved in lymphomas, but only in leukemias, so we focused our attention on c-*myc*, *bcl*-2 oncogenes, and *bcl*-1 locus.

Chromosomic translocations of the 10q24 band are quite frequent in lymphoid neoplasias, involving T cell receptor (TCR) and JH regions (Dube et al. 1986; Hatano et al. 1991). Recently, in a case of B non-Hodgkin lymphoma, a new putative oncogene, t(10;14)(q24;q32), was isolated and named *lyt*-10 (lymphocyte translocation chromosome 10; Neri et al. 1991).

In recent years cellular genes, whose function consists in a negative regulation of cellular growth and differentiation, have been found. These genes are altered in many human cancers and are called "tumor suppressor genes." Human p53 gene is one of these genes; it lies on chromosome 17p13 and has been examined in a wide spectrum of primary tumors (Mackay et al. 1988; Baker et al. 1989; Nigro et al. 1989; Takahashi et al. 1989; Kelman et al. 1989; Gaidano et al. 1991). Usually the mechanisms that lead to the loss of p53 function are allelic delections following by mutations of surviving allele, which lead to functional inactivation of genic product. However, in some cases, p53 gene behaves as a dominant negative oncogene (Baker et al. 1989; Lavinguer et al. 1989; Milner and Medcalf 1991). Mutations in the p53 gene are turning out to be the most common genetic alterations in human cancers.

The aim of the present study was to investigate the pathogenetic role of c-*myc* and *bcl*-2 oncogenes, *bcl*-1 and *lyt*-10 (Neri et al. 1991) loci, and p53 tumor suppressor gene in a representative panel of cutaneous lymphomas including 25 cases of CBCL (analyzed for all the genes cited above) and 29 cases of CTCL (analyzed only for p53 and *lyt*-10).

Material and Methods

We have studied 54 cases of cutaneous lymphomas, 29 of which were CTCL analyzed exclusively for p53 gene and *lyt*-10 locus and 25 cases of CBCL analyzed for c-*myc*, *bcl*-2, *bcl*-1, *lyt*-10, and p53 gene. Pathologic skin biopsies have been taken during normal diagnostic procedures.

The 29 cases of CTCL were represented by 16 cases of MF (seven in tumoral stage, seven not tumoral, and two erythrodermic variants), five cases of medium and large pleomorphic T cell lymphoma Ki-1+ (PTL), four cases of ALCL Ki-1^+, two cases of $CD8^+$ CTCL, and two cases of lymphomatoid papulosis (Lyp).

The 25 cases of CBCL included three cases of centroblastic–centrocytic, follicular, and diffuse (CbCcF/D), 12 cases of CbCc, eight cases of Cb, one case of Cc, and one case of lymphoplasmocytoid IC. Of these, one Cc and two CbCc lymphoma were not primary cutaneous lymphomas, but secondary localizations in patients with a nodal lymphoma.

High molecular weight genomic DNA was obtained from fresh or frozen samples owing to digestion with proteinase K, extraction with phenol chloroform, and precipitation with ethanol.

Southern Blot Hybridization

Southern blot hybridization was used for immunoglobulin heavy chain (IgH), TCR, c-*myc*, *bcl*-2, *bcl*-1, and *lyt*-10 rearrangements analysis.

Eight to ten micrograms DNA was completely digested with the restriction enzymes *Eco*RI, *Bam*HI, *Hind*III, and, in selected instances, *SACI*. The digested DNA was electrophoresed through 0.7% agarose gel, put in denaturing solution (NaOH 0.5 *M*; NaCl 1.5 *M*) for 45 min, then in neutralizing solution (TRIS 0.5 *M*; NaCl 3.0 *M*; pH 7.4) for 60 min, and finally transferred to nylon membranes (Hybond-N+). Prehybridization and hybridization was carried out in a solution of TRIS HCl (pH 7.4) 0.1 *M*, formamide 50%, standard saline citrate (SSC) 3X, sodium dodecyl sulphate (SDS) 0.1%, Denhardt's 5%, ss-DNA 10 mg/ml, Dextran sulfate 10%; 3×10^6 cpm/ml labeled probe were added to the hybridization solution. Filters were prehybridized for 3 h at 37°C and hybridized for 15–20 h at the same temperature. The probes used were:

- For IgH locus, a 6.0-kb *Bam*HI–*Hind*III fragment specific for the joining region (JH)
- For TCR-β locus, a 0.8-kb Pst I insert specific for the constant β_1 region
- For TCR-γ locus, a 0.7-kb *Eco*RI–*Hind*III fragment JTγ
- For c-*myc*, an *Eco*RI–*Cla*I fragment specific for the third exon
- For *bcl*-2, the 1.5-kb *Hind*III–*Eco*RI insert from the pFL-1 specific for the major breakpoint cluster region (MBR)

- For *bcl*-1, the probe specific for the major translocation cluster (MTC) breakpoint, a 1.8-kb *Sac*I fragment, and the additional probe designated p94 PS (p94), a 460-bp *Pvu*II–*Sma*I genomic fragment that lies approximately 23.4 kb 5′ of the MTC
- For *lyt*-10, three probes, namely PV/H 1.4 kb, Pst 1.5 kb, and *Eco*RI 3 kb specific for the 5′ and 3′ regions of the gene

Each probe was labeled with $\alpha[^{32}P]$dCTP using the random priming method (Feinberg and Vogelstein 1984). Following hybridization, filters were washed three times at room temperature and subsequently twice for 30 min at 60°C with a solution of SSC 1X/ SDS 1X and exposed to XAR-5 film with two intensifying screen at −80°C for 2–7 days.

Polymerase Chain Reaction, Single-Strand Conformation Polymorphism Analysis and Direct Sequencing

Analysis of mutations in exons 5–9 of p53 gene was performed in CBCL and CTCL by polymerase chain reaction (PCR; Saiki et al. 1988), single strand conformation polymorphism (SSCP; Orita et al. 1989a,b), and direct sequencing of amplyified fragment (Sanger et al. 1977).

Oligonucleotide Primers

All the oligonucleotides used for PCR amplification in this study were synthesized by the solid-phase triester method (Neri et al. 1988). Names and sequences of p53 primers are as follows:

1. P5-5, 5′-TTCCTCTTCCTGCAGTACTC-3′ (nucleotides 911–930)
2. P6-3, 5′-AGTTGCAAACCAGACCTCAG-3′ (nucleotides 1249–1268)
3. P7-5, 5′-GTGTTGTCTCCTAGGTTGGC-3′ (nucleotides 1269–1288)
4. P8-5, 5′-TATCCTGAGTAGTGGTAATC-3′ (nucleotides 1411–1430)
5. P9-3, 5′-AAGACTTAGTACCTGAAGGGT-3′ (nucleotides 1654–1674)
6. P5-3, 5′-ACCCTGGGCAACCAGCCCTGT-3′ derived from intron 5 sequence
7. P6-5, 5′-ACAGGGCTGGTTGCCCAGGGT-3′, derived from intron 5 sequence
8. P7-3, 5′-GTCAGAGGCAAGCAGAGGCT-3′, derived from intron 7 sequence
9. P8-3, 5′-AAGTGAATCTGAGGCATAAC-3′, derived from intron 8 sequence
10. P9-5, 5′-GCAGTTATGCCTCAGATTCAC-3′, derived from intron 8 sequence

Single-Strand Conformation Polymorphism Analysis

SSCP analysis was accomplished according to an adapted version of a previously reported method (Orita et al. 1989). Briefly, PCR were performed with 100 ng genomic DNA, 5 pmol of each primer, 2.5 μ*M* dNTP, 1 μCi of α[^{32}P]dCTP, 10 m*M* TRIS-HCl (pH 8.8), 50 m*M* KCl, 2 m*M* $MgCl_2$, 0.01% gelatine, 0.05 units Taq polymerase (Cetus), in a final volume of 10 μl. Thirty cycles of denaturation (94°C), annealing (63°C for reactiones amplifying exons 5,6,7, and 9; 58°C for exon 8), and extension (72°C) were done on an automated heat block (DNA thermal cycler; Perkin-Elmer/Cetus). The reaction mixture (6 μl) was diluted in 25 μl 0.1% SDS/10 m*M* EDTA (pH 8.0) solution; 4 μl of the obtained solution was mixed 1:1 with a sequencing stop solution (Sambrook et al. 1989) containing 20 m*M* NaOH. Samples were heated at 95°C for 5 min, chilled on ice, and immediately loaded onto a 6% acrylamide/TBE gel containing 10% (Vol/Vol) glycerol. Gels were run at 8 W for 12–15 h at room temperature. Autoradiography was performed with an intensifying screen for 6–8 h.

Direct Sequencing of Polymerase Chain Reaction Products

Direct sequencing of the amplified product was performed as described by Sanger et al. (1977).

Results

Southern Blot Hybridization Analysis

DNA extracted from 25 biopsies of CBCL was analyzed for rearrangements of the immunoglobulin heavy chain (JH), c-*myc*, *bcl*-2, *bcl*-1, and *lyt*-10 genes. DNA extracted from 29 biopsies of CTCL was analyzed for rearrangement of TCR-β and TCR-γ genes and *lyt*-10 locus. The results are listed in Tables 1 and 2.

Analysis of Cutaneous B cell lymphoma. By using JH probe for the immunoglobulin heavy chain gene, monoclonal rearrangement bands were found in 23 out of 25 cases (Fig. 1a). Rearrangements of c-*myc* gene were not present in any of the samples examined (data not shown).

Four cases out of 25 CBCL (two cases of secondary and two cases of primary cutaneous follicular lymphomas) were found rearranged for *bcl*-2 gene using the probe pFL1, and two cases (a case of secondary Cc and a case of primary cutaneous CbCc lymphoma) were found rearranged for *bcl*-1 locus using the probe for the MTC breakpoint, a 1.8-kb *Sac*I fragment (Fig. 1b) and the P94 probe.

Only in one Cb case was *lyt*-10 rearrangement detected.

Table 1. Summary of Southern blot analysis of 25 cases of cutaneous B cell lymphoma (CBCL)

Case no.	Diagnosis	JH	*bcl*-1 MTC	*bcl*-1 P94	*bcl*-2 PFL-1	*bcl*-2 PFL-2	c-*myc*	*lyt*-10
B1	CBCC	R	G	G	G	G	G	G
B2	CB	R	G	G	R	G	G	G
B3	CBCC[a]	R	G	G	R	G	G	G
B4	CBCC	R	G	G	G	G	G	G
B5	CBCC	R	G	G	G	G	G	G
B6	CBCC[a]	R	G	G	R	G	G	ND
B7	CBCC F/D	R	G	G	G	G	G	G
B8	CB	R	G	ND	G	ND	ND	ND
B9	CBCC	R	G	G	G	ND	G	ND
B10	CBCC	R	G	G	G	ND	G	ND
B11	CBCC	R	ND	ND	ND	ND	G	ND
B12	LPC	R	G	G	G	G	G	G
B13	CB	R	G	G	ND	G	ND	ND
B14	CB	R	G	G	G	G	G	ND
B15	CB	R	G	G	G	G	G	R
B16	CB	R	G	G	G	G	G	G
B17	CBCC	R	G	G	G	G	G	G
B18	CB	R	G	ND	G	G	ND	ND
B19	CB	R	G	G	G	G	G	ND
B20	CBCC F/D	R	G	G	G	G	G	G
B21	CBCC	R	G	G	G	G	G	G
B22	CBCC F/D	G?	G	R	G	ND	G	G
B23	CBCC	R	G	G	G	G	G	G
B24	CC[a]	R	R	G	G	G	G	G
B25	CBCC	G?	G	G	R	G	G	G

JH, c-*myc*, *bcl*-2, *bcl*-1, and *lyt*-10 configurations were assessed on *Eco*RI and *Bam*HI DNA digests. In addition, case B2 was also digested with *Sac*I and case B12 also with *Hind*III. *bcl*-1 results derive from hybridization with a 1.8-kb *Sac*I fragment specific for major translocation cluster (MTC) breakpoint and p94 probes.
CbCc, centroblastic–centrocytic diffuse; CbCcFD, centroblastic–centrocytic follicular and diffuse; Cb, centroblastic diffuse; Cc, centrocytic diffuse; LPC, lymphoplasmocytoid; R, rearranged; G, germline; ND, not done.
[a] Secondary lesion in patients with a previous or simultaneous nodal B lymphoma.

Analysis of Cutaneous T Cell Lymphoma. Rearrangements of TCR-β and/or TCR-γ were detected in all cases (Table 2). *Lyt*-10 rearrangement was found in two cases of tumoral MF.

Single-Strand Conformation Polymorphism Analysis and Direct Sequencing for p53 Gene Analysis

Analysis of p53 gene, performed both in CBCL and CTCL cases, showed a mutation in one case out of 54. The mutation involved a case of MF in

Table 2. Summary of Southern blot analysis of 25 cases of cutaneous T cell lymphoma (CTCL)

Tumor type	Case no.	TCR-B			TCR-γ			*lyt*-10	
		E	B	H	E	B	H	E	B
Tumoral MF	T1	R	R	R	R	R	R	R	
	T2	R	R	R	R	R	R	R	
	T3	R	G	G	G	R	R	G	
	T4	R	R	R	R	R	R	G	
	T5	R	ND	R	R	ND	R	G	
	T6	R?	ND	G?	R?	ND	R	G	
	T7	R	R	ND	R	R	ND	G	
Nontumoral MF	T8	R	R	G	R	R	R	G	
	T9	R	R	R	R	R	R	G	
	T10	R	R	R	R	R	R	G	
	T11	R?	G	G	R	G	R?	G	
	T12	R	R	G	R	R	R	G	
	T13	R	R	R	R	ND	R	G	
	T14	R	G?	ND	R	R	ND	G	
	T15	R	ND	ND	R?	ND	ND	G	
	T16	R	G?	ND	R?	G	ND	G	
Pleom./Ki-1+	T17	R	ND	G	R	ND	R	G	
	T18	R	R	ND	ND	ND	ND	G	
	T19	R	R	ND	ND	ND	ND	G	
	T20	R	R	ND	ND	ND	ND	G	
	T21	R	R	ND	ND	ND	ND	G	
ALCL-Ki-1+	T22	R	ND	G	G	ND	G	G	
	T23[a]	R	ND	ND	R	ND	R	G	
	T24	G	G	G	G	G	R	G	
	T25	R	R	ND	R	R	ND	G	
CD8$^+$ LY	T26	R	R	ND	R	R	ND	G	
	T27	R	R	ND	R	R	ND	ND	
Lyp	T28	R	R	R	R	ND	R	G	
	T29	R?	R	ND	R	ND	ND	G	

E, *Eco*RI; B, *Bam*HI; H, *Hing*III; R, rearranged; G, germline; ND, not done; MF, mycosis fungoides; Pleom, pleomorphic T cell lymphoma; CD8$^+$ LY, CD8$^+$ CTCL; Lyp, lymphomation papulosis; ALCL, anaplastic large cell lymphoma; TCR, T cell receptor.

[a] Lymph nodal biopsy.

tumoral stage (one out of seven) at codon 163 of p53 gene (TAC → CAC; Tyr → Asp). The results SSCP analysis are summarized in Table 3, while representative results and the case presenting mutation are shown in Fig. 2.

Discussion

In the present paper we have examined the involvement of several oncogenes in a representative group of 54 CTCL and CBCL.

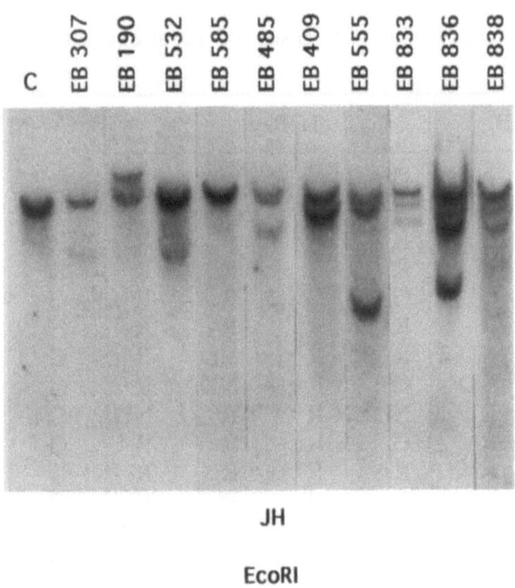

a

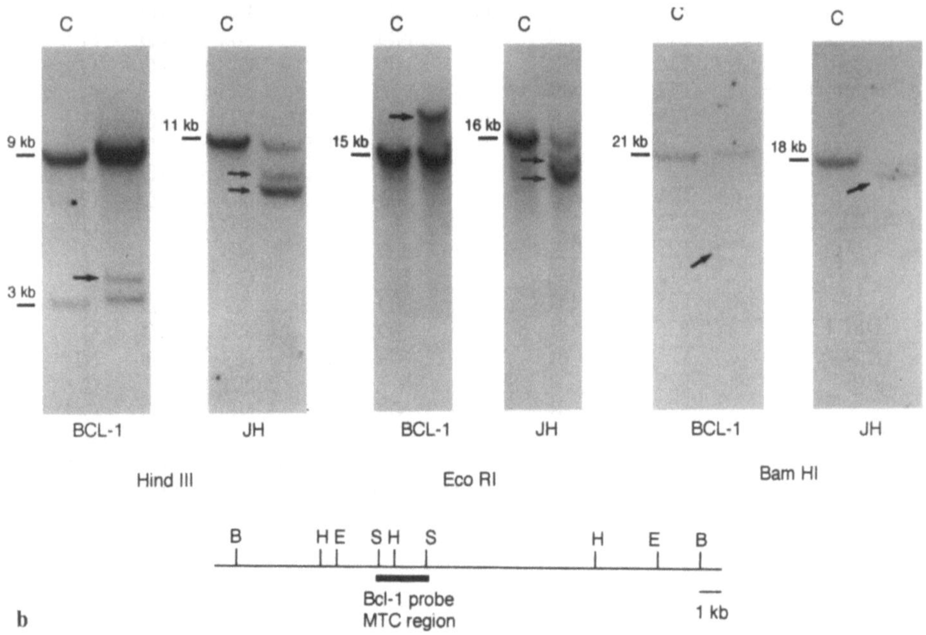

b

Fig. 1. a Southern blot analysis of the immunoglobulin heavy chain gene rearrangement. DNA from ten representative cases of cutaneous B cell lymphoma (CBCL) was digested with *Eco*RI restriction enzyme, fractionated in 0.8% agarose gel, transferred to Nylon membrane, and hybridized to JH probe. *C*, human placental DNA. Germline band is indicate by *dash*. **b** Southern blot analysis of the *bcl*-1 locus. DNA from case B24 (see Table 1) was digested with following restriction enzymes: *Hin*DIII, *Eco*RI, *Bam*HI, fractionated in 0.8% agarose gel, and transferred to Nylon membranes. Filters were subsequently hybridized to JH and *bcl*-1 probes. *Dashes* indicate germline bands and *arrows* indicate rearranged bands. *C*, human placental DNA. In the *lower* panel are shown the *bcl*-1 locus and *bcl*-1 probe used

Table 3. Frequency of p53 mutations (exons 5–9) in cutaneous lymphomas

Diagnosis	Positive	Tested
CBCL	0	25
CbCc	0	12
CbCcF/D	0	3
Cb	0	8
Cc	0	1
LPC	0	1
CTCL	1	29
Tumoral MF	1	7[a]
Nontumoral MF	0	9
Pleomophic/Ki-1+	0	5
ALCL-Ki-1+	0	4
CD8^{+} CTCL	0	2
Lyp	0	2

CBCL, cutaneous B cell lymphoma; CbCc, centroblastic–centrocytic; F/D, follicular and diffuse; LPC, lymphoplasmocytoid; CTCL, cutaneous T cell lymphoma; MF, mycosis fungoides; ALCL, anaplastic large cell lymphoma; Lyp, lymphomatoid papulosis.
[a] Mutation was found in exon 5, codon 163 (TAC → CAC; Tyr → Asp).

In all except two cases, it was possible to demostrate the presence of rearranged bands with JH or TCR-β or TCR-γ probes using Southern blot analysis.

As regards CBCL, recent literature data, particularly some immunohistochemical and genotypical studies, have suggested that primary CBCL are a quite peculiar type of B cell lymphoma, biologically different from their nodal counterpart. Nevertheless, the overall prognosis of CBCL is better than that of their nodal counterpart. The absence of *bcl*-2 rearrangement and the weak cytoplasmic expression or the absence of *bcl*-2 protein, or the negativity of the CD10-CALLA B cell marker (Delia et al. 1989; Volkenandt et al. 1992), for instance, were considered as a marker to differentiate primary cutaneous center cell-derived B lymphomas from nodal lymphomas, in which all these markers are very frequent. It is of interest that analogous results were obtained at the same time from other authors analyzing mucosa-associated lymphoid tissue (MALT)-derived B cell lymphomas, in which a derivation from monocytoid B cells was hypothesized on the basis of cytotype, phenotype, and genotype (Pan et al. 1989; Isaacson et al. 1991; Vandenberghe et al. 1992; Ortiz-Hidalgo and Wright 1992). In MALT-derived B cell lymphomas, the absence of *bcl*-1 locus rearrangement was also reported (Wotherspoon et al. 1990). Our previous immunohistochemical studies (personal communication at the World Congress on Dermatology,

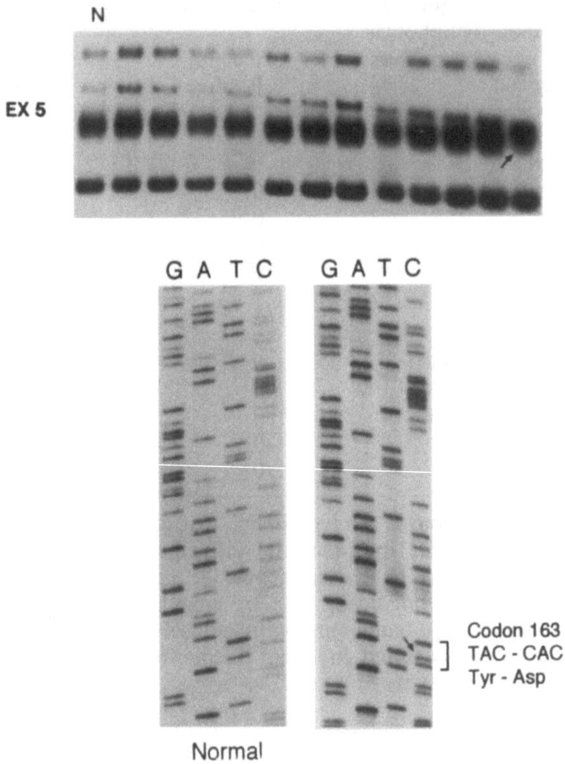

Fig. 2. *Upper panel*, polymerase chain reaction–single-strand contormation polymorphism (PCR-SSCP) analysis of cutaneous T cell lymphoma (CTCL). *N*, human placental DNA. Arrow indicates the abnormal band of case no. 5. *Lower panel*, direct sequencing analysis of exon 5 of p53 gene in placental DNA (normal) and in the SSCP-mutated case. Mutated codon with amino acid substitution is indicated; mutated band is indicated by an *arrow*

New York 1992) showed that primary CBCL are phenotypically heterogeneous and show a variable expression of the B cell markers specific for the different B subsets of the follicle (CD20, CD21, IGD, L-selectin, CD23, CD69, CD72–CD78). In the present study we aimed to complete our previous analysis on *bcl*-2 and c-*myc* involvement in CBCL (Delia et al. 1989). We confirmed the absence of c-*myc* and the rare rearrangement of *bcl*-2. Two primary and two secondary B cell lymphomas, in fact, showed a *bcl*-2 rearrangement which is specific for the follicular nodal B cell lymphomas. This event, very rare in CBCL, should be considered for the evaluation of the possible secondary origin of CBCL.

The histopathological features of primary CBCL might be very heterogeneous; in some cases it is possible to observe neoplastic infiltrate formed by small to medium lymphoid centrocytic-like cells, suggesting intermediate differentiation lymphomas (IDL-Cc), in which the *bcl*-1 locus was found to be frequently involved (Rimokh et al. 1990; Medeiros et al. 1990). In our study we included 25 CBCL, some of which suggesting IDL. Only one of the primary CBCL analyzed showed a rearranged band with the two probes used for the detection of the *bcl*-1 locus. In contrast, in the secondary CBCL case of IDL-Cc lymphoma the presence of a rearranged band was easily detected. These data, even if not conclusive, suggest that the involvement of the *bcl*-1 locus is not relevant in most primary CBCL; they also confirm the specificity of the *bcl*-1 locus for IDL-Cc nodal lymphomas.

The analysis of p53 gene using the PCR technique was also performed to detect the presence of specific mutation, starting out from the literature data, which suggested an involvement of p53 in some cases of malignant lymphomas, mainly in very aggressive forms or in transformed phases as cited in the introduction. We studied several cases of CBCL. In none of these cases did we detect p53 mutation using PCR. These results were not suprising, considering the overall good prognosis of CBCL in comparison with the same nodal cytotype.

Furthermore, we analyzed 29 cases of primary CTCL, including cases of MF in different stages, Lyp, $CD8^+$ CTCL, ALCL, and PTL. We exptected a high incidence of mutations in the more aggressive forms, such as $CD8^+$ CTCL, ALCL, and PTL or in the cases of transformed MF. The results of our analysis showed a mutation in one out of 16 cases of MF. The patient presenting with the mutation was in tumoral stage and histologically showed an immunoblastic transformation. Therefore, in CTCL the event of p53 mutation seems to be rare. This result could be in agreement with previous reports on the presence of p53 mutation in case of "transformed" lymphomas.

Finally, the analysis of the role of a new putative oncogene *lyt*-10, involved in cytogenetics aberration involving region 10q24, showed the presence of rearrangements in three cases: two cases of MF and one case of centroblastic diffuse lymphoma. An extensive study on the expression of *lyt*-10 in several hematological malignancies has been recently reported (Fracchiolla et al. 1993). The significance of the quite frequent *lyt*-10 involvement in cutaneous lymphomas (50% of all hematological malignancies studied) in comparison with other hematological malignancies is unknown.

References

Baker SJ, Fearon ER, Nigro JM et al (1989) Chromosome 17 delections and p53 mutations in colorectal cancer. Science 244:217–221

Berti E, Alessi E, Caputo R (1991) Reticulohistiocytoma of the dorsum (Crosti's disease) and other B-cell lymphomas. Semin Diagn Pathol 8(2):82–90

Dalla Favera R, Ceserman E (1986) Human genes and diseases. In: Blasi F (ed) Genes and diseases, vol 8. Wiley, New York, p 503

Delia D, Borrello MG, Berti E, Pierotti MA et al (1989) Clonal immunoglobulin gene rearrangements and normal T-cell receptor, bcl-2 and c-myc genes in primary cutaneous B-cell lymphomas. Cancer Res 49:4901–4905

Dube ID, Raimondi SC, Kalouser DK (1986) A new translocation, t(10;14) (q24; q11), in T-cell neoplasia. Blood 67:1182–1184
Feinberg AP, Vogelstein B (1984) A technique for radiolabelling DNA restriction endonuclease fragments to high specific activity. Ann Biochem 132:6–13, 266–267
Fracchiolla NS, Lombardi L, Salina M et al (1993) Structural alteration of NF-Kb transcription-factor lyt-10 in lymphoid malignancies. Oncogene 8:2839–2845
Gaidano G, Ballerini P, Gong JZ et al (1991) P53 mutations in human lymphoid malignancies: association with Burkitt lymphoma and chronic lymphocytic leukemia. Proc Natl Acad Sci USA 88:5413–5417
Hatano M, Roberts WM, Minden M et al (1991) Novel homeobox gene, hox 11, is deregulated by the t(10;14) in T-cell leukemia. Science 253:79–82
Isaacson PG, Wotherspoon AC et al (1991) Bcl-2 expression in lymphomas. Lancet 337:175–176
Kelman Z, Prokocinur M, Peller S (1989) Rearrangements in the p53 gene in Philadelphia chromosome positive chronic myelogeneous leukemia. Blood 74: 2318–2324
Kerl H, Cerroni L, Burg G (1991) The morphologic spectrum of T-cell lymphomas of the skin: a proposal for a new classification. Semin Diagn Pathol 8(2):55–61
Krolewski JJ, Dalla Favera R (1989) Molecular genetic approaches in the diagnosis and classification of lymphoid malignancies. Hematol Pathol 3(2):45–61
Lavinguer A, Maltby V, Mock D et al (1989) High incidence of lung, bone, and lymphoid tumors in transgenic mice overexpressing mutant alleles of the p53 oncogene. Mol Cell Biol 9:3982–3991
Le Boit PE (1991) Variants of mycosis fungoides and related cutaneous T-cell lymphomas. Semin Diagn Pathol 8(2):73–81
Mackay J, Steel CM, Elder PA et al (1988) Allele loss on short arm of chromosome 17 in breast cancer. Lancet:1384–1385
Medeiros LJ, Van Krieken JH, Jaffe ES et al (1990) Association of bcl-1 rearrangements with lymphocytic lymphoma of intermediate differentiation. Blood 76(10): 2086–2090
Milner J, Medcalf EA (1991) Cotranslation of activated mutant p53 with wild type drivers the wild-type p53 protein into the mutant conformation. Cell 65:765–774
Neri N, Knowles DM, Greco A et al (1988) *ras* gene mutations in human lymphoid malignancies. Proc Natl Acad Sci USA 85:9268–9272
Neri A, Chih-Chao C, Lombardi L et al (1991) B-cell lymphoma. Associated chromosomal translocation involves candidate oncogene lyt-10 homologous to NF-kBp50. Cell 67:1075–1087
Nigro JM, Baker SJ, Preisinger AC et al (1989) Mutations in the p53 gene occur in diverse human tumor types. Nature 342:705–708
Orita M, Suzuky Y, Sekiya T et al (1989a) Rapid and sensitive detection of point mutation and DNA polymorphisms using the polymerase chain reaction. Genomics 5:874–879
Orita M, Jwahana H, Kanazawa H et al (1989b) Detection of polymorphisms of human DNA by gel electrophoresis as single-strand conformation polymorphisms. Proc Natl Acad Sci USA 86:2766–2767
Ortiz-Hidalgo C, Wright DH (1992) The morphological spectrum of monocytoid B-cell lymphoma and its relationship to lymphomas of mucosa-associated lymphoid tissue. Histopathology 21(6):555–561
Pan L, Diss TC, Cunningham D et al (1989) The bcl-2 gene in primary B-cell lymphoma of mucosa-associated lymphoid tissue (MALT). Am J Pathol 135: 7–11
Raffeld M, Jaffe ES (1991) Bcl-1, t(11;14), and mantle cell derived lymphoma. Blood 78:259

Rimokh R, Berger F, Cornillet P et al (1990) Break in the bcl-1 locus is closely associated with intermediate lymphocytic lymphoma subtype. Genes Chrom Cancer 2:223–226
Saiki RK, Gelfand DH, Stoffel S et al (1988) Primer-directed enzymatic amplification of DNA with a thermostable DNA polymerase. Science 23:487–491
Sambrook J, Fritch EF, Maniatis T (1989) Molecular cloning: a laboratory manual. Cold Spring Harbor Laboratory, Cold Spring Harbor, New York
Sanger F, Nicklen S, Coulson AR (1977) DNA sequencing with chain terminating inhibitors. Proc Natl Acad Sci USA 74:5463
Takahashi T, Nau MM, Chibaa I et al (1989) P53: a frequent target for genetic abnormalities in lung cancer. Science 246:491
Tsujimoto Y, Yunis J, Onorato-Showe L et al (1984) Molecular cloning of chromosomal breakpoint of B-cell lymphomas and leukemia with the t(11;14) chromosome translocation. Science 224:1403–1406
Vandenberghe E, De Wolf Peeters C et al (1992) Chromosome 11q rearrangements in B non-Hodgkin's lymphoma. Br J Haematol 81(2):212–217
Volkenandt M, Cerroni L, Rieger E et al (1992) Analysis of the 14;18 translocation in cutaneous lymphomas using the polymerase chain reaction. J Cutan Pathol 19:353–356
Weisenburg DD, Sanger WG, Armitage JO et al (1987) Intermediate lymphocytic lymphoma. Immunophenotypic and cytogenetic finding. Blood 69:1617
Willemze R, Meijer CJM, Scheffer E et al (1987) Diffuse large cell lymphomas of follicular center origin presenting in the skin. Am J Pathol 126:325–333
Wotherspoon AC, Pan LX, Diss TC et al (1990) A genotypic study of low grade B cell lymphomas including lymphomas of mucosa associated lymphoid tissue (MALT). J Pathol 162(2):135–140

IV. Other Skin Cancers

Trends in Nonmelanoma Skin Cancer in Japan

M. Ichihashi[1], K. Naruse[1], S. Harada[2], T. Nagano[1], T. Nakamura[1], T. Suzuki[1], N. Wadabayashi[1], and S. Watanabe[3]

[1] Department of Dermatology, Kobe University School of Medicine, Kobe, Japan
[2] Department of Dermatology, Kasai Municipal Hospital, Kasai, Japan
[3] Epidemiology Division, National Cancer Research Institute, Tokyo, Japan

Abstract

We compared the prevalence of skin cancer and solar keratosis (SK) in patients who attended 26 Japanese university hospitals between 1976–1980 with those who attended between 1986–1990 to investigate whether the incidence of skin cancer has increased or not. Age-adjusted incidence rates of basal cell carcinomas (BCC) and SK, but not squamous cell carcinomas (SCC), from 1986–1990 were higher than those from 1976–1980. In addition, a population-based incidence study was conducted in Kasai City, Hyogo prefecture, to establish the frequency of skin cancer and SK. A total of 4736 people over 20 years of age were examined. Two BCC and 36 SK patients were identified clinically and histopathologically. SCC was not found. Age-adjusted incidence rates of BCC and SK per 100000 were 16.5 and 486.1, respectively. The BCC incidence rate in Kasai City was significantly higher than the incidence of Japanese nonmelanoma skin cancer (NMSC) reported by Gordon in 1976. Further, subjects classified as skin type I showed statistically higher SK prevalence rates compared to skin types II and III.

The present study indicates that the prevalences of NMSC and SK in Japanese have increased during the last three decades and that skin type I may be a risk factor for NMSC in Japanese.

Introduction

Studies on the relationship between environmental ultraviolet (UV) dose and skin cancer development in Caucasians have been extensively carried out almost for 100 years, and various risk factors for UV-induced skin cancer have been proposed (Urback et al. 1974; Scotto et al. 1982; Urback 1987; Jung 1991). For Japanese, however, sunlight was not considered to be a serious cause of malignant skin tumors, since an epidemiological survey conducted a few decades ago estimated the incidence rate of nonmelanoma skin cancer (NMSC) on sun-exposed area in Japanese to be a few cases per 100 000 (Quisenberry 1963).

Tada and Miki (1984) showed an increase in Japanese skin cancer patients through a survey of patients who visited Japanese university hospitals in Japan between 1970 and 1975 by comparing their data with Miyaji's survey in the 1960s (Miyaji 1960). They also showed an apparent increase in basal cell carcinoma (BCC) in comparison with squamous cell carcinoma (SCC).

A depletion of the atmospheric ozone layer would undoubtedly result in an increase of harmful UVB flux and annual dose at ground level (Dahlback et al. 1989). This may in turn result in an increase in skin cancers and precancerous lesions on sun-exposed skin (Urback 1989). Furthermore, there are many studies suggesting an increase of NMSC in Japanese, although all studies have been conducted in patients who visited hospital dermatology clinics.

We conducted two kinds of analytical surveys on the frequency of NMSC and precancerous lesion in sun-exposed areas in Japanese.

One was in patients who visited the dermatology department of 26 Japanese university hospitals, the other in citizens who participated in health-screening examination by trained dermatologists. The objective of the studies was to elucidate a reliable incidence rate of skin cancers in Japanese and to clarify the trend in skin cancer incidence over the last two decades.

Comparative studies of 26 university clinics on the prevalence rate of NMSC revealed that BCC and solar keratoses (SK) have increased significantly in the period 1986–1990 compared with the incidence during 1976–1980, whereas our research did not show any increase in SCC between these two times.

Furthermore, we confirmed that exposure to sunlight was a major factor influencing the prevalence of skin cancer in Japanese, since people who live in the southern part of Japan, who are exposed to an approximately twofold higher annual dose of sunlight, have a nearly four- to sixfold higher incidence rate of BCC and SCC compared with those who live in the northern part of Japan. Our health screening examination, which was performed for the first time in Japan, showed a unexpectedly high frequency of SK in Japanese. Furthermore, our results strongly suggest that skin type I is an important risk factor for skin cancer in Japanese.

Patients and Methods

Skin Cancer Patients in University Hospitals

Records of malignant skin tumors diagnosed clinically and histopathologically at the dermatology departments of 26 university hospitals between

1976 and 1980 and between 1986 and 1990 were collected and analyzed at Kobe University. The tumor sites examined were limited to the face, ear, back of the hands, extensor aspect of forearms, and scalp with sparse or no hair. Cancers on the lips were also included. The university hospitals participating in this study ranged from the northern part to the southern part of Japan: Sapporo Medical College (MC), Tohoku University (U), Hirosaki U, Fukusima MC, Niigata U, Keio U, Tokyo Medical and Dental U, Shinshu U, Tokai U, Nagoya City U, Kanazawa U, Osaka U, Nara MC, Kinki U, Wakayama MC, Osaka MC, Kobe U, Okayama U, Hiroshima U, Yamaguchi U, Tokushima U, Ehime U, Kurume U, Nagasaki U, Miyazaki MC, and Ryukyu U.

The occupation of the patients was not evaluated, because detailed descriptions of each case were not obtained. Xeroderma pigmentosum and albinism were excluded from the study.

Skin Cancer Prevalence in Health Examination in Kasai City

The total number of residents in Kasai City was 52837 at the time of the study. There was little difference between men (25969) and women (26868). The age distribution of the male and female population in Kasai City is shown in Fig. 1. Kasai City is situated at 34°56′ North latitude. The study was conducted from 18 May 1992 to 21 November 1992. Each subject in the survey was examined by well trained dermatologists. In all subjects skin examination was confined to sun-exposed area of the face including the ears,

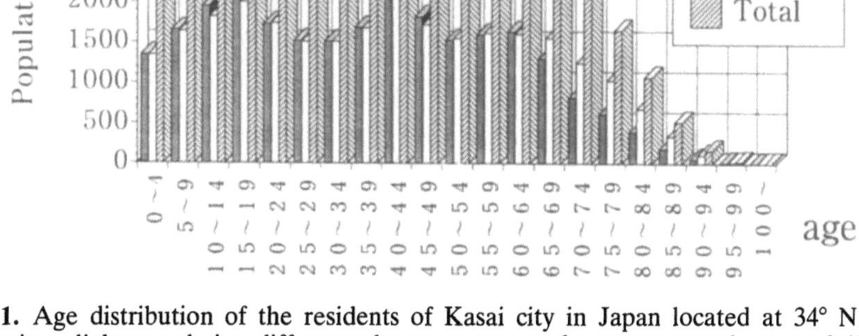

Fig. 1. Age distribution of the residents of Kasai city in Japan located at 34° N. There is a slight population difference between men and women over the age of 65 years

the back of the hands, the extensor surface of the forearms, and the scalp if partially or entirely bald. A total of 4736 residents, more than 90% of the participants in the municipal regional health examination, were surveyed in this skin cancer examination.

Subjects diagnosed as having or suspected of having malignant skin cancers or SK were biopsied at the Department of Dermatology at Kasai Municipal Hospital.

Participants were asked to complete a short questionnaire. The following information was obtained: acute reaction of sun-exposed areas and pattern of occupational sun exposure, indoors or outdoors. A guideline from the first questionnaire to each participant was made to classify subjects as belonging to one of three categories: (1) skin type I, mostly burning and scarcely tanning; (2) skin type II, moderately burning and moderately tanning; (3) skin type III, mostly tanninng and scarcely burning (Satoh and Kawada 1986). The population data of Kasai City in 1992 was used in this study.

Results

The number of patients who visited 26 Japanese university hospitals between 1976 and 1980 and between 1986 and 1990 was 501 789 and 538 112, respectively. The prevalence of BCC, SCC, and SK of the dermatological patients who lived in the southern part of Japan (Nagasaki, Miyazaki, Okinawa) was approximately 3.5 times higher than that in the northern part of Japan (Hokkaido, Tohoku, Fukushima) in both first and second time periods (Fig. 2).

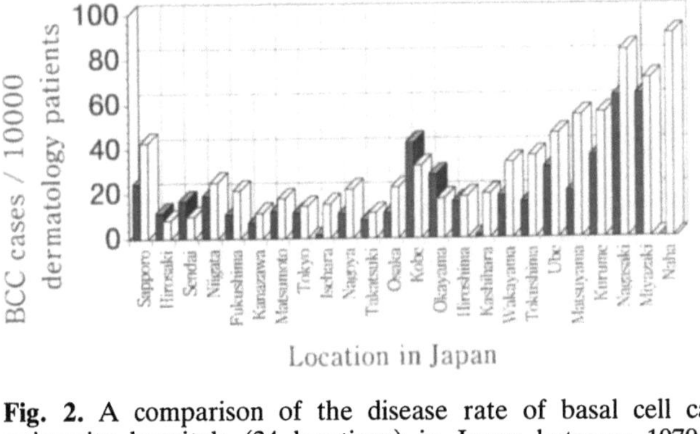

Fig. 2. A comparison of the disease rate of basal cell carcinoma (*BCC*) at 26 university hospitals (24 locations) in Japan between 1970–1980 and 1986–1990. Locations are plotted from Sapporo (North) to Naha (South) in reversed latitudinal degrees (North latitude). There is an apparently higher disease rate of BCC in the southern part of Japan compared to the north. BCC/10 000 dermatology patients in 1976–1980 (■) and in 1986–1990 (□)

Prevalence rates of BCC, SCC, and SK in the two time periods were calculated per 100000 patients, and the rates in the first time period were age-adjusted according to the different age distribution between 1979 and 1989 (Table 1). The prevalence rates of BCC without age adjustment of the first and second time periods were 152.3 and 234.0, respectively. After age adjustment, the prevalence rates of BCC in the first and second time periods were 200.9 and 234.0, respectively. The prevalence rate of BCC in the second time period was significantly higher than in the first time period. The prevalence rates of SCC in the first and second time periods were 119.7 and 136.4, respectively, without age adjustment, and 152.6 and 136.4, respectively, after age adjustment, showing that there was no increasing trend of SCC during the two time periods.

The prevalence rate of SK in the first and second time periods was 76.6 and 141.0, respectively, after age adjustment, showing an approximately 1.8 times higher incidence of SK in the second period than in the first time period.

The age distribution of both male and female populations examined for skin cancer screening in Kasai city is shown in Fig. 3. Of the total subjects who participated in the skin cancer examination, 75.0% were between 40 and 69 years of age. A total of two BCC and 36 SK were diagnosed histopathologically among 4736 persons over 20 years of age. We could not identify any SCC or malignant melanoma (MM) in the subjects examined.

The two BCC patients were aged 66 and 69 years, respectively. The prevalence rate of BCC per 100000 Kasai residents was 36.1 for men and 16.5 for both men and women. The number of SK patients in Kasai City is plotted against age distribution in Fig. 4. There were 24 and 12 female patients. In men, the incidence increased sharply at the age of 60–64 years, whereas in women SK increased sharply at the age of 70–74 years. The youngest SK patients was 44 years old, and more than 90% of SK patients were older than 60 years of age. The mean age of SK at diagnosis was 70.4 years.

Table 1. Diseases rates of squamous cell carcinoma (SCC), basal cell carcinoma (BCC), and solar keratosis (SK) among dermatology patients in two time periods 1976–1980 and 1986–1990

	Disease rate					
	BCC		SCC		SK	
	1st	2nd	1st	2nd	1st	2nd
Not age adjusted	157.3	234.0	119.7	136.4	58.0	141.0
Age adjusted	200.9	234.0	152.6	136.4	76.6	141.0

Disease rates were calculated per 100000 patients. The rates in the first time periods were age adjusted according to the different age distribution between 1979 and 1989.

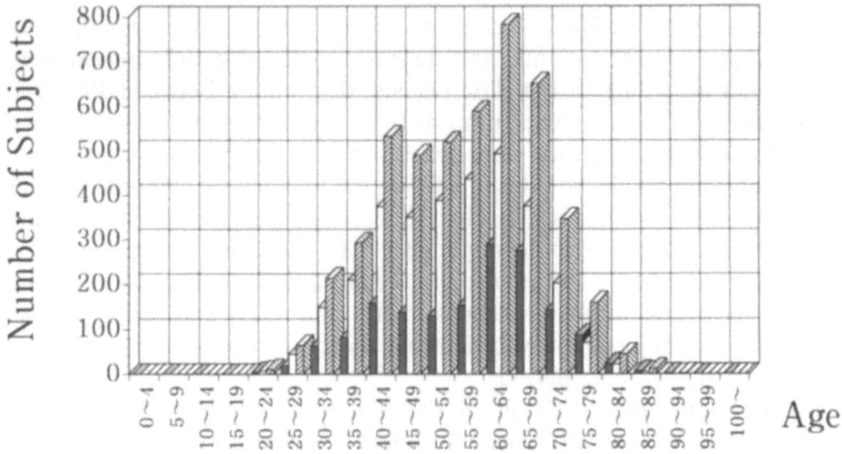

Fig. 3. Age distribution of subjects examined for nonmelanoma and melanoma skin cancer in Kasai City. People aged between 40 and 69 made up approximately 75% of the total participants of 4736. There were approximately twice as many female participants (□) as male (■)

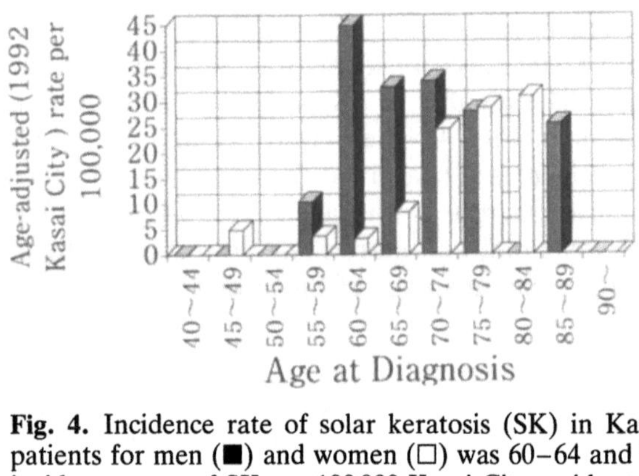

Fig. 4. Incidence rate of solar keratosis (SK) in Kasai City. The peak age of SK patients for men (■) and women (□) was 60–64 and 70–74 years, respectively. The incidence rates of SK per 100 000 Kasai City residents were 678.1 for men and 388.9 for women. The SK incidence in men was statistically higher than that in women

The age- and sex-adjusted prevalence rates for SK in Kasai City in 1992 were 678.1 for men, 388.9 for women, and 486.9 for both men and women. The SK prevalence in men was statistically 1.7-fold higher than that in women ($p < 0.005$).

The prevalence of SK was statistically higher in outdoor workers than in indoor workers (Table 2). The number of subjects divided into skin types I, II, and III was 804, 2973, and 540, respectively. The population rate among

Table 2. Incidence of solar keratosis (SK) with respect to sunlight exposure

Group	Participants (*n*)	SK patients (*n*)	Incidence per 100 000
Outdoor workers	1524	24	505.5
Indoor workers	2867	12	267.2

Population was age and sex adjusted to the Japanese census in 1991.
There is a significant difference between the two groups ($p < 0.01$).

Table 3. Relationship between incidence of solar keratosis (SK) and skin type

Skin type	Participants[a]	Patients[b]		Patients/100 000	
		(*n*)	(%)	Kasai	Japan
I	804	10	1.2	1112.7[c]	894.4[d]
II	2973	23	0.8	419.2	351.7
III	540	3	0.6	524.2	426.3

Prevalence rate of SK in skin type I was significantly higher than that of skin type III ($p < 0.005$) and skin type II ($p < 0.01$).
[a] A total of 4317 subjects out of 4736 participants answered the questionnaire.
[b] All the patients were diagnosed clinically and histopathologically.
[c] Age and sex were adjusted to the Kasai City population in 1992.
[d] Age and sex were adjusted to the Japanese population in the 1991 census.

4736 residents belonging to skin type I, II, and III was 18.6%, 68.9%, and 12.5%, respectively.

Subjects with skin type I had the highest prevalence rate of SK prevalence in skin type I had a twofold higher incidence than in skin type III (Table 3).

Discussion

The intensity of UVB radiation reaching the surface of the earth is limited by the ozone lying predominantly in the stratosphere. The stratospheric ozone layer has been found to be depleted by chlorofluorocarbons (CFC) in the last 20 years. Recent findings on ozone depletion have prompted concerns about the relationship between the level of solar UVB radiation that reach the earth's surface and incidence rates of NMSC and MM.

Recently, incidence rates of skin cancer have been reported to be increasing over time in Europe (Levi et al. 1988), the United States (Scotto et al. 1983), Canada, Australia (Gallagher et al. 1990), and Japan (Ichihashi 1992). The incidence rate of NMSC in dermatological patients who visited Japanese university hospitals has been reported to have increased between 1971–1975 compared to that of 1956–1960. The incidence rate of NMSC between 1971–1975 was 0.171%, whereas it was as low as 0.025% between 1956 and 1960. In the 1980s, there were many reports from individual dermatology departments of Japanese hospitals of the apparent increase in NMSC patients during the last 10–20 years.

We started a nationwide survey of NMSC incidence rates among dermatological patients of university hospitals during two time periods, 1976–1980 and 1986–1990, in order to clarify a possible increasing trend in NMSC in Japan (Ichihashi 1992). The age-adjusted prevalence rate of BCC between 1986 and 1990 was 1.4 times greater than the BCC prevalence between 1976 and 1980, whereas the prevalence rate of SCC during the two time periods has not changed significantly in spite of a sharp increase in SK, the precancerous lesions of SCC in the second time period compared to the first.

Furthermore, a latitudinal and UVB gradient was clearly evident in our survey, with high NMSC incidence rates in the Kyushuu district in the southern part of Japan and a lower incidence rate in Tohoku in the northern part of Japan, although the incidence rate of NMSC in Hokkaido, the most northern part of Japan, was higher than in Tohoku and Fukushima, which are further south than Sapporo.

The results suggest that factors other than surface UVB may contribute to the development of skin cancers on sun-exposed skin, since UVB measured in the United States by Scotto et al. (1988). did not change from 1973 to 1984. Further, calculated surface UVB in Japan based on whole solar radiation also did not change during our two time periods.

The causative factors responsible for the high incidence rate of NMSC in the second time period may be as follows:

1. A sharp increase in the aged population in the second time period
2. Increased concern about NMSC and MM in the public, resulting in early and frequent visit to doctors
3. Increased opportunities for outdoor recreations such as boating, fishing, swimming, and skiing
4. Lack of shade at public outdoor recreation sites
5. Desire to sunbathe
6. Earlier recognition and diagnosis by well-trained professionals
7. Chemicals in food and the environment

We performed the first population-based study in this health-screening examination to clarify the prevalence rate of skin cancer and precancerous lesion on sun-exposed skin.

Based on a total of 36 SK (24 men and 12 women) identified by health-screening examination in Kasai city, prevalence rate of SK per 100000 population was 486.86. The incidence rate of SK over 40 and 60 years of age was 995.32 and 2069.84, respectively. These values were much higher than that we expected from the study on NMSC and precancer lesions in the dermatological patients of university hospitals, even though these values are significantly lower than the 56.9% of Caucasians over 40 years of age who lived in Victoria (Marks et al. 1983).

Men had a statistically higher incidence rate of SK than women in our study. The incidence rate of NMSC, particularly SCC, has been reported to be substantially higher in men than women. This can be explained by behavioral and occupational differences. Men work outdoors and take part in more outdoor leisure activities than women. In addition, most women use sun-protective cosmetics when they go out in the middle of the day.

Outdoor workers showed an approximately twofold higher SK incidence rate compared with indoor workers, and SK incidence in rural residents was higher than that in the urban residents. These results clearly indicate that lifetime UV dose plays a pivotal role in the development of skin cancer in Japanese. Our present results coincide well with others reported previously.

The main factors contributing to the incidence of NMSC are grouped into two categories: one is the physical characteristics of the individual in the population surveyed and the other is the dose of sunlight or the way in which th individuals in the population are exposed (Marks and Sober 1993). Skin color is the major physical characteristic which determines the development of NMSC: the darker the constitutive untanned color of the skin, the lower the incidence of NMSC. The untanned skin color of Japanese ranges between a light and dark complexion.

The annual incidence rate of NMSC in black South Africas has been reported to be low as one per 100000 populations, whereas in white Australians, whose exposure to sunlight is similar to people in South Africa, the annual incidence rate is greater than 800 per 100000 populations (Marks and Sober 1993; Giles et al. 1988). The annual incidence rate of NMSC in Japanese was expected to be as low as 3.5 per 100000, based on a survey of Japanese people in Hawaii (Quisenberry 1963). The incidence rate of BCC in Kasai City was as high as 16.5 per 100000 population. This is nearly four times higher than NMSC incidence rate in Japanese in Hawaii. Although it is not a convincing result, as we identified only two BCC patients by examining 4736, the result still suggests an increasing trend of NMSC in Japanese.

In addition to constitutive skin color, the ability to tan when exposed to sunlight is also a predictor of the risk of NMSC in fair-skinned people. The highest risk is among those who only burn and never tan when exposed, whereas the lowest risk is among those who only tan and never burn.

In the present study, there was a statistically significant difference in SK incidence between skin types I and II, and I and III: the incidence in skin type I was about twofold higher than in skin type III. The result strongly indicates that Japanese skin type I is a risk factor for skin cancer development.

Another possible risk factor for NMSC development may be genetically determined immune suppression induced by UVB radiation. Mice exposed to low-dose UVB radiation allowed the development of transplanted UV-induced tumor from genetically identical mice, whereas genetically identical normal mice without UV irradiation rejected implanted UV-induced tumors. Further, it was revealed that a tumor-specific population of T cells was responsible for suppressing immune response to reject skin cancers (Fisher and Kripke 1978, 1982). Further, UV radiation caused immune suppression of allergic contact hypersensitivity in mice by inducing suppressor T cells, which are specific for antigen applied to the mice skin after UV irradiation (Elmets et al. 1983; Glass et al. 1990).

In addition, Yoshikawa et al. (1990) have demonstrated a marked difference of the susceptibility to UVB-induced suppression of allergic contact hypersensitivity between cancer-bearing and cancer-free people exposed to low-dose UVB: 92% of patients with skin cancer on sun-exposed areas were susceptible to UV-induced immunosuppression, whereas only 40% of normal individuals were UV susceptible. It seems to be important to examine whether Japanese with UV-induced skin cancer are UV susceptible in local allergic contact hypersensitivity.

Further clinical and population-based epidemiological studies in Japanese may contribute to clarifing the risk factors for UV-induced skin cancer in both Japanese and other Asian peoples.

Acknowledgements. This study was supported in part by grants from the Environmental Agency for "Human Effect UVB" and from the Lydia O'Leary Memorial Foundation for Biomedical Research.

References

Dahlback A, Henriksen T, Larsen SHH, Stamnes K (1989) Biological UV-dose and effect of an ozone layer depletion. Photochem Photobiol 49:621–625

Elmets CA, Bergstresser PR, Tigelaar RE, Wood PJ, Streilein JW (1983) Analysis of the mechanism of unresponsiveness produced by haptens painted on skin exposed to low dose ultraviolet radiation. J Exp Med 158:781–794

Fisher MS, Kripke ML (1978) Further studies on the tumor specific suppressor cells induced by ultraviolet radiation. J Immunol 121:1139–1144

Fisher MS, Kripke ML (1982) Suppressor T lymphocytes control the development of primary skin cancer in ultraviolet-irradiated mice. Science 216:1133–1134

Gallagher RP, Ma B, McLean D, Yang CP, Ho V, Carruther JA, Warshawski LM (1990) Trend in basal cell carcinoma, squamous cell carcinoma, and melanoma of the skin from 1973 through 1987. J Am Acad Dermatol 23:413–421
Giles GG, Marks R, Foley P (1988) Incidence of non-melanocytic skin cancer treated in Australia. Med J 296:13–17
Glass MJ, Bergstresser PR, Tigelaar RE, Streilein JW (1990) UVB radiation and DNFB skin painting induced suppressor cell universally in mice. J Invest Dermatol 94:273–278
Ichihashi M (1992) UV-induced skin cancer in Japanese. Rinsho Hifu 34:11–23 (in Japanese)
Jung EG (1991) Photocarcinogenesis in the skin. J Dermatol 18:1–10
Levi F, la Vecchia C, Te V-C, Mezzanotte G (1988) Descriptive epidemiology of skin cancer in the Swiss Canton of Vaud. Int J Cancer 42:811–816
Marks R, Sober AJ (1993) Skin cancer. In: Eds Lim HW, Soter NA (eds) Clinical photomedicine. Dekker, New York, PP 113–135
Marks R, Ponsford MW, Selwood TS, Goodman G, Manson G (1983) Non-melanotic skin cancer and solar keratoses in Victoria. Med J Aust 2:619–622
Miyaji T (1963) Skin cancers in Japan: a nationwide 5-year survey, 1956–1960. Conference on biology of cutaneous cancer. Natl Cancer Inst Monogr 10:55–70
Quisenberry WB (1963) Ethinic difference in skin cancer in Hawaii. Conference on biology of cutaneous cancer. Natl Cancer Inst Monogr 10:181
Satoh Y, Kawada A (1986) Action spectrum for melanin pigmentation to ultraviolet light, and Japanese skin typing. In: Fitzpatrick TB, Wick MM, Tada K (eds) Brown melanoderma: biology and disease of epidermal pigmentation. University of Tokyo, Tokyo, pp 85–95
Scotto J, Fears TR, Franmeni JF (1982) Solar radiation. In: Schottenfeld D, Fraumeni JF (eds). Cancer epidemiology and prevention. Saunders, Philadelphia, pp 254–276
Scotto J, Fears TR, Fraumeni JF (1983) Incidence of non-melanoma skin cancer in the United States. US Department of Health and Human Services, Public Health Servise National Cancer Institute, NIH Publ 83–2433
Scotto J, Cotton G, Urback F, Berger D, Fears T (1988) Biologically effective ultraviolet radiation: surface measurement in the United States, 1974 to 1985. Science 239:762–764
Tada M, Miki Y (1984) Malignant skin tumors among dermatology patients in university hospitals of Japan: a statistical survey 1971–1975. J Dermatol 11: 313–321
Urback F (1987) Man and ultraviolet radiation. In: Passchier WF, Bosn Jakovic BFM (eds) Human exposure to ultraviolet radiation. Risks and regulation. Excepta Medica, Amsterdam, pp 3–16
Urback F (1989) Potential effects of altered solar ultraviolet radiation on human skin cancer. Photochem Photobiol 50:507–513
Urback F, Epstein JH, Forbes PD (1974) Ultraviolet carcinogenesis: experimental, global, and genetic aspects. In: Pattrak MI, Harber LC, Seiji M, Kukita A (eds) Sunlight and man 1974, University of Tokyo Press, Tokyo, pp 259–283
Yoshikawa Y, Rae V, Bruins-Slot W, Van den Berg J-W, Taylar R, Streilein W (1990) Susceptibility to effects of UVB radiation on induction of contact hypersensitivity as a risk factor for skin cancer in humans. J Invest Dermatol 95:530–536

Kaposi's Sarcoma: A Reevaluation

C.E. Orfanos, R. Husak, U. Wölfer, and C. Garbe

Department of Dermatology, University Medical Center Steglitz,
The Free University of Berlin, Hindenburgdamm 30, 12200 Berlin, Germany

Abstract

Kaposi's sarcoma (KS) is a multicentric neoplasia of microvascular origin arising during development of immunodeficiency in human immunodeficiency virus (HIV)-infected individuals. More than 130 patients with HIV-associated KS (98% male homosexuals; median age, 35 years) have been diagnosed at the Department of Dermatology, University Medical Center Steglitz, Berlin, during the years 1982–1992. Mucocutaneous and visceral involvement was a common finding in patients with HIV-associated KS, increasing from 39% at the first visit to 65% at the last observation. In 90% of the patients significant immunosuppression was found (75% had a $CD4^+$ count < 200/mm^3) at the time of first diagnosis. However, immunosuppression was not a prerequisite for the development of KS, since the tumor had been diagnosed before severe immunosuppression was present in about 10% of the patients. Significant prognostic predictors for the final outcome were: (a) the degree of immunosuppression, (b) the presence of mucosal and visceral manifestation, and (c) the past history of opportunistic infections. The median survival time was 28 months in KS patients with more than 300 $CD4^+$ lymphocytes ($n = 18$), but only 14 months in immunosuppressed (less than 300 $CD4^+$ lymphocytes) individuals with KS ($n = 70$). The median survival time in the entire group evaluated ($n = 89$ patients) was 17 months after first diagnosis. In 71 HIV-infected individuals who died at the Berlin Department during the last 8 years, disseminated KS was the major direct or indirect cause of death (49% of cases).

Therapeutic benefit for KS patients was observed after long-term administration of recombinant interferon alpha (rIFN-α; 9–18 million IU s.c. every 2 days) alone or combined with antiretroviral drugs such as zidovudine over several months. Prolongation of survival was found after such treatment modalities in 30%–40% of treated patients. Bleomycin and vincristine

Recent Results in Cancer Research, Vol. 139

and other systemically used cytostatics have also been applied with moderate results.

The etiology of HIV-associated KS is still unknown and coinfection with herpes simplex virus (HSV), cytomegalovirus (CMV), or human papillomavirus (HPV) as well as certain growth-stimulating cytokines (transforming growth factors, TGF; tumor necrosis factor alpha, TNF-α; interleukin-6, IL-6; tat; vascular endothelial growth factors, VEGF; oncostatin M) produced by HIV-infected cells may be cofactors. Overall, KS was found to be a tumor with high malignant potential, and the median survival times were short. In spite of the poor prognosis, management and treatment results were improved by use of IFN-α, antiretroviral and cytotoxic drugs, and by the growing experience of the medical community with this HIV-associated tumor.

Introduction

Human immunodeficiency virus (HIV)-associated Kaposi's sarcoma is a multicentric systemic vascular tumor derived from endothelial cells with malignant course. It occurs as multiple inflammatory lesions with angioproliferation leading to angioneoplasia. They are usually first located in the skin, where they appear as purple macules, plaques, or nodular infiltrates, which may cause lymphatic obstruction.

HIV-associated Kaposi's sarcoma was first noted in 1981 and is the most common neoplasm associated with HIV infection (Friedman-Kien et al. 1981). Among HIV patients, Kaposi's sarcoma is one of the most frequent medical problems. The tumor occurs almost exclusively in homosexual males with well-developed immune deficiency; however, it may also appear in early stages, approximately 1.5–2 years after seroconversion, without any measurable alteration of the immunological criteria (Orfanos et al. 1988). The incidence of Kaposi's sarcoma has dropped continuously within the risk group of HIV-infected individuals from 50% at the beginning of the 1980s to the current rate of approximately 20% (Beral et al. 1990; Rutherford et al. 1989). This appears partly due to the fact that the tumor had been a marker for the diagnosis of acquired immunodeficiency syndrome (AIDS) and HIV infection during that time. HIV-associated Kaposi's sarcoma is a severe illness which disseminates to the mucosa and other organs and is frequently fatal. In contrast to its decreasing incidence, an increasing proportion of deaths due to wide-spread HIV-associated Kaposi's sarcoma has been registered (Peters et al. 1991).

More than 130 patients with HIV-associated Kaposi's sarcoma were documented in the HIV follow-up clinics at the Department of Dermatology, University Medical Center Steglitz, Berlin, during the years 1982–1992. It is the aim of this report to present some epidemiological data and give a detailed reevaluation of the documented cases of Kaposi's sarcoma, the most life-threatening tumor among HIV patients.

Material and Methods

Since 1982, more than 130 patients have presented with HIV-associated Kaposi's sarcoma at the Department of Dermatology, UMC Steglitz, Berlin. In all patients the presence of HIV antibodies was determined by enzyme-linked immunosorbent assay (ELISA) and confirmed by the western Blot technique. Punch biopsy specimens of Kaposi's sarcoma lesions were taken from all patients and histological examination revealed Kaposi's sarcoma in each case. All the relevant information, including the demographical data of the patients, data of the diagnosis, and the course of the $CD4^+$ cell values, was documented by the attending physicians using a form suitable for computer evaluation. The risk group and the level of immune suppression were completed through further information obtained from other physicians and clinical settings. To characterize the immune status of the patients, we determined the lymphocytic subpopulations at the time of the first visit and consecutively every 3 months in the HIV follow-up clinic. For evaluating the immune status, the absolute $CD4^+$ lymphocyte counts and the $CD4^+/CD8^+$ lymphocyte ratio were analyzed.

For our computerized documentation, we used the database program dBASE IV. Frequency calculations and statistical comparison of frequency distributions were done with the PC program SPSS/PC+ version 4.0. Median survival times were calculated according to the method of Kaplan-Meier, using the SPSS/PC+ statistical program.

Results

HIV-associated dermatological disorders in 456 patients were documented in the HIV follow-up clinics at the Department of Dermatology, University Medical Center Steglitz, Berlin, during the time period from 1982 to 1992. Among them only oral candidiasis (45%), seborrheic dermatitis (39%), and folliculitis (33%) were more frequent than Kaposi's sarcoma (24%; Fig. 1). Epidemiological data and the therapeutical use of recombinant interferon alpha (rIFN-α) and of zidovudine (AZT), alone or in combination, were documented separately in patients with HIV-associated Kaposi's sarcoma. The impact of the absolute $CD4^+$ count and of clinical features of Kaposi's sarcoma on the median survival time of the patients were also analyzed.

Patients

All patients with HIV-associated Kaposi's sarcoma were males and 98% of them were homosexuals. The risk behavior remained unknown in only 2%.

More than 90% of the patients were between 20 and 50 years old. The median age of the patients was 35 years (Fig. 2). The mean time between

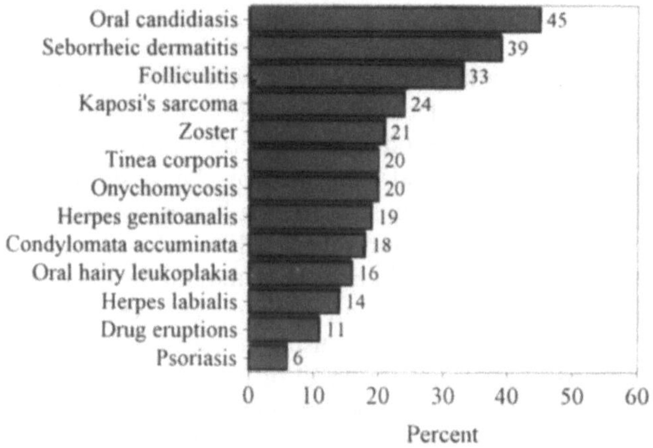

Fig. 1. Prevalence of dermatological disorders in 456 human immunodeficiency virus (HIV)-infected individuals during the time period 1982–1992

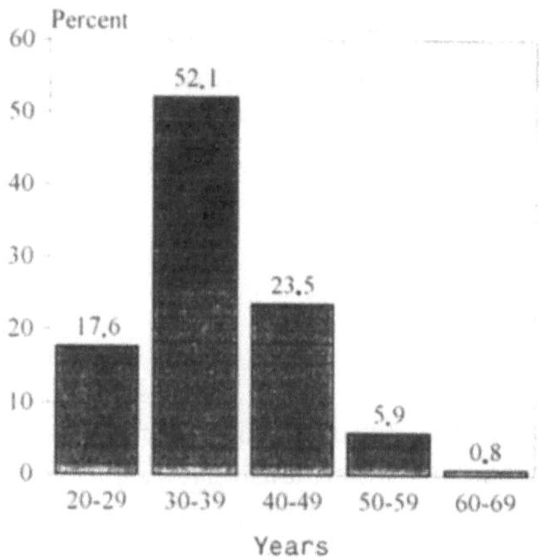

Fig. 2. Age distribution of 119 patients with human immunodeficiency virus (HIV)-associated Kaposi's sarcoma. Median age, 35 years

their first visit and the last follow-up examination was 18 months, ranging between 3 months and 7 years.

The staging of Kaposi's sarcoma patients according to Mitsuyasu was documented during their first visit and during the last observation. At the first visit, 56% of the patients had cutaneous Kaposi's sarcoma only, in 39% mucocutaneous Kaposi's sarcoma-lesions were found, and only 3% had additional visceral involvement. In comparison, during their last observation 31% of the patients showed cutaneous involvement, 65% showed mucocutaneous lesions, and in 36% visceral dissemination was detected (Tables 1, 2).

Table 1. Staging of Kaposi's sarcoma according to Mitsuyashu (as percentages)

	First visit (n = 96)	Last observation (n = 83)
Stage I Cutaneous limited (<10 lesions or in only one anatomical region)	28	10
Stage II Cutaneous disseminated (>10 lesions or in more than one region)	65	49
Stage III Visceral only	1	2
Stage IV Cutaneous and visceral	6	39

Table 2. Physical manifestations of Kaposi's sarcoma (as percentages)

	First visit (n = 121)	Last observation (n = 89)
Skin only	56	31
Mucosa only	3	3
Visceral only	2	1
Mucocutaneous	36	29
Mucocutaneous and visceral	3	36

In the large majority of the patients with HIV-associated Kaposi's sarcoma the immunological parameters showed significant deterioration over the follow-up period. More than 50% of the 111 patients with complete immune status had $CD4^+$ counts less than $100/mm^3$ and nearly 75% had $CD4^+$ counts less than $200/mm^3$. However, nearly 10% of the patients who developed Kaposi's sarcoma had more than $500/mm^3$ $CD4^+$ cells, i.e., they were in a stage with no significant reduction of the circulating $CD4^+$ lymphocytes (Fig. 3). The reduced immune status at the time of diagnosis of Kaposi's sarcoma was confirmed if the $CD4^+/CD8^+$ lymphocyte ratio was calculated. More than 75% of our AIDS patients with Kaposi's sarcoma had a $CD4^+$ to $CD8^+$ ratio of less than 0.4 at the first diagnosis (Fig. 4).

During the follow-up period, the presence of opportunistic infections in our Kaposi's sarcoma patients was documented; 41% of the HIV-infected individuals registered had developed primarily KS and then an opportunistic infection during their further follow-up, in comparison to 29% of patients in whom first an opportunistic infection was diagnosed and then the neoplasm

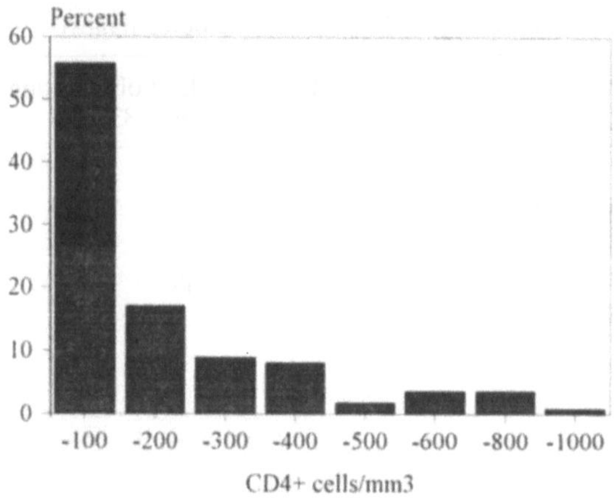

Fig. 3. CD4$^+$ cells of 111 patients with human immunodeficiency virus (HIV)-associated Kaposi's sarcoma at their first examination

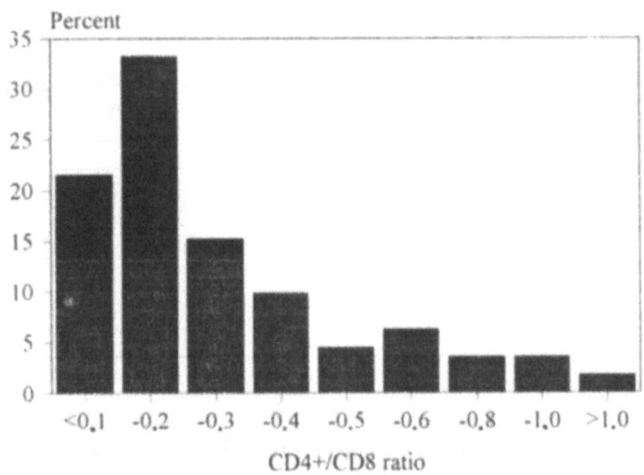

Fig. 4. CD4$^+$ to CD8$^+$ ratio of 111 patients with human immunodeficiency virus (HIV)-associated Kaposi's sarcoma at their first examination

appeared. Kaposi's sarcoma was the only AIDS-defining disease in 23% of the patients, as classified according to the definition given by the Centers for Disease Control (CDC) in 1987; finally, in 7% of our patients Kaposi's sarcoma appeared in the presence of an opportunistic infection.

Survival Times and Prognosis

A total of 71 HIV-infected patients with Kaposi's sarcoma have died at the University Medical Center Steglitz, Berlin, during the last 8 years. Disseminated tumor was found by autopsy in nearly 50% of the patients and was regarded as a major cause of death, followed by pneumocystic pneumonia (PCP) and other opportunistic infections responsible for the death of another 20% of the patients. In the remaining 30%, various causes were found responsible for the lethal outcome (including suicide in one case; Fig. 5).

The median survival time after first diagnosis of Kaposi's sarcoma in the entire group evaluated (n = 89 patients) was 17 months. These findings indicate the highly malignant potential of disseminated HIV-associated Kaposi's sarcoma, although the survival rates of patients with Kaposi's sarcoma obviously depended on the absolute $CD4^+$ number. AIDS patients with Kaposi's sarcoma and an absolute peripheral blood $CD4^+$ count of more than $300/mm^3$ had a much better prognosis, with a median survival time of 27.9 months (n = 16). The majority of the patients (n = 70), however, had developed Kaposi's sarcoma with a $CD4^+$ count below $300/mm^3$ and their prognosis was poor, with a median survival time of 14.4 months (Fig. 6). Similar findings resulted when relating the prognostic outcome to the $CD4^+$ to $CD8^+$ ratio. In the group of patients with a $CD4^+$ to $CD8^+$ ratio higher than 0.3, a median survival time of 27 months was calculated (n = 25), whereas the median survival time in the group with a $CD4^+$ to $CD8^+$ ratio below 0.3 was only 13 months (n = 60).

As a further parameter, the importance of cutaneous and mucocutaneous involvement on the outcome and prognosis of the patients was analyzed. The median survival time of patients with Kaposi's sarcoma limited to the skin at the first presentation (n = 51) was 24 months. In patients with mucocutaneous involvement (n = 34; e.g., oral mucosa), however, the

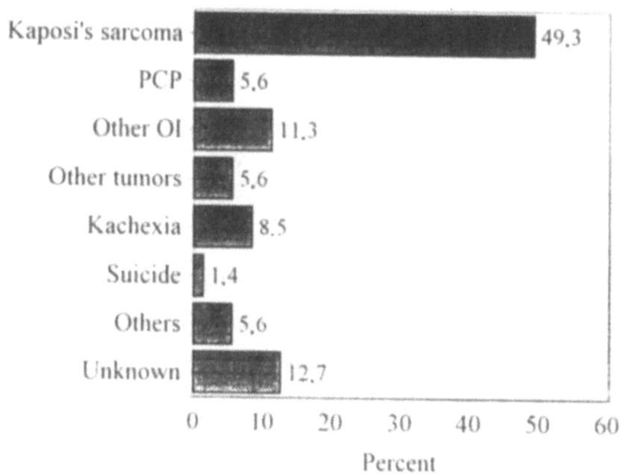

Fig. 5. Causes of death among 71 human immunodeficiency virus (HIV)-patients with Kaposi's sarcoma who died during the follow-up period. *PCP*, pneumocystic pneumonia; *OI*, opportunistic infection

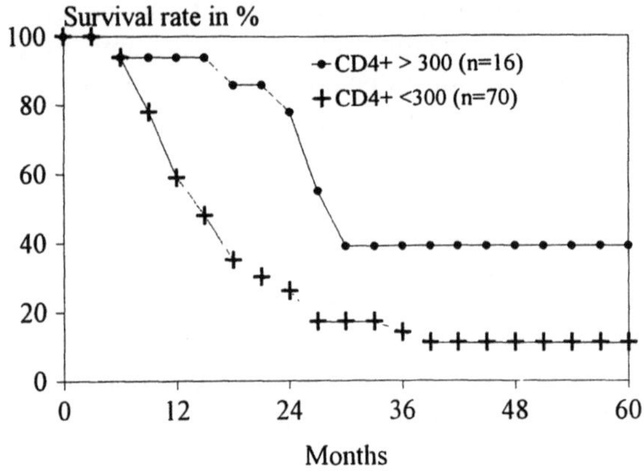

Fig. 6. Five-year survival rate of Kaposi's sarcoma depending on the absolute $CD4^+$ count. Median survival time was 27.9 months for the group with more than $300/mm^3$ and 14.4 months for the group with less than $300/mm^3$

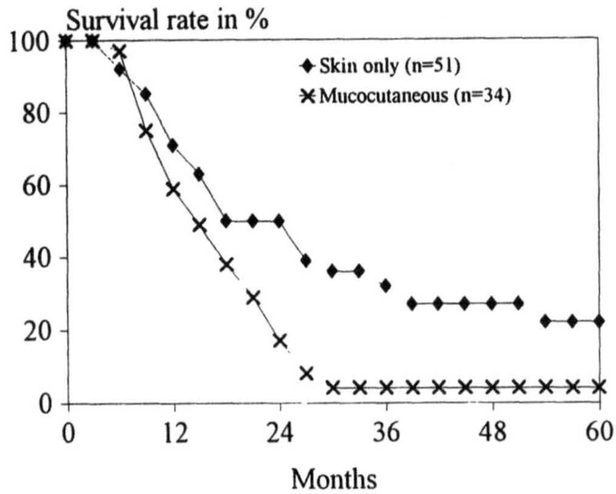

Fig. 7. Five-year survival rate of Kaposi's sarcoma depending on the clinical manifestation. Median survival time was 24 months for the group in which it was limited to the skin and 15 months for the group with mucocutaneous involvement

calculated median survival time was only 15 months, indicating that the presence of mucosal involvement during the first visit may serve as an additional prognostic parameter, related with unfavorable prognosis and shortened life expectation time (Fig. 7).

Therapy

HIV-associated Kaposi's sarcoma has been treated with local radiation therapy, cryosurgery, intralesional injections of rIFN-α, or intralesional chemotherapy (e.g., vinblastine). Patients with disseminated Kaposi's sarcoma received a combination of AZT and systemic rIFN-α, or systemic chemotherapy including agents such as vincristine and vinblastine.

During, recent years two studies have been performed in our department using rIFN-α, alone or in combination with AZT, in the management of disseminated HIV-associated Kaposi's sarcoma. The agent rIFN-α enhances cytotoxic T cell and natural killer cell activity and was reported to exert direct antiproliferative and antiviral properties. Treatment with rIFN-α, consisting of i.m. or s.c. injections of 3–18 million IU every 2 days usually required 6–8 weeks for initial response. Experiences with the use of rIFN-α indicate that it is more effective in patients with an absolute $CD4^+$ lymphocyte count over 200/mm^3 and without life-threatening opportunistic infections. Because tumor activity is related to the degree of immunosuppression, the additional use of AZT was investigated. A preliminary evaluation of the patients treated revealed complete response in 17% of the patients in both groups (rIFN-α, $n = 25$, versus rIFN-α plus AZT, $n = 42$). Partial response was obtained in 13% of the group treated with rIFN-α monotherapy versus 17% of the group treated with rIFN-α and AZT. Progressive disease was observed in 29% of the group with rIFN-α versus 36% of the group with combination therapy (Fig. 8).

The duration of remissions under treatment significantly differed between the two treatment regiments. The duration of remissions was 13–18 months in one third of the patients treated with the combined schedule, whereas another 20% remained free of tumor relapse over 7–12 months. In the group treated with rIFN-α monotherapy, the percentage of patients who had tumor remission over 7–12 months or over 13–18 months was clearly lower (6% and 19%; Fig. 9).

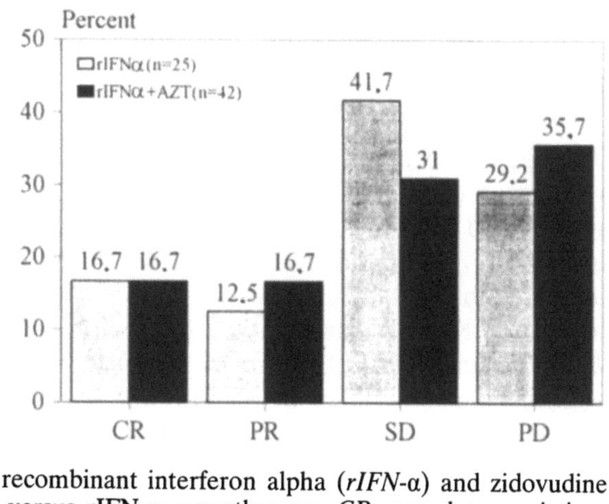

Fig. 8. Clinical response to recombinant interferon alpha (*rIFN-α*) and zidovudine (*AZT*) combination therapy versus rIFN-α monotherapy. *CR*, complete remission; *PR*, partial remission; *SD*, stable disease; *PD*, progressive disease

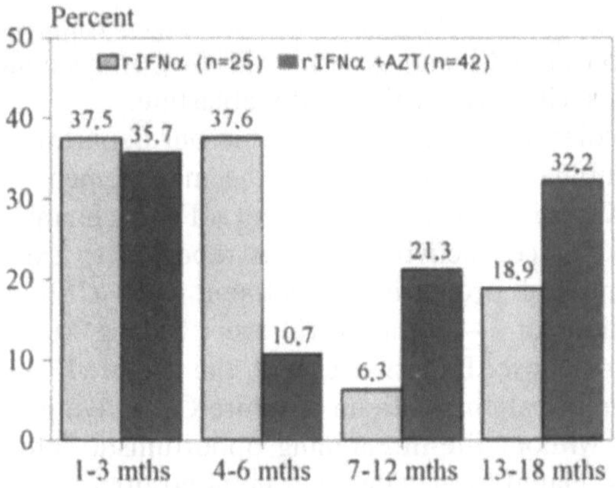

Fig. 9. Duration of remissions by recombinant interferon alpha (*rIFN*-α) and zidovudine (*AZT*) combination therapy versus rIFN-α monotherapy

A smaller percentage of patients with Kaposi's sarcoma refused any systemic therapy and the skin lesions were treated with X-ray radiation and topical modalities only. The survival time of this group without systemic therapy ($n = 8$) was evaluated in comparison to the groups of patients treated with rIFN-α with ($n = 21$) and without AZT ($n = 34$).

In the group without systemic therapy, the median survival time was significantly lower (11 months) in comparison to the two groups treated systemically. In particular, the group which received combined rIFN-α and AZT had the best prognosis with more than 24 months survival time (Fig. 10). These findings emphasize the treatment option in patients with HIV-associated Kaposi's sarcoma, particularly those in early stages without mucosal involvement and preserved immune response.

Discussion

The epidemic variant of disseminated Kaposi's sarcoma was one of the first recognized manifestations of AIDS; the Center for Disease Control (CDC) reported 26 cases of Kaposi's sarcoma in homosexual men in New York City and California (Friedman-Kien et al. 1981). After 1–2 years, this tumor also appeared in several European cities, and in 1982 the first patient with HIV-associated Kaposi's sarcoma was seen by us in Germany (Vossmann et al. 1983; Orfanos 1983; Bratzke et al. 1987). Prior to AIDS epidemic, the angiosarcoma multiplex of Kaposi was a relatively rare tumor observed mostly in males in the mediterranean area of Eastern European or Jewish ancestry as a slowly growing tumor with multiple hyperpigmented lesions usually located on the lower legs. In the late 1950s and the early 1960s, a different type of Kaposi's sarcoma was reported in young Africans, men and

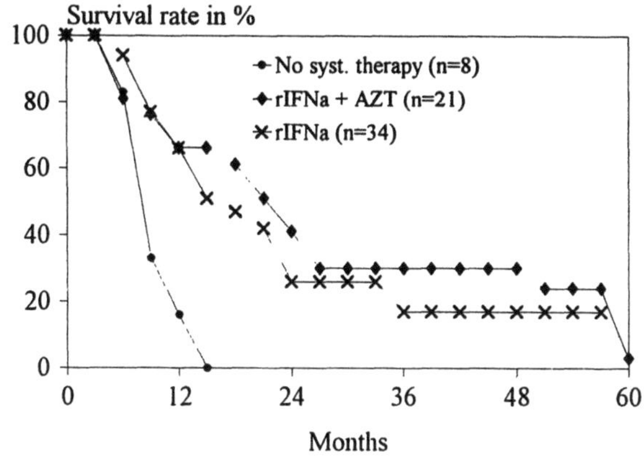

Fig. 10. Five-year survival rate depending on different therapeutical regimens. Median survival time was 24.2 months with recombinant interferon alpha (*rIFN-α*) and zidovudine (*AZT*) combination therapy, 18.8 months with rIFN-α monotherapy, and 11 months without systemic therapy

women and also in young children. This variety was called endemic African Kaposi's sarcoma, showing various clinical subtypes (Kestens et al. 1985; Friedman-Kien and Saltzmann 1990). During the last two to three decades, an increasing number of Kaposi's sarcoma have been seen among organ transplant recipients and in other patients receiving immunosuppressive therapy (Klein et al. 1974; Harwood et al. 1979).

Epidemiology

The spread of the HIV disease in the 1980s was associated with an explosion of epidemic Kaposi's sarcoma, which is now the most common malignant tumor in AIDS patients (Haverkos 1987). Beral and coworkers (1990) calculated that the overall risk of developing Kaposi's sarcoma in patients with AIDS is 20000 times more common than in the general population an 300 times more common than in other immunosuppressed groups. Our observations confirmed again that HIV-associated Kaposi's sarcoma occurs almost exclusively in homosexual and bisexual males infected with the virus. This has been repeatedly reported by other authors too (Haverkos 1987; Beral et al. 1990). The prevalence of Kaposi's sarcoma in HIV-infected individuals has dropped continuously since the early 1980s from approximately 40% at the beginning of the epidemic to the current rate of less than 20% (Beral et al. 1990; Rutherford et al. 1989; Bunikowski et al. 1992). Interestingly, the prevalence of HIV-associated Kaposi's sarcoma among the main risk group of homosexual men varies in different geographical areas. Investigations limited to the USA showed that HIV-related Kaposi's sarcoma is more common in California (28%) and in New York (25%); these rates are significantly higher than in other areas of the United States (median value for all other states, 17%; Beral et al. 1990; Archibald et al. 1990). Thus far we do not know whether this type of geographic distribution also exists in other countries, particularly in Germany, due to the lack of corresponding data. However, we should consider that the overall rate of patients diagnosed with HIV-associated Kaposi's sarcoma continues to rise as more HIV-infected patients are diagnosed with AIDS (Beral et al. 1990). Although the proportion of AIDS patients diagnosed with Kaposi's sarcoma may be lower in recent years, Peters and coworkers (1991) registered in a retrospective analysis of medical records in the UK an increasing proportion of deaths due to AIDS-related Kaposi's sarcoma, from 12% in 1986 to 32% in 1989. These findings correlate with our own investigations: among 71 patients with HIV-associated Kaposi's sarcoma who died during the years 1982–1992, disseminated tumor was the cause of death in nearly 50% of the cases. A possible explanation for the increasing impact of Kaposi's sarcoma as the cause of death in HIV-infected individuals may be the rapid improvement of our therapeutic panoply in treating opportunistic infections and the large scale establishment of prophylactic schedules against PCP and toxoplasmosis. The significance of these infections as causes of death have significantly decreased during recent years (Peters et al. 1991).

Pathogenesis and Etiology

Although etiology and pathogenesis of HIV-related Kaposi's sarcoma still remains unclear, several contributing factors have been implicated:

1. There is some evidence that the HIV virus plays an indirect role in the development of HIV-associated Kaposi's sarcoma. Ensoli and colleagues (1990, 1991) showed that HIV-infected T cells carrying the $CD4^{+}$ antigen promote the growth of cells derived from HIV-associated Kaposi's sarcoma lesions and that the HIV tat gene, introduced into the germline of mice, induces vascular skin lesions histologically resembling human Kaposi's sarcoma. These findings suggest that tat protein may play an important role in the development or progression of Kaposi's sarcoma in HIV-infected individuals.
2. HIV-associated Kaposi's sarcoma cells have been shown to produce angiogenic growth factors and cytokines including fibroblast growth factors (FGF), TNF-α, IL-6, tat, and recently identified VEGF factors (VEGF) and oncostatin M, a major growth factor for Kaposi's sarcoma cells (Ensoli et al. 1989; Delli-Bovi et al. 1987; Huang et al. 1992a; Xerri et al. 1991; Miles et al. 1990; Weindel et al. 1992; Nair et al. 1992). Nakamura and coworkers (1992) found a noncytotoxic bacterial cell wall complex which inhibits the angiogenesis of Kaposi's sarcoma cell cultures

and Kaposi's sarcoma lesions. Summarizing these studies, it is suggested that cytokines and endothelial growth factors may be involved in the pathogenesis of HIV-associated Kaposi's sarcoma and their investigation may be useful for the development of new therapeutic agents.

3. Genetic predisposition appears as a contributing factor in the etiology of HIV-associated Kaposi's sarcoma, showing increased incidence of HLA DR5 in individuals with classic Kaposi's sarcoma as well as in those with iatrogenic Kaposi's sarcoma (Tebbe et al. 1991). This hypotheses are supported by the fact that the overwhelming majority of patients with Kaposi's sarcoma are men (95% of all cases of AIDS-related Kaposi's sarcoma in the United States in Europe occur in homosexual and bisexual men) and that in mice transfected with the tat gene, only male animals develop the tumor (Friedman-Kien and Saltzman 1990; Vogel et al. 1988).
4. Although no infectious agent could be detected in cultured cells derived from Kaposi's sarcoma lesions, there is some evidence for a sexually transmitted Kaposi's sarcoma agent. This could explain the increased prevalence of Kaposi's sarcoma in homosexual and bisexual men compared with other risk groups and also the presence of Kaposi's sarcoma in female partners of bisexual men in contrast to partners of intravenous drug users and to hemophiliacs. The declining incidence of Kaposi's sarcoma coincides with changes in sexual behavior and safer sex practices among the homosexual community (Friedman-Kien and Saltzman 1990; Beral et al. 1990; Couturier et al. 1990; Bary et al. 1991; Peterman et al. 1993). Several viral agents have been investigated as a possible cause; among them were hepatitis A and B viruses, herpesviruses, and particularly CMV, which has a high prevalence of serum antibodies in all types of Kaposi's sarcoma (Wahman et al. 1991; Giraldo et al. 1978; Drew et al. 1982). Up to now, however, no consistent association between any viral agent and Kaposi's sarcoma has been established and all efforts to detect CMV DNA sequences in HIV-related Kaposi's sarcoma tissue have failed (Delli-Bovi et al. 1986). Recently, HPV-16-related DNA fragments have been isolated from tissue specimens of Kaposi's sarcoma patients with and without HIV infection; whether this virus plays a role in the etiology of the neoplasm remains to be determined (Huang et al. 1992b).

Clinical Course

Cutaneous Kaposi's sarcoma lesions in HIV patients are seen initially as an ecchymotic-like macule with red, pink, tan, or mostly violaceous color. They are usually asymptomatic, but are felt to represent a significant cosmetic stigma. After some weeks or months the lesions become palpable, sometimes firm to hard, and develop into flat nodules; these may be of any shape, although they are initially often oval and tend to grow along the lines of skin cleavage (Rendon et al. 1988). The overlying epidermis is usually intact, but it may become necrotic with formation of erosions or ulcers and crusting. Some lesions may enlarge and become confluent, forming tumorous plaques with lymphedema. Large lesions on palms or soles may impede function of the extremities. Oral involvement HIV-associated Kaposi's sarcoma has been described in 40% of patients; in the group presented here, 36% of our patients had mucocutaneous lesions at their first visit (Silverman et al. 1986; Ficarra et al. 1988).

Lemlich and coworkers (1987) reported visceral Kaposi's sarcoma involvement in 29% of 24 AIDS patients they reviewed postmortem, even without cutaneous lesions; this finding should be considered in the differential diagnosis of HIV-related illnesses, e.g., gastrointestinal bleeding. Visceral involvement, including the gastrointestinal tract, abdominal lymph nodes, and the lungs, is frequently seen, particularly in late stages of HIV disease, being responsible for systemic complications leading to death in some cases (Lemlich et al. 1987; Barrison et al. 1988; McKenzie et al. 1991). There is some evidence that disseminated HIV-associated Kaposi's sarcoma with visceral involvement is increasingly responsible for the lethal outcome in HIV patients, probably because of the reasons we discussed above.

The differential diagnosis of HIV-associated Kaposi's sarcoma include dermatofibroma, pyogenic granuloma, hemangioma, bacillary angiomatosis, ecchymosis, granuloma anulare, blue nevus, insect bite reactions, malignant melanoma, and cutaneous lymphoma. Sometimes these lesions can occur concurrently with Kaposi's sarcoma in HIV patients and make the diagnosis difficult.

There are some reports that skin trauma or prior cutaneous disease may contribute to the development of Kaposi's sarcoma as Koebner's phenomenon (Janier et al. 1990; Plettenberg et al. 1990a), and occasionally Kaposi's sarcoma lesions may resolve spontaneously (Real and Krown 1985).

Prognosis

The prognosis of all patients with HIV-associated Kaposi's sarcoma is variable; it appears to be related to: (a) the mucosal and visceral involvement of the tumor, (b) the activity of HIV infection, and (c) the degree of underlying immunosuppression. The tumor may develop at any stage of HIV infection, but in the large majority of cases it occurs after significant reduction of the immune status parameter. The influence of $CD4^+$ counts on the outcome and prognosis of HIV-associated Kaposi's sarcoma has been investigated in a prospective study of 212 patients seen by a group in New York from 1981 to 1986; with a median survival time of 32 months, Kaposi's sarcoma patients with more than 300 $CD4^+$ cells in their peripheral blood had the best prognosis (Chachoua et al. 1989). These findings are in accordance with our own data and the data of other authors (Spornraft et al. 1988). In addition to this parameter, we found that mucocutaneous involvement was a marker for poor prognosis. The prevalence of such lesions and the presence of systemic opportunistic infection prior or at the time of presentation will worsen the prognosis of Kaposi's sarcoma substantially, in comparison to patients who developed Kaposi's sarcoma early after HIV infection (Krown et al. 1989; Feigal et al. 1991). Finally, poor prognosis was found for patients with older age at the time of diagnosis of HIV-associated Kaposi's sarcoma and with later diagnosis. This indicated that age and year of diagnosis may also serve as predictors of survival (Payne et al. 1990).

Management and Treatment

Overall, treatment for HIV-associated Kaposi's sarcoma appears helpful, but is rarely curative. Treatment schedules remain focused on palliative goals and are usually directed towards individual lesions which are cosmetically disturbing, bulky, and hemorrhagic and cause functional disturbance such as lymphatic obstruction and lymphedema. Moreover, visceral Kaposi's sarcoma, e.g., in the lungs or the gastrointestinal tract, can produce significant functional impairment requiring immediate and effective treatment. Therapeutic strategies should consider the $CD4^+$ counts, the number of Kaposi's sarcoma lesions, the presence of mucosal and visceral involvement, and the history of prior opportunistic infections in addition to the individual requirements of the patients.

Different local modalities for treating HIV-associated Kaposi's sarcoma have been employed with varying success, including local radiation therapy (8–30 Gy), cryosurgery, laser surgery, excisional surgery, and electrocauterization (Schöfer et al. 1991; Plettenberg et al. 1991; Tappero et al. 1991, 1992; Cooper 1990; de Wit et al. 1990).

Also the use of intralesional IFN or intralesional application of chemotherapeutic agents, mainly vinblastine and bleomycin, has been shown to be effective on Kaposi's sarcoma lesions both in cutaneous localization and in the oral cavity (Sulis et al. 1989; Epstein et al. 1989; Boudreaux et al. 1993; Epstein and Scully 1989; Dupuy et al. 1993).

IFN is known to exert antiviral and antiproliferative activities, as demonstrated by tumor regression in various malignancies, and also to display some immune-modulating effects (Krown 1991; Lane et al. 1988; Borden and Ball 1981; Borden et al. 1982). IFN-α is able to inhibit angiogenic lesions induced in mice and to modulate growth factor production (Sidky and Borden 1987). Light and electron microscopic investigations performed in our laboratories revealed cytotoxic effects of rIFN-α-2a on proliferating cells in vivo expressing endothelial cell markers (Mayer da Silva et al. 1987; Ruszczak et al. 1987), and similar findings were obtained on human dermal microvascular cells growing in vitro (Ruszczak et al. 1991). Because of these characteristics, IFN-α became a candidate as a therapeutic agent in HIV-associated Kaposi's sarcoma. In the first series treated with IFN-α monotherapy, 33%–67% responses in patients with HIV-associated Kaposi's sarcoma were reported (Groopmann et al. 1984; Volberding et al. 1984; Rios et al. 1985). Further studies revealed response rates between 27% and 38%, in accordance with our own observations (Gelmann et al. 1985; Abrams and Volberding 1986; Krown et al. 1986; Real et al. 1986; Rozenbaum et al. 1990; Plettenberg et al. 1990). Systemic IFN therapy appears particularly effective in slowly growing nodular tumors in patients with minor systemic symptoms, absence of prior opportunistic infection, and a $CD4^+$ lymphocyte count of more than $200/mm^3$ (Gelmann et al. 1985). We have observed long-term responses with stable disease over 2–5 years (Stadler et al. 1989; Schaart et al. 1991). We also found significant therapeutic improvement under the combined administration of IFN-α and AZT (Kovacs et al. 1989; Krown et al. 1989; Stadler et al. 1990; Fischl et al. 1991; Scadden et al. 1991a). Under this regimen, response rates between 40% and 50% were obtained, showing greater efficacy than IFN-α monotherapy. Experimental evidence indicates synergistic activities between IFN-α and AZT, leading to inhibition of HIV replication by different mechanisms (Fischl 1991; Hartshorn et al. 1987; Ruprecht et al. 1990).

Side effects such as hematologic toxicity and neutropenia were frequent in all combination studies, and several authors advocated the application of colony-stimulating factors (CSF) in order to prevent neutropenia. The addition of granulocyte-macrophage (GM)-CSF and granulocyte (G)-CSF was found beneficial in this respect and did not affect the antitumor activity (Scadden et al. 1991b; Schröder et al. 1992; Krown et al. 1992).

In summary, IFN-α alone or in combination with AZT has an undoubtable benefit in cutaneous and mucocutaneous Kaposi's sarcoma in patients with a peripheral $CD4^+$ count of more than $200/mm^3$ and the absence of opportunistic infections. Furthermore, we found a measureable effect on the prolongation of the median survival times of patients with HIV-associated Kaposi's sarcoma, as discussed above.

As soon as visceral involvement of Kaposi's sarcoma occurs, treatment with combined cytostatic regimens should be considered. Systemic chemotherapy induces regression of HIV-associated Kaposi's sarcoma, even in patients with poor prognostic indicators. Traditional chemotherapeutic agents, such as vinblastine and etoposide, produce high tumor response rates, but their use is often complicated by bone marrow suppression and potentially immunosuppressive effects (Gelmann et al. 1987; Gill et al. 1990b, 1991). The chemotherapeutic agents of choice are vincristine and bleomycin, as both are relatively marrow-sparing agents. In any systemic therapy for HIV-associated Kaposi's sarcoma, antiretroviral therapy appropriate prophylaxis for opportunistic infections, and also hematological support should be available. Promising new therapeutic approaches for

HIV-associated Kaposi's sarcoma include angiogenesis inhibitors, retinoids, anti-tat-compounds, and cytokine antagonists (Lilenbaum and Ratner 1994). Such remedies will hopefully improve the clinical management of this potentially life-threatening tumor and increase the quality of life of people with HIV-associated Kaposi's sarcoma.

References

Abrams DI, Volberding PA (1986) Alpha interferon therapy of AIDS-associated Kaposi's sarcoma. Semin Oncol 13 [3 Suppl 2]:43–47

Archibald CP, Schechter MT, Craib KJ, Le TN, Douglas B, Willoughby B, O'Shaughnessy M (1990) Risk factors for Kaposi's sarcoma in the Vancouver Lymphadenopathy-AIDS Study. J Acquir Immune Defic Syndr 3 [Suppl 1]:S18–S23

Barrison IG, Foster S, Harris JW, Pinching AJ, Walker JG (1988) Upper gastrointestinal Kaposi's sarcoma in patients positive for HIV antibody without cutaneous disease. Br Med J Clin Res Ed 296:92–93

Bary M, Vittecoq D, Liotier JY, Calamy G (1991) Heterosexual transmission of the aetiological agent of Kaposi's sarcoma. Lancet 337:234

Beral V, Peterman TA, Berkelman RL, Jaffe HW (1990) Kaposi's sarcoma among persons with AIDS: a sexually transmitted infection? Lancet 335:123–128

Border EC, Ball LA (1981) Interferons: biochemical, cell growth, inhibitory, and immunological effects. Prog Hematol 12:299–239

Border EC, Hogan TF, Voelkel JG (1982) Comparative antiproliferative activity in vitro of natural interferons α and β for diploid and human cells. Cancer Res 42:4948–4953

Boudreaux AA, Smith LL, Cosby CD, Bason MM, Tappero JW, Berger TG (1993) Intralesional vinblastine for cutaneous Kaposi's sarcoma associated with acquired immunodeficiency syndrome. A clinical trial to evaluate efficacy and discomfort associated with infection. J Am Acad Dermatol 28:61–65

Bratzke B, Stadler R, Eichhorn R, Ehlers G, Orfanos CE (1987) Disseminiertes mukokutanes Kaposi-Sarkom bei AIDS. Klinische und therapeutische Erfahrungen an 13 Patienten. Hautarzt 38:286–294

Bunikowski R, Estermann J, Koch MA (1992) AIDS in der Bundesrepublik Deutschland: die klinische Manifestation von AIDS. Med Klin 87:1–7

Chachoua A, Krigel R, Lafleur F, Ostreicher R, Speer M, Laubenstein L, Wernz J, Rubenstein P, Zang E, Friedman Kien A (1989) Prognostic factors and staging classification of patients with epidemic Kaposi's sarcoma. J Clin Oncol 7:774–780

Cooper JS (1990) Optimal treatment of epidemic Kaposi's sarcoma Int J Radiat Oncol Biol Phys 19:807–808

Couturier E, Ancelle Park RA, de Vincenzi I, Downs AM, Brunet JB (1990) Kaposi sarcoma as a sexually transmitted disease. Lancet 335:1105

de Wit R, Smit WG, Veenhof KH, Bakker PJ, Oldenburger F, Gonzalez DG (1990) Palliative radiation therapy for AIDS-associated Kaposi's sarcoma by using a single fraction of 800 cGy. Radiother Oncol 19:131–136

Delli-Bovi P, Curatola AM, Kern FG, Greco A, Ittmann M, Basilico C (1987) An oncogene isolated by transfection of Kaposi's sarcoma DNA encodes a growth factor that is a member of the FGF family. Cell 50:729–737

Delli-Bovi P, Donti E, Knowles DM Jr, Friedman Kien A, Luciw PA, Dina D, Dalla Favera R, Basilico C (1986) Presence of chromosomal abnormalities and

lack of AIDS retrovirus DNA sequences in AIDS-associated Kaposi's sarcoma. Cancer Res 46:6333–6338
Drew WL, Conant MA, Miner RC et al (1982) Cytomegalovirus and Kaposi's sarcoma in young homosexual men. Lancet 2:125–127
Dupuy J, Price M, Lynch G, Bruce S, Schwartz M (1993) Intralesional interferon-alpha and zidovudine in epidemic Kaposi's sarcoma. J Am Acad Dermatol 28:966–972
Ensoli B, Nakamura S, Salahuddin SZ, Biberfeld P, Larsson L, Beaver B, Wong Staal F, Gallo RC (1989) AIDS-Kaposi's sarcoma-derived cells express cytokines with autocrine and paracrine growth effects. Science 243:223–226
Ensoli B, Barillari G, Salahuddin SZ, Gallo RC, Wong Staal F (1990) Tat protein of HIV-1 stimulates growth of cells derived from Kaposi's sarcoma lesions of AIDS patients. Nature 345:84–86
Ensoli B, Barillari G, Gallo RC (1991) Pathogenesis of AIDS-associated Kaposi's sarcoma. Hematol Oncol Clin North Am 5:281–295
Epstein JB, Lozada Nur F, McLeod WA, Spinelli J (1989) Oral Kaposi's sarcoma in acquired immunodeficiency syndrome. Review of management and report of the efficacy of intralesional vinblastine. Cancer 64:2424–2430
Epstein JB, Scully C (1989) Intralesional vinblastine for oral Kaposi sarcoma in HIV infection. Lancet 2:1100–1101
Feigal DW, Katz MH, Greenspan D, Westenhouse J, Winkelstein W Jr, Lang W, Samuel M, Buchbinder SP, Hessol NA, Lifson AR et al (1991) The prevalence of oral lesions in HIV-infected homosexual and bisexual men: three San Francisco epidemiological cohorts. AIDS 5:519–525
Ficarra G, Berson AM, Silverman S Jr, Quivey JM, Lozada Nur F, Sooy DD, Migliorati CA (1988) Kaposi's sarcoma of the oral cavity: a study of 134 patients with a review of the pathogenesis, epidemiology, clinical aspects, and treatment. Oral Surg Oral Med Oral Pathol 66:543–550
Fischl MA (1991) Antiretroviral therapy in combination with interferon for AIDS-related Kaposi's sarcoma. Am J Med 90:2S–7S
Fischl MA, Uttamchandani RB, Resnick L, Agarwal R, Fletcher MA, Patrone Reese J, Dearmas L, Chidekel J, McCann M, Myers M (1991) A phase I study of recombinant human interferon-alpha 2a or human lymphoblastoid interferon-alpha n1 and concomitant zidovudine in patients with AIDS-related Kaposi's sarcoma. J Acquir Immune Defic Syndr 4:1–10
Friedman Kien AE, Saltzman BR (1990) Clinical manifestations of classical, endemic African, and epidemic AIDS-associated Kaposi's sarcoma. J Am Acad Dermatol 22:1237–1250
Friedman Kien L, Lauberstein L, Marmor M et al (1981) Kaposi's sarcoma and pneumocystis pneumonia among homosexual men – New York City and California. MMWR 30:305–308
Gelmann EP, Preble OT, Steis R, Lane HC, Rook AH, Wesley M, Jacob J, Fauci A, Masur H, Longo D (1985) Human lymphoblastoid interferon treatment of Kaposi's sarcoma in the acquired immune deficiency syndrome. Clinical response and prognostic parameters. Am J Med 78:737–741
Gelmann EP, Longo D, Lane HC, Fauci AS, Masur H, Wesley M, Preble OT, Jacob J, Steis R (1987) Combination chemotherapy of disseminated Kaposi's sarcoma in patients with the acquired immune deficiency syndrome. Am J Med 82:456–462
Gill PS, Rarick M, Bernstein Singer M, Harb M, Espina BM, Shaw V, Levine A (1990a) Treatment of advanced Kaposi's sarcoma using a combination of bleomycin and vincristine. Am J Clin Oncol 13:315–319
Gill PS, Rarick MU, Espina B, Loureiro C, Bernstein Singer M, Akil B, Levine AM (1990b) Advanced acquired immune deficiency syndrome-related Kaposi's

sarcoma. Results of pilot studies using combination chemotherapy. Cancer 65: 1074–1078

Gill PS, Rarick M, McCutchan JA, Slater L, Parker B, Muchmore E, Bernstein Singer M, Akil B, Espina BM, Krailo M et al (1991) Systemic treatment of AIDS-related Kaposi's sarcoma: results of a randomized trial. Am J Med 90:427–433

Giraldo G, Beth E, Henle W et al (1978) Antibody patterns to herpesviruses in Kaposi's sarcoma. II. Seological association of American Kaposi's sarcoma with cytomegalovirus. Int J Cancer 22:126–131

Groopman JE, Gottlieb MS, Goodman J, Mitsuyasu RT, Conant MA, Prince H, Fahey JL, Derezin M, Weinstein WM, Casavante C et al (1984) Recombinant alpha-2 interferon therapy for Kaposi's sarcoma associated with the acquired immunodeficiency syndrome. Ann Intern Med 100:671–676

Hartshorn KL, Vogt MW, Chou TC, Blumberg RS, Byington R, Schooley RT, Hirsch MS (1987) Synergistic inhibition of human immunodeficiency virus in vitro by azidothymidine and recombinant alpha A interferon. Antimicrob Agents Chemother 31:168–172

Harwood AR, Osoba D, Hofstader SL et al (1979) Kaposi's sarcoma in recipients of renal transplants. Am J Med 67:759–765

Haverkos HW (1987) Factors associated with the pathogenesis of AIDS J Infect Dis 156:251–257

Huang YQ, Li JJ, Nicolaides A, Zhang WG, Freidman Kien AE (1992a) Fibroblast growth factor 6 gene expression in AIDS-associated Kaposi's sarcoma. Lancet 339:1110–1111

Huang YQ, Li JJ, Rush MG, Poiesz BJ, Nicolaides A, Jacobson M, Zhang WG, Coutavas E, Abbott MA, Friedman Kien AE (1992b) HPV-16-related DNA sequences in Kaposi's sarcoma. Lancet 339:515–518

Janier M, Morel P, Civatte J (1990) The Koebner phenomenon in AIDS-related Kaposi's sarcoma. J Am Acad Dermatol 22:125–126

Kestens L, Melbye M, Biggar RJ, Stevens WJ, Piot P, De Muynck A, Taelman H, De Feyter M, Paluku L, Gigase PL (1985) Endemic African Kaposi's sarcoma is not associated with immunodeficiency. Int J Cancer 36:49–54

Klein MB, Pereira FA, Kantor I (1974) Kaposi's sarcoma complicating systemic lupus erythematosus treated with immunosuppression. Arch Dermatol 110:602–604

Kovacs JA, Deyton L, Davey R, Falloon J, Zunich K, Lee D, Metcalf JA, Bigley JW, Sawyer LA, Zoon KC et al (1989) Combined zidovudine and interferon-alpha therapy in patients with Kaposi sarcoma and the acquired immunodeficiency syndrome (AIDS). Ann Intern Med 111:280–287

Krown SE (1991) Interferon and other biological agents for the treatment of Kaposi's sarcoma. Hematol Oncol Clin North Am 5:311–322

Krown SE, Real FX, Vadhan Raj S, Cunningham Rundles S, Krim M, Wong G, Oettgen HF (1986) Kaposi's sarcoma and the acquired immune deficiency syndrome. Treatment with recombinant interferon alpha and analysis of prognostic factors. Cancer 57 [Suppl 8]:1662–1665

Krown SE, Metroka C, Wernz JC (1989) Kaposi's sarcoma in the acquired immune deficiency syndrome: a proposal for uniform evaluation, response, and staging criteria. AIDS Clinical Trials Group Oncology Committee. J Clin Oncol 7:1201–1207

Krown SE, Pareoles J, Bundow D, Polsky B, Gold JW, Flomenberg N (1992) Interferon alpha, Zidovudine, and granulocyte-macrophage colony-stimulating factor: a phase I AIDS Clinical Trials Group study in patients with Kaposi's sarcoma associated with AIDS. J Clin Oncol:1344–1351

Lane HC, Kovacs JA, Feinberg J, Herpin B, Davey V, Walker R, Deyton L, Metcalf JA, Baseler M, Salzman N et al (1988) Anti-retroviral effects of

interferon-alpha in AIDS-associated Kaposi's sarcoma. Lancet 2:1218–1222
Lemlich G, Schwam L, Lebwohl M (1987) Kaposi's sarcoma and acquired immunodeficiency syndrome. Postmortem findings in twenty-four cases. J Am Acad Dermatol 16:319–325
Lilenbaum RC, Ratner E (1994) Systemic treatment of Kaposi's sarcoma: current status and future directions. AIDS 8:141–151
Mayer-da Silva A, Stadler R, Imcke E, Bratzke B, Orfanos CE (1987) Disseminated Kaposi's sarcoma in AIDS: histogenesis-related populations and influence of long-term treatment with rIFN-αA. J Invest Dermatol 89:618–624
McKenzie R, Travis WD, Dolan SA, Pittaluga S, Feuerstein IM, Shelhamer J, Yarchoan R, Masur H (1991) The causes of death in patients with human immunodeficiency virus infection: a clinical and pathologic study with emphasis on the role of pulmonary diseases. Medicine (Baltimore) 70:326–343
Miles SA, Rezai AR, Salazar Gonzalez JF, Vander Meyden M, Stevens RH, Logan DM, Mitsuyasu RT, Taga T, Hirano T, Kishimoto T et al (1990) AIDS Kaposi sarcoma-derived cells produce and respond to interleukin 6. Proc Natl Acad Sci USA 87:4068–4072
Nair BC, DeVico AL, Nakamura S, Copeland TD, Chen Y, Patel A, O'Neil T, Oroszlan S, Gallo RC, Sarngadharan MG (1992) Identification of a major growth factor for AIDS-Kaposi's sarcoma cells as oncostatin M. Science 255:1430–1432
Nakamura S, Sakurada S, Salahuddin SZ, Osada Y, Tanaka NG, Sakamoto N, Sekiguchi M, Gallo RC (1992) Inhibition of development of Kaposi's sarcoma-related lesions by a bacterial cell wall complex. Science 255:1437–1440
Orfanos CE (1983) Acquired immune deficiency syndrome (AIDS) und disseminiertes Kaposi-Sarkom. Eine neue Infektionskrankheit? Hautarzt 34:319–321
Orfanos CE, Bratzke B, Lehmann FM (1988) Das HIV-1-assoziierte mukokutane Kaposi-Sarkom. AIFO 3:561–569
Payne SF, Lemp GF, Rutherford GW (1990) Survival following diagnosis of Kaposi's sarcoma for AIDS patients in San Francisco. J Acquir Immune Defic Syndr 3 [Suppl 1]:S14–S17
Peterman TA, Jaffe HW, Beral V (1993) Epidemiologic clues to the etiology of Kaposi's sarcoma. AIDS 7:605–611
Peters BS, Beck EJ, Coleman DG, Wadsworth MJ, McGuinness O, Harris JR, Pinching AJ (1991) Changing disease patterns in patients with AIDS in a referral centre in the United Kingdom: the changing face of AIDS. BMJ 302:203–207
Plettenberg A, Engelmann L, Meigel W (1990a) Pathogenese des HIV-assoziierten Kaposi-Sarkoms – das Koebner-Phänomen als moglicher Auslösemechanismus. Z Hautkr 65:684–686, 689
Plettenberg A, Kern P, Dietrich M, Meigel W (1990b) Rekombinantes Interferon alpha 2A n der Behandlung des HIV-assoziierten Kaposi-Sarkoms. Langzeitergebnisse. Med Klin 85:647–652
Plettenberg A, Janik I, Kolb H, Meigel W (1991) Lokaltherapeutische Massnahmen beim HIV-assoziierten Kaposi-Sarkom mit besonderer Berucksichtigung der Rontgenweichstrahltherapie. Strahlenther Onkol 167:208–213
Real FX, Krown SE (1985) Spontaneous regression of Kaposi's sarcoma in patients with AIDS. N Engl J Med 313:1659
Peal FX, Oettgen HF, Krown SE (1986) Kaposi's sarcoma and the acquired immunodeficiency syndrome: treatment with high and low doses of recombinant leukocyte A interferon. J Clin Oncol 4:544–551
Rendon MI, Roberts LJ, Tharp MD (1988) Linear cutaneous lesions of Kaposi's sarcoma: a clinical clue to the diagnosis of acquired immunodeficiency syndrome. Arch Dermatol 124:327–329

Rios A, Mansell PW, Newell GR, Reuben JM, Hersh EM, Gutterman JU (1985) Treatment of acquired immunodeficiency syndrome-related Kaposi's sarcoma with lymphoblastoid interferon. J Clin Oncol 3:506–512

Rozenbaum W, Gharakhanian S, Navarette MS, De Sahb R, Cardon B, Rouzioux C (1990) Long-term follow-up of 120 patients with AIDS-related Kaposi's sarcoma treated with interferon alpha-2a. J Invest Dermatol 95 [Suppl 6]:161S–165S

Ruprecht RM, Chou TC, Chipty F, Sosa MG, Mullaney S, O'Brien L, Rosas D (1990) Interferon-alpha and 3′-azido-3′-deoxythymidine are highly synergistic in mice and prevent viremia after acute retrovirus exposure. J Acquir Immune Defic Syndr 3:591–600

Ruszczak Z, Mayer-da-Silva A, Orfanos CE (1987) Kaposi's sarcoma in AIDS. Multicentric angioneoplasia in early skin lesions. Am J Dermatopathol 9:388–398

Ruszczak Z, Stadler R, Orfanos CE (1991) Immunphenotyping of HIV-associated Kaposi's sarcoma cells in vivo and in vitro: influence of rIFN-alpha and rIFN-gamma. J Invest Dermatol 96(6):1005

Rutherford GW, Schwarcz SK, Lemp GF, Barnhart JL, Rauch KJ, Warner WL, Piland TH, Werdegar D (1989) The epidemiology of AIDS-related Kaposi's sarcoma in San Francisco. J Infect Dis 159:569–572

Scadden DT, Bering HA, Levine JD, Bresnahan J, Evans L, Epstein C, Groopman JE (1991a) GM-CSF as an alternative to dose modification of the combination zidovudine and interferon-alpha in the treatment fo AIDS-associated Kaposi's sarcoma. Am J Clin Oncol 14 [Suppl 1]:S40–S44

Scadden DT, Bering HA, Levine JD, Bresnahan J, Evans L, Epstein C, Groopman JE (1991b) Granulocyte-macrophage colony-stimulating factor mitigates the neutropenia of combined interferon alfa and zidovudine treatment of acquired immune deficiency syndrome-associated Kaposi's sarcoma. J Clin Oncol 9:802–808

Schaart FM, Bratzke B, Ruszczak Z, Stadler R, Ehlers G, Orfanos CE (1991) Long-term therapy of HIV-associated Kaposi's sarcoma with recombinant interferon alpha-2a. Br J Dermatol 124:62–68

Schöfer H, Ochsendorf FR, Hochscheid I, Milbradt R (1991) Kaposi-Sarkome im Gesicht. Palliative Behandlung mit Kryochirurgie, intraläsionaler Chemotherapie, Röntgenweichstrahltherapie und Camouflage. Hautarzt 42:492–498

Schröder K, Garbe C, Waibel M, Reupke H, Detmar M, Dallenbach F, Orfanos CE (1992) Granulozyten-Koloniestimulierender Faktor (G-CSF) in der Behandlung von Patienten mit HIV-assoziiertem mukokutanem Kaposi-Sarkom. Erfolgreicher Einsatz bei virus- bzw. medikamenteninduzierter Leukopenie. Hautarzt 43:700–706

Sidky YA, Borden EC (1987) Inhibition of angiogenesis by interferons: effects on tumor- and lymphocyte-induced vascular responses. Cancer Res 47:5155–5161

Silverman S Jr, Migliorati CA, Lozada Nur F, Greenspan D, Conant MA (1986) Oral findings in people with or at high risk for AIDS: a study of 375 homosexual males. J Am Dent Assoc 112:187–192

Spornraft P, Froschl M, Ring J, Meurer M, Goebel FD, Ziegler Heitbrock HW, Riethmuller G, Braun Falco O (1988) T4/T8 ratio and absolute T4 cell numbers in different clinical stages of Kaposi's sarcoma in AIDS. Br J Dermatol 119:1–9

Stadler R, Bratzke B, Mayer-da-Silva A, Carbe C, Orfanos CE (1989) Interferons in dermatology. J Am Acad Dermatol 20:650–656

Stadler R, Bratzke B, Schaart F, Orfanos CE (1990) Long-term combined rIFN-alpha-2a and zidovudine therapy for HIV-associated Kaposi's sarcoma: clinical consequences and side effects. J Invest Dermatol 95 [Suppl 6]:170S–175S

Sulis E, Floris C, Sulis ML, Zurrida S, Piro S, Pintus A, Contu L (1989) Interferon administered intralesionally in skin and oral cavity lesions in heterosexual drug

addicted patients with AIDS-related Kaposi's sarcoma. Eur J Cancer Clin Oncol 25:759–761
Tappero JW, Berger TG, Kaplan LD, Volberding PA, Kahn JO (1991) Cryotherapy for cutaneous Kaposi's sarcoma (KS) associated with acquired immune deficiency syndrome (AIDS): a phase II trial. J Acquir Immune Defic Syndr 4:839–846
Tappero JW, Grekin RC, Zanelli GA, Berger TG (1992) Pulsed-dye laser therapy for cutaneous Kaposi's sarcoma associated with acquired immunodeficiency syndrome. J Am Acad Dermatol 27:526–530
Tebbe B, Mayer da Silva A, Garbe C, von Keyserlingk HJ, Orfanos CE (1991) Genetically determined coincidence of Kaposi sarcoma and psoriasis in an HIV-negative patient after prednisolone treatment. Spontaneous regression 8 months after discontinuing therapy. Int J Dermatol 30:114–120
Vogel J, Hinrichs SH, Reynolds RK, Luciw PA, Jay G (1988) The HIV tat gene induces dermal lesions resembling Kaposi's sarcoma in transgenic mice. Nature 335:606–611
Volberding P, Valero R, Rothman J, Gee G (1984) Alpha interferon therapy of Kaposi's sarcoma in AIDS. Ann NY Acad Sci 437:439–446
Vossmann D, Thies W, Bauer R, Orfanos CE (1983) Disseminiertes Kaposi-Sarkom der Haut bei einem jungen Homosexuellen mit Drogenabus. Hautarzt 34:339–345
Wahman A, Melnick SL, Rhame FS, Potter JD (1991) The epidemiology of classic, African, and immunosuppressed Kaposi's sarcoma. Epidemiol Rev 13:178–199
Weindel K, Marme D, Weich HA (1992) AIDS-associated Kaposi's sarcoma cells in culture express vascular endothelial growth factor. Biochem Biophys Res Commun 183:1167–1174
Xerri L, Hassoun J, Planche J, Guigou V, Grob JJ, Parc P, Birnbaum D, deLapeyriere O (1991) Fibroblast growth factor gene expression in AIDS-Kaposi's sarcoma detected by in situ hybridization. Am J Pathol 138:9–15

Human Leukocyte Antigens and Multiple Basal Cell Carcinomas

R. Rompel[1], J. Petres[1], K. Kaupert[2], and G. Müller-Eckhardt[2]

[1] Department of Dermatology, Municipal Clinics of Kassel, Kassel, Germany
[2] Institute for Clinical Immunology and Transfusion Medicine, University of Gießen, Gießen, Germany

Abstract

This study presents data on human leukocyte antigen (HLA) phenotypes of 49 unrelated patients with multiple basal cell carcinomas (five or more BCC). Previous investigators noted an association with HLA-DR1 and a negative association with HLA-DR4. However, the previously found association was weak. HLA typing for class I (HLA-A, -B, -C) and class II antigens (HLA-DR, -DQ) was done from acid citrate dextrose (ACD)-stabilized peripheral blood using the modified lymphocytotoxicity test after T/B cell separation by immunobeads. Antigen frequencies of the patient group were compared to those of healthy individuals of a local German population ($n = 716$). Chi-square test and Fisher's exact test were used for statistical evaluation. While a significant association with HLA-DR1 was not observed in our study, we were able to confirm a significant decrease of HLA-DR4 in the patient group (12.2% versus 25.1%; $p < 0.05$; relative risk, RR, 0.48). In addition, HLA-Cw7 was significantly increased in the patient group (61.2% versus 40.8%; $p < 0.01$; RR, 2.29). In a subgroup of patients with multiple BCC located on the trunk ($n = 25$), the negative association with HLA-DR4 was even stronger (4% versus 25.1%; $p < 0.02$; RR, 0.12), whereas HLA-Cw7 was not significant (60.0% versus 40.8%; $p = 0.06$). Our results showed decreased frequencies of HLA-DR4 and increased frequencies of HLA-Cw7 in cases of multiple BCC, although statistical evaluation revealed only a weak association. This might be due to possible heterogeneity in this disease, e.g., BCC of the trunk versus BCC of the face, or any other cofactors. However, HLA-CR4 may be a protective factor against the development of multiple BCC.

Recent Results in Cancer Research, Vol. 139

Introduction

Basal cell carcinoma (BCC) is the most common malignancy in humans (Miller 1991), and it accounts for more than 75% of all malignant skin tumors (Giles et al. 1988; Yiannias et al. 1988). Several conditions preferentially favor the development of BCC, such as ultraviolet (UV) light (Granstein and Sober 1982), X-ray radiation (Davis et al. 1989), scars (Lawrence 1952), nevus sebaceus (Jones and Heyl 1970), ingestion of arsenic (Shannon and Strayer 1989), and immunosuppression (Miller 1991). Furthermore, some genetic syndromes are associated with the development of multiple BCC, such as Bazex's syndrome (Mehta and Potdar 1985), xeroderma pigmentosum (Kraemer et al. 1984), and nevoid BCC syndrome (Gorlin 1987). However, in the majority of patients with multiple BCC, none of these predisposing conditions are found. Previous investigators noted an association of multiple BCC with human leukocyte (HLA) antigens which might play a role in etiopathogenesis (Gerimele et al. 1988; Czarmecki et al. 1991a,b, 1992; Myskowski et al. 1985). However, these findings were contradictory and the associations were only weak. We have, therefore, investigated HLA class I and class II phenotypes in a cohort of 49 German patients with multiple BCC.

Patients and Methods

HLA typing was done in 49 unrelated patients with multiple BCC who attended the Department of Dermatology, Municipal Clinics of Kassel, Germany. The patients had five or more BCC. Underlying predisposing conditions for the development of multiple BCC, as mentioned above, had been excluded by anamnesis and physical examination as well as laboratory or imaging techniques.

HLA typing for class I (HLA-A, -B, -C) and class II antigens (HLA-DR, -DQ) was done from acid citrate dextrose (ACD)-stabilized peripheral blood using the modified lymphocytotoxicity test after T/B cell separation by immunobeads (Vartdal et al. 1986). Local, commercial, and international antisera were used, including those of international histocompatibility workshops. Antigen frequencies of the patient group were compared to those of healthy individuals of a local German population ($n = 716$). In addition, the patient group was subdivided into two groups according to the main localization of the BCC: BCC on the trunk ($n = 25$) and facial BCC ($n = 24$). The chi-square test and Fisher's exact test were used for statistical evaluation. The p values were corrected by multiplication with the number of antigens tested (class I, 55; class II, 15). The relative risks (RR) were determined in cases of significance.

Results

Phenotype frequencies of HLA class I and class II antigens are shown in Tables 1 and 2, respectively. Regarding the total patient group, a markedly increased frequency of HLA-Cw7 was noted (61.2 versus 40.8%; $p < 0.005$, corrected p not significant; RR, 2.29). HLA-DR4 was observed in 12.2% as compared with 25.1% of the controls ($p < 0.05$, corrected p not significant; RR, 0.48).

The subgroup of patients with multiple BCC of the face also showed an increased frequency of HLA-Cw7 (62.5 versus 40.8%; $p < 0.05$, corrected p not significant; RR, 2.42). No difference was noted for HLA-DR4 in this group.

In the subgroup of patients with multiple BCC mainly on the trunk, HLA-DR4 was even more decreased, to 4.0% as compared with 25.1% of the controls ($p < 0.05$, corrected p not significant; RR, 0.12). Further deviations of antigen frequencies in this group were noted for HLA-A11 (28.0 versus 10.6%; $p < 0.01$), HLA-B17 (24.0 versus 9.1%; $p < 0.05$), HLA-Bw22 (16.0 versus 4.2%; $p < 0.05$), and HLA-Cw3 (44.0 versus 24.4%; $p < 0.05$). However, none of those findings remained significant after correction of p values.

Discussion

Our data first describe a positive association of HLA-Cw7 with multiple BCC. We also confirmed the negative association of HLA-DR4, as previously reported by Czarnecki et al. (1991a). However, statistical evaluation revealed only a weak association with these antigens, while the corrected p values were not significant.

Previous reports on HLA phenotypes in patients with multiple BCC were controversial. An early study by Dellon et al. did not demonstrate any association with antigens of the HLA-A and -B locus in a group of 26 patients (Dellon et al. 1975). Myskowski et al. (1985) first investigated HLA class II antigens with special respect to ethnic groups. The association of HLA-DR1 in non-Irish and non-Ashkenazi patients is questionable, because only 14 patients formed that patient collective. Subsequent studies also noted increased frequencies of HLA-DR1 in multiple BCC. However, the association was only weak, while corrected p values showed no significance (Cerimele et al. 1988; Czarnecki et al. 1991b, 1992). A negative association with HLA-DR4 was only reported by Czarnecki et al. (1991a). The same working group reported a positive association with HLA-DR7 and no association with HLA-DR1 in a collective of 34 patients with five or more BCC and squamous cell carcinomas (Czarnecki et al. 1991b). Weak associations with class I antigens were reported by Cerimele et al. for HLA-B17

Table 1. Human leukocyte (HLA) antigen class I frequencies in patients and controls (subspecificities not listed)

HLA	All BCC ($n = 49$; %)	BCC of the face ($n = 24$; %)	BCC of the trunk ($n = 25$; %)	Controls ($n = 716$; %)
A1	32.7	33.3	32.0	27.7
A2	51.0	58.3	44.0	50.8
A3	32.7	29.2	36.0	29.8
A9	20.4	20.8	20.0	22.6
A10	16.3	20.8	12.0	12.0
A11	16.3	4.2	28.0**	10.6
A19	10.2	12.5	8.0	19.8
A28	4.1	4.2	4.0	8.66
B5	8.2	8.3	8.0	13.8
B7	36.7	37.5	36.0	24.3
B8	16.3	16.7	16.0	18.7
B12	14.3	20.8	8.0	25.1
B13	2.0	0.0	4.0	6.8
B14	4.1	8.3	0.0	6.1
B15	10.2	0.0	20.0	12.0
B16	8.2	8.3	8.0	7.0
B17	16.3	8.3	24.0*	9.1
B18	8.2	4.2	12.0	8.8
B21	6.1	8.3	4.0	5.0
B22	12.2	8.3	16.0*	4.2
B27	10.2	20.8	0.0	8.5
B35	18.4	20.8	16.0	18.3
B37	4.1	8.3	0.0	3.1
B40	14.3	8.3	20.0	13.1
B41	0.0	0.0	0.0	2.1
B47	0.0	0.0	0.0	0.3
B53	2.0	4.2	0.0	1.3
B70	0.0	0.0	0.0	0.6
B73	0.0	0.0	0.0	0.1
Bw4	49.2	70.8	48.0	62.9
Bw6	91.8	87.5	96.0	83.7
Cw1	4.1	4.2	4.0	7.3
Cw2	8.2	12.5	4.0	12.4
Cw3	30.6	16.7	44.0*	24.4
Cw4	16.3	20.8	12.0	21.0
Cw5	10.2	16.7	4.0	13.3
Cw6	22.5	16.7	28.0	19.4
Cw7	61.2***	62.5*	60.0, n.s.	40.8
Cw8	4.1	8.3	0.0	4.8

BCC, basal cell carcinoma.
* $p < 0.05$, corrected p not significant.
** $p < 0.01$, corrected p not significant.
*** $p < 0.005$, corrected p not significant.

Table 2. Human leukocyte (HLA) antigen class II frequencies in patients and controls (subspecificities not listed)

HLA	All BCC ($n = 49$; %)	BCC of the face ($n = 24$; %)	BCC of the trunk ($n = 25$; %)	Controls ($n = 716$; %)
DR1	16.3	16.7	16.0	20.5
DR2	36.7	33.3	40.0	32.4
DR3	26.5	29.2	24.0	18.6
DR4	12.2*	20.8	4.0*	25.1
DR5	28.6	29.2	28.0	26.9
DR6	30.6	29.2	32.0	27.2
DR7	24.5	20.8	28.0	21.9
DR8	2.0	0.0	4.0	4.8
DR9	0.0	0.0	0.0	2.0
DR10	0.0	0.0	0.0	1.4
DR52	75.5	75.0	76.0	64.4
DR53	30.6	29.2	32.0	44.1
DQ1	23.4	70.8	76.0	68.9
DQ2	40.8	41.7	40.0	36.6
DQ3	40.8	45.8	36.0	52.1

BCC, basal cell carcinoma.
*$p < 0.05$, corrected p not significant.

(negative) and HLA-Cw3 (positive association; Cerimele et al. 1988). An increased frequency of HLA-Cw3 also emerged in our subgroup of patients with BCC on the trunk, although this patient group was rather small.

It cannot be ruled out that weak associations with HLA really exist, which might be due to possible heterogeneity of the disease (e.g., BCC of the trunk versus BCC of the face, or any other cofactors). However, on the basis of the literature results and our own findings, the role of HLA antigens in the etiopathogenesis of multiple BCC remains questionable. If a real association of certain HLA antigens does actually exist, it is thought to play only a minor role for the development of multiple BCC. As discussed by Czarnecki et al. (1991a), it appears that environmental factors, especially UV light, override heredity.

Acknowledgements. This work was supported by the Deutsche Forschungsgemeinschaft (DFG MU 725/1–4).

References

Cerimele D, Contu L, Carcassi C et al (1988) HLA and multiple skin carcinomas. Dermatologica 176:176–181

Czarnecki D, Lewis A, Nicholson I, Tait B (1991a) Multiple basal cell carcinomas and HLA frequencies in southern Australia. J Am Acad Dermatol 24:559–561

Czarnecki D, Lewis A, Nicholson I et al (1991b) Multiple nonmelanoma skin cancer associated with HLA DR 7 in southern Australia. Cancer 68:439–440

Czarnecki D, Lewis A, Nicholson I et al (1992) HLA-DR1 is not a sign of poor prognosis for the development of multiple basal cell carcinomas. J Am Acad Dermatol 26:717–719

Davis MM, Hanke CW, Zollinger TW et al (1989) Skin cancer in patients with chronic radiation dermatitis. J Am Acad Dermatol 20:608–616

Dellon AL, Potvin C, Chretein PB (1975) The immunobiology of skin cancer. Plast Reconstr Surg 55:341–352

Giles GG, Marks R, Foley P (1988) Incidence of non-melanocytic skin cancer treated in Australia. Br Med J 296:13–17

Gorlin RJ (1987) Nevoid basal-cell carcinoma syndrome. Medicine (Baltimore) 66:98–113

Granstein RD, Sober AJ (1982) Current concepts in ultraviolet carcinogenesis. Proc Soc Exp Biol Med 170:115–125

Jones EW, Heyl T (1970) Naevus sebaceus. A report of 140 cases with special regard to the development of secondary malignant tumours. Br J Dermatol 82:99–117

Kraemer KH, Lee MM, Scotto J (1984) Xeroderma pigmentosum. Cutaneous, occular, and neurologic abnormalities in 830 published cases. Arch Dermatol 123:241–250

Lawrence EA (1952) Carcinoma arising in the scars of thermal burns. Surg Gynecol Obstet 95:579–588

Mehta VR, Potdar R (1985) Bazex syndrome. Follicular atrophoderma and basal cellopitheliomas. Int J Dermatol 24:444–446

Miller SJ (1991) Biology of basal cell carcinoma, part II. J Am Acad Dermatol 24:161–175

Myskowski PL, Pollack MS, Schorr E et al (1985) Human leukocyte antigen associations in basal cell carcinoma. J Am Acad Dermatol 12:997–1000

Shannon RL, Strayer DS (1989) Arsenic induced skin toxicity. Hum Toxicol 8:99–104

Vartdal F, Gaudernack G, Funderud S et al (1986) HLA class I and II typing using cells positively selected from blood by immunomagnetic isolation – a fast and reliable techique. Tissue Antigens 28:301–312

Yiannias JA, Goldberg LH, Carter-Campbell S et al (1988) The ratio of basal cell carcinoma to squamous cell carcinoma in Houston, Texas. J Dermatol Surg Oncol 14:886–889

Immunohistochemistry of Eccrine Poroma and Porocarcinoma – More Than Acrosyringeal Tumors?

U. Wollina[1], E. Castelli[2], and D. Rülke[1]

[1]Department of Dermatology, Friedrich Schiller University of Jena, 07740 Jena, Germany
[2]Clinica Dermatologica, Universitá de Palermo, Palermo, Italy

Abstract

Sweat gland tumors have been classified according to their presumed physiological counterpart of the sweat apparatus. Both benign poroma and malignant porocarcinoma are thought to be acrosyringeal tumors. In order to specify this general assumption, we performed histochemistry and immunohistochemistry on paraffin sections of 29 poromas and eight porocarcinomas. In detail, we used Lapham's stain, Masson's silver impregnation, and immunoperoxidase staining with glandular marker antibodies against glycoproteins (CEA, LS59, NKI/C-3) and intermediate filament proteins (wide spectrum keratin, Cam 5.2, Vim 9(1)).

Poromas disclosed some scattered S100-positive dendritic cells, red-stained cells in Lapham's method, several silver impregnated dendritic cells, and numerous cells surrounding poromas which were positive for LS59 and NKI/C-3. The labeling with wide spectrum keratin antiserum was low compared to epidermal keratinocytes.

Porocarcinomas made some difference. CEA-positive single vacuolated cells could be observed, and S100-positive cells failed to show dendrites as in poromas. Some tumor cell clusters were stained weakly with LS59 and NKI/C-3 in addition to surrounding cells in both tumor entities. Three out of eight porocarcinomas disclosed sparsely distributed scattered cells weakly reactive with antiboides Cam 5.2 or Vim 9(1).

In general, malignant porocarcinomas expressed a greater variety of cellular markers than benign poromas. The differentiation of both tumors, however, was directed toward inner duct cells and myoepithelium. Since myoepithelial cells are missing in normal acrosyringium, poromas and porocarcinomas are thought to be sweat gland tumors related to the distal portion of the dermal duct.

Recent Results in Cancer Research, Vol. 139

Introduction

The eccrine sweat gland tumors of skin are a group of neoplasias resembling more or less the mature sweat apparatus. Both dedifferentiation from preexisting structures and emergence from pluri- or oligopotential precursor cells have been considered in their formal pathogenesis (Abenoza and Ackerman 1990; Hashimoto et al. 1987; Lever and Schaumburg-Lever 1990; Massa and Medenica 1987).

The concept of histogenesis, however, has been questioned, since even cells with a stable phenotype are capable of changing it either with or without proliferation (Beresford 1990). The change in cellular phenotype depends upon cell type-specific and microenvironmental factors, which are now becoming more and more recognized. This view gains support from clinical data suggesting the existence of fields of neoplasia for adnexal tumors in skin (see Hashimoto et al. 1987; Lever and Schaumburg-Lever 1990). Therefore, tumors may mimic ceertain parts of the sweat apparatus without intimate histogenetic, primary relationship to mature stuctures (Wollina 1993).

In this chapter we will discuss eccrine differentiation of so-called acrosyringeal tumors and the possible role of neuroendocrine cells. A major class comprises benign poroma and the malignant counterpart, porocarcinoma.

Eccrine Poroma

Eccrine poroma was first described by Pinkus et al. (1956) on palmoplantar skin, which is rich in eccrine sweat glands. However, poromas may also, though less frequently, occur in other anatomical regions and occasionally within chronic radiation dermatitis. These dome-shaped or verrucous lesions are often crusted or eroded, easily bleeding but otherwise asymptomatic.

The tumor consists of solid basaloid epithelial cells creating a network that grows downwards from the epidermis. Its stroma is angiomatous. Subgroups of poromas can form cystic spaces within solid masses (solid cystic hidradenoma). Vacuolated or clear cells dominate in clear cell hidradenoma or eccrine acrospiroma (Abenoza and Ackerman 1990; Hashimoto et al. 1987; Massa and Medenica 1987). If the tumor predominates in the dermis, the term dermal duct tumor is commonly used. The formation of cystic areas is more pronounced than in "classical" poromas (Winkelmann and McLeod 1966). Among others, Wick and Swanson (1991) suggested that the above-mentioned subtypes should be classified as poromas, since all of them share significant histopathologic features despite minor variations.

Pinkus et al. (1956) have pointed to the fact that the poroma is never a part of the epidermis, but develops within its boundaries in connection with a 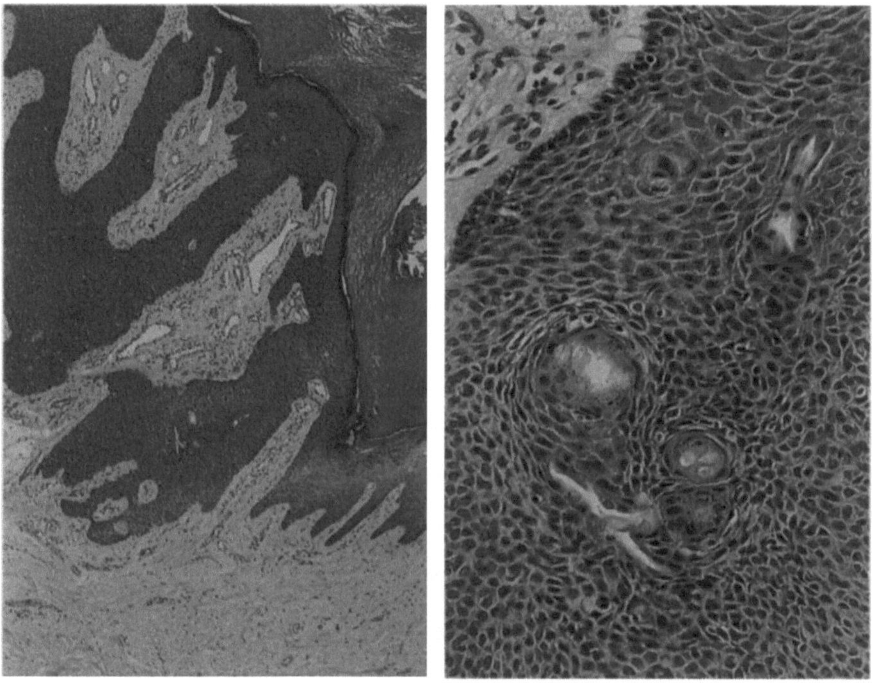 b

Fig. 1a,b. Poroma. Architectural features suggestive of dermal duct involvement. **a** Overview. **b** Dermal duct-like structures and intercellular spaces (hematoxylin-eosin)

(abnormal) sweat ducts. This view opens at least two possible differentiation patterns, i.e., towards the acrosyringium and the dermal duct (Fig. 1).

In dermatopathologic textbooks and reviews on this topic, poromas have been classified as benign acrosyringeal tumors (see Massa and Medenica 1987; Hashimoto et al. 1987; Pinkus et al. 1956). However, there is ultrastructural evidence for separation between tumor cells as in embryonic dermal ducts (Lever and Schaumburg-Lever 1990).

Eccrine Porocarcinoma

The porocarcinoma is a rare adnexal tumor of human skin and was originally described by Pinkus and Mehregan (1963). About 50% of the lesions occur on the lower limbs, followed by the trunk, the upper limbs, and the head. They may present as nodule, plaque, or ulcerated tumors (Fig. 2). Metastastases have been documented (Abenoza and Ackerman 1990; Hashimoto et al. 1987).

The histopathologic picture of the tumor consists of solid masses of anaplastic epithelial cells extending from the epidermis downward into the dermis and occasionally dropping to the subcutaneous fat.

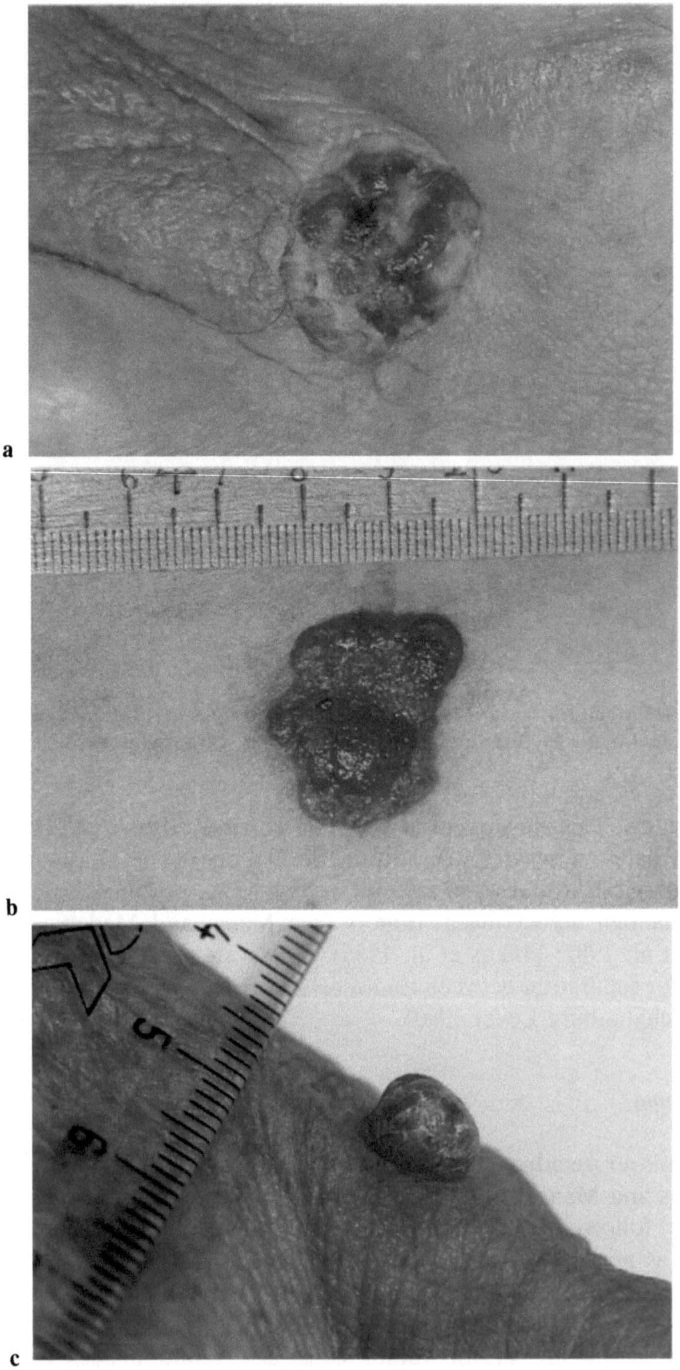

Fig. 2a–c. Clinical variability of porocarcinoma. **a** Ulcerated nodule. **b** Eroded plaque. **c** Exophytic nodule

A remarkable feature of growth is the presence of sharply outlined nests and islands of atypical cells in intraepidermal location (Pinkus and Mehregan 1963). Both in the intraepidermal and in the dermal nests, ducts and duct-like cystic lumina may be seen, which are formed either by vacuolated cells or by separation of neighboring cells.

The tumor masses are composed of large and sometimes multinucleated giant cells with irregularly shaped nuclei and large, variable periodic acid-Schiff (PAS)-reactive cytoplasm, or small cells with hyperchromatic nuclei and scanty cytoplasm. These cells are devoid of tonofibrils but show desmosomes. Mitotic figures are common (Pinkus and Mehregan 1963; Abenoza and Ackerman 1990; Lever and Schaumburg-Lever 1990; Hashimoto et al. 1987; Shaw et al. 1982; Wick and Swanson 1991).

Based upon histopathology, poroma and porocarcinoma have been classified as acrosyringeal tumors (see Hashimoto et al. 1987; Massa and Medenic 1987; Akiyoshi et al. 1991; Mehregan et al. 1983; Snow and Reizner 1992; Shaw et al. 1982). In the present study, we have investigated poromas and porocarcinomas by histochemistry and immunohistochemistry in order to elucidate possible differentiation pathways.

Materials and Methods

Porocarcinomas

A total of 29 poromas and eight porocarcinomas were obtained from the dermatopathologic files of the Clinica Dermatologica dell' University Palermo and the Division of Dermatopathology of the Department of Dermatology, Friedrich Schiller University of Jena.

Tissue Processing and Staining

Routine processed, formalin-fixed tissue was available. Paraffin sections were deparaffinized, rehydrated, and used for histochemical staining (Lapham's method for myoepithelial cells, myelin, and keratin; Masson's silver impregnation for melanocytes) and immunoperoxidase staining with aminoethyl carbazole as described in detail elsewhere (Wollina et al. 1992a,c). The primary antibodies are summarized in Table 1.

Results

By immunohistochemistry, porocarcinomas disclosed a remarkable variability in antigen expression. In general, the cellular phenotypes showed a greater diversification than in the benign poromas.

Table 1. Antibodies

Antibody	Manufacturer/Supplier	
(Neuro-)glandular antigens		
CEA	Dakopatts	Rabbit anti-carcinoembryonal antigen (1:300)
S100A	Dakopatts	Rabbit anti-S100A (prediluted)
LS59	Dr. L.M. Jerry (Calgary/Canada)	IgG2a against NGA (1:100)
NKI/C-3	Monosan	IgG1 against NGA (1:20)
Intermediate filaments		
Wide-spectrum keratin	Dakopatts	Rabbit wide-spectrum antikeratin (1:100)
Cam 5.2	Becton-Dickinson	IgG2a against simple-type keratins (1:2)
Vim 9(1)	Monosan	IgG1 against vimentin (1:10)

CEA, Carcinoembryonic antigen; NGA, neuroglandular antigen.

Lumen formations and single vacuolated cells of porocarcinomas were strongly reactive with CEA (Fig. 3). In several slides, some single CEA-positive cells have been found just beneath the tumor masses within the stroma. Though in single poromas limited lumen formations were observed, the scattered intratumoral and dermal CEA-positive cells were missing.

S100A staining (Fig. 4) of scattered not clustered cells was obvious in both types of tumors. Whereas in poromas these cells clearly formed dendrites, in porocarcinomas more polygonal or irregularly shaped cells were seen. S100A-reactive cells were abundant within the tumor stroma and around small vessels.

In poromas and porocarcinomas, some red-stained cells could be identified with Lapham's method (Fig. 5). They were different from the melanocytes sparsely distributed among these eccrine tumors, which had been identified with silver impregnation (Masson).

LS59 (Fig. 6) and NKI/C-3 (Fig. 7) labeled numerous mast cells around poromas and porocarcinomas. In the latter, there were areas with intratumoral mast cells, too. Intratumoral granulated mast cells were identified in close contact with lumen formations (cuticular cells; Fig. 7). Furthermore, polygonal tumor cell clusters, squamous islands, or lumen formations have been detected in limited malignant cases showing a weak diffuse cytoplasmic staining with LS59 or NKI/C-3.

Immunostaining (Table 2) with broad-spectrum antikeratin was markedly diminished in both tumor entities when compared to adjacent epidermal keratinocytes. In three out of eight porocarcinomas, small, sparsely distributed, scattered cells were weakly reactive with Vim 9(1) or Cam 5.2. In only one case could Cam 5.2-positive epidermal Merkel cells be identified. Two malignant tumors expressed simple-type keratins in circumscribed luminal formations, and another disclosed a weak cytoplasmic Cam 5.2

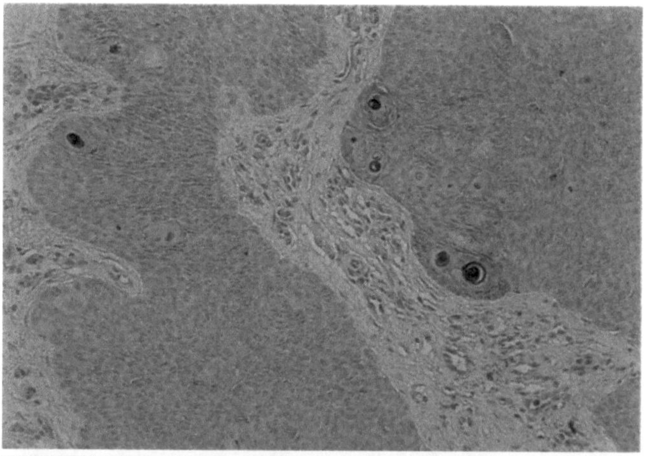

a

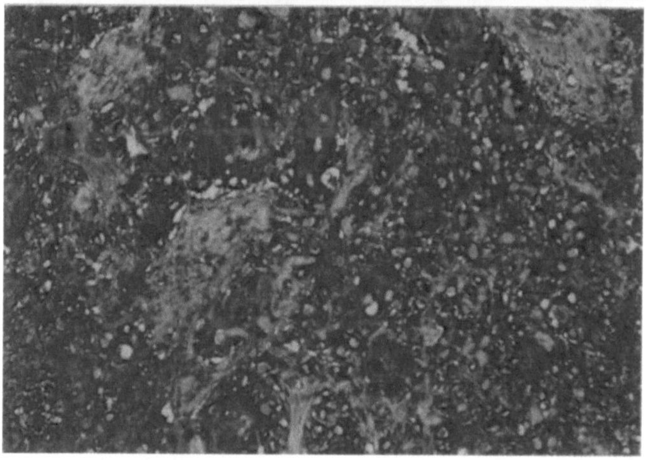

b

Fig. 3a,b. Poroma (**a**) and porocarcinoma (**b**). Immunostaining for carcinoembryonic antigen (CEA). **a** Labeling of eccrine dermal duct. **b** Variable diffuse cytoplasmic staining of tumor cells

reactivity of clusters of polygonal cells without any lumen. Poromas remained unstained with Vim 9(1) and Cam 5.2.

Discussion

Histochemistry and immunostaining of adnexal tumors may not only facilitate diagnosis, but also provides additional information on the eccrine differentiation pathways within these sophisticated skin tumors (Hashimoto et al. 1987; Wick and Swanson 1991; Wollina et al. 1992a,b).

In the present study we have focused on so-called acrosyringeal tumors: poroma and porocarcinoma. Poromas disclosed some red-stained cells with a

b

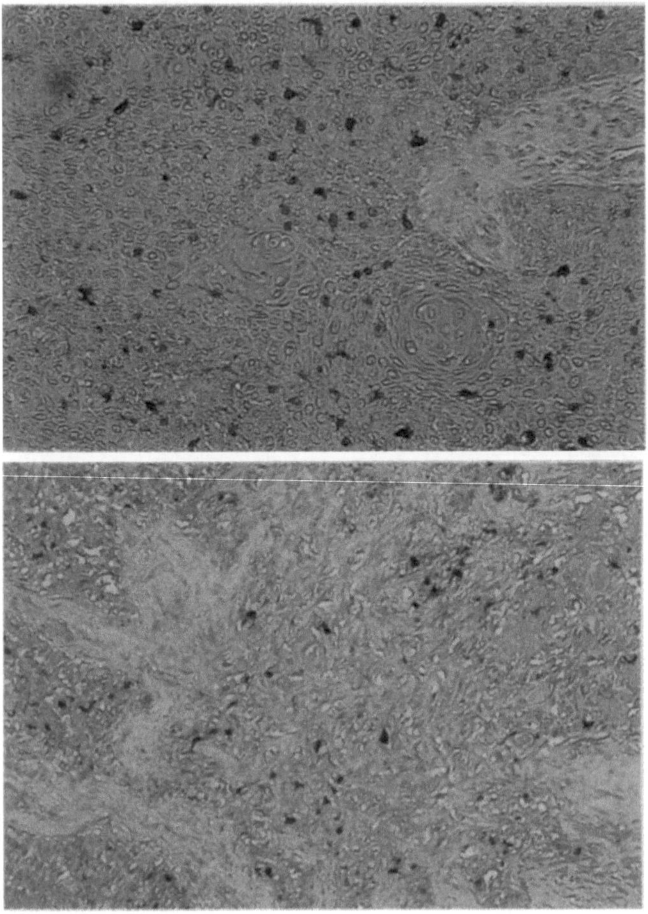

Fig. 4a,b. Poroma (**b**) and porocarcinoma (**b**). Immunostaining for S100A. Note the dendritic cell shape of S100A-positive cells in **b** and the irregular shape of polygonal tumor cells in **a**

Lapham's method, but only a few positively silver-impregnated (Masson) pigment granules. Immunostainings were almost completely negative. In cases with more mature adenoid structures, LS59 and Cam 5.2 were fixed. S100-positive dendritic cells have been classified as melanocytes.

The porocarcinoma is a rare entity of eccrine neoplasms. CEA was expressed by lumen-forming vacuolated cells as well as more mature duct equivalents (Mita et al. 1989; Requena et al. 1990). In some cases we observed a dropping of CEA-positive cells from the tumor masses into the stroma. S100A was almost limited to scattered, irregularly shaped cells – probably related to dendritic cells within eccrine poromas (Mita et al. 1989) or to myoepithelial cells (Guelstein et al. 1988; Wollina et al. 1991; Wollina

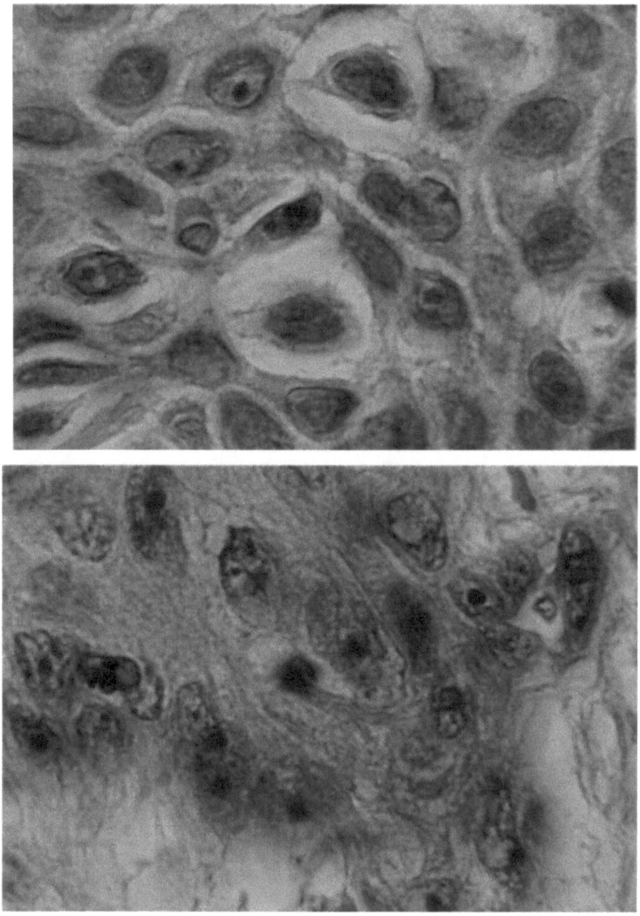

a

b

Fig. 5a,b. Poroma (**a**) and porocarcinoma (**b**). Lapham's stain shows myoepithelial cells (reddish) in both tumor types

and Castelli 1993; McGuire et al. 1988). Requena et al. (1990) observed interdigitating S100-positive cells of the surrounding epidermis, but not within a periungual porocarcinoma.

The expression of neuroglandular antigens detected by the monoclonal antibodies NKI/C-3 and LS59 was very limited in our material. Squamous islands or lumen formations were stained. On the other hand, we observed a variable amount of immunoreactive cells with a granulated cytoplasm, which are thought to represent mast cells (Sikora et al. 1987; Wollina et al. 1992a).

Simple-type, glandular keratins recognized by monoclonal antibody Cam 5.2 were found in traces among very sparsely distributed malignant tumor cells, whereas in a study on mucinous sweat gland carcinomas all tumors

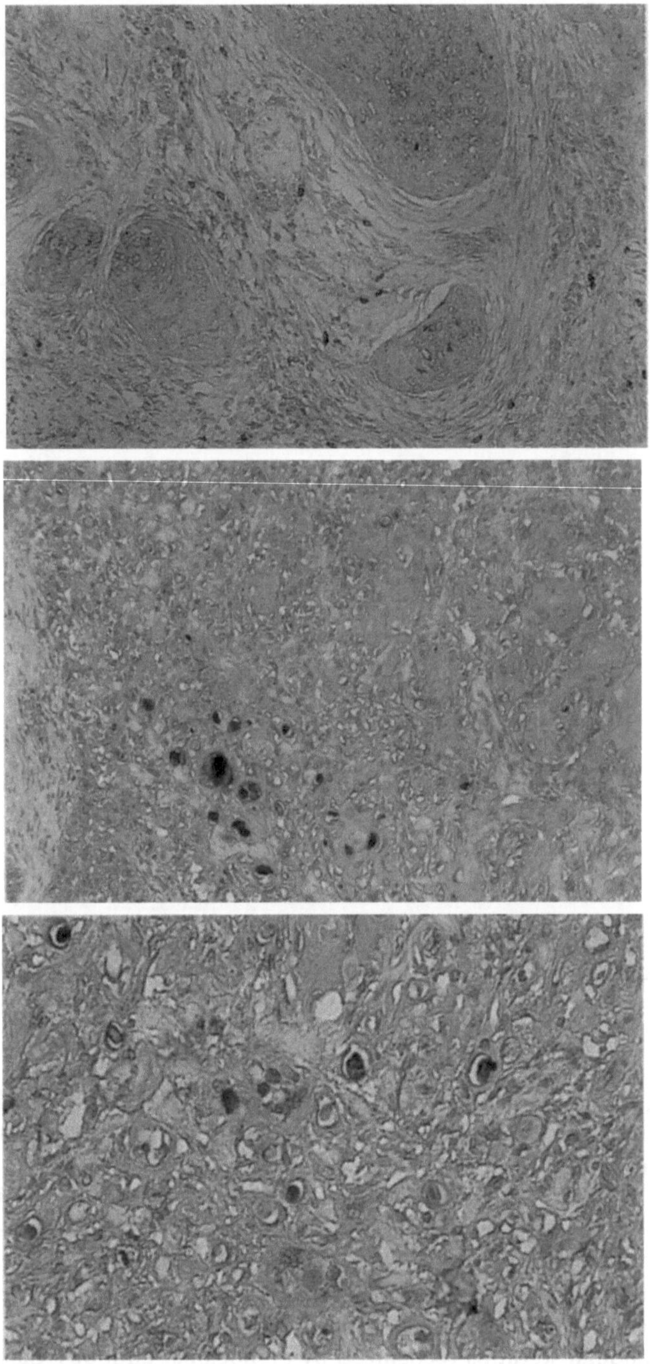

a

b

c

Fig. 6a–c. Poroma (**a**) and porocarcinoma (**b, c**). Immunostaining for LS59. **a** Variable staining of stromal and intratumoral mast cells. **b, c** Strong cytoplasmic staining of mast cells in close relation to cuticular tumor cells

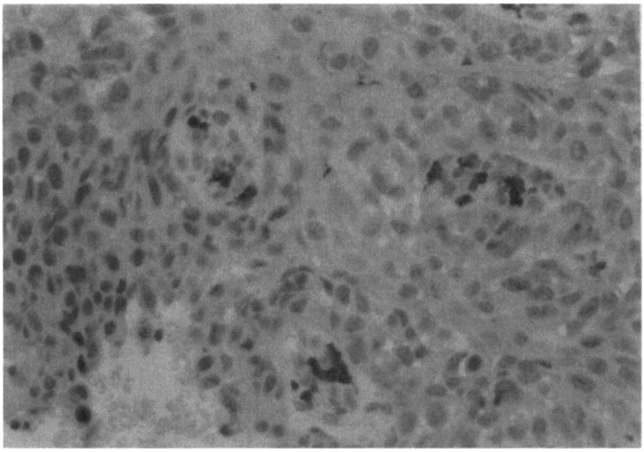

Fig. 7. Porocarcinoma, immunostaining with NKI/C-3. Numerous granulated mast cells in close contact to cuticular cells

Table 2. Immunostaining patterns of porocarcinomas (PC), poromas (PO), and the normal human sweat gland apparatus (SG) (see Wollina 1993; Wollina et al. 1991)

Antibodies	PC	PO	SG
CEA	++/−	++/−	++ (Secretory coil and inner duct cells)
S100A duct	+/−	−	+/++ (Inner cells and myoepithelium)
LS59	+/+	(+)/−	+ (Secretory coils)
NKI/C-3	+/−	−	− (Secretory coils)
Wide-spectrum keratin	(+)	−	++ (Myoepithelium, secretory and outer duct cells)
Cam 5.2	++/−	−	++ (Myoepithelium and secretory coils)
Vim 9(1)	(+)/−	−	+ (Myoepithelium)

CEA, Carcinoembryonic antigen.

specimens reacted with antibodies to keratins nos. 7, 8, 18, and 19 (Eckert et al. 1993).

Vimentin reactivity was weak and limited to some scattered cells within porocarcinomas. The expression of vimentin, S100A, and glandular keratins by components of porocarcinomas suggests myoepithelial differentiation (Mita et al. 1989; Wollina 1991). This has gained further support by histochemical stains, which demonstrated scattered red cells by Lapham's method. Eckert et al. (1992), however, failed to detect myoepithelial cells in 14 cases of poroma stained for alpha-smooth muscle actin. Concerning the increasing literature on myoepithelial differentiation in glandular tumors, there is no uniformity in the expression of so-called marker antigens (S100, actin, keratin, vimentin) among myoepithelial cells with possible coexpression of intermediate filaments (Eckert et al. 1992; McGuire et al. 1988; Guelstein et al. 1988; Wollina 1991; Wollina et al. 1992b). The variability in phenotype is remarkable and may represent a limited degree of commitment.

If we compare immunoreactivity of poroid and cuticular cells of both poroma and porocarcinoma, the latter seem the more differentiated. Indeed, none of the antibodies selectively labeled poroid cells (see Abenoza and Ackerman 1990).

Winkelmann and McLeod (1966) stated with regards to differentiating poroma and dermal duct tumor that "a dermal tumor of the pore is a paradox." Our immunohistochemical data suggest that poroma and porocarcinoma are eccrine tumors with a variable differentiation towards both inner duct epithelium and myoepithelium. Mita et al. (1989) reported ultrastructural findings resembling neurosecretory granules of anaplastic cells, pointing to a neuroendocrine differentiation in porocarcinoma.

In the normal sweat gland, there is no evidence of myoepithelial cells in the acrosyringium (Hashimoto et al. 1965) or the dermal duct, in contrast to the secretory coils (Hashimoto et al. 1966). This raises doubts about whether poromas and porocarcinomas are acrosyringeal tumors, as suggested previously, since they may contain a dermal component of eccrine glands, the myoepithelial cell. Additionally, these tumors show variable numbers of neuroendocrine cells of skin – melanocytes (in poromas only), mast cells, and probably Merkel cells – within the tumor masses.

In conclusion, poroma and porocarcinoma are composed of poroid, undifferentiated and cuticular, fairly well differentiated cells. By histochemistry and immunohistochemistry, classification of poroma and porocarinoma as eccrine tumors with a variable differentiation toward the eccrine duct epithelium and myoepithelium and neuroendocrine cells is supposed, resolving the paradox mentioned by Winkelmann and McLeod (1966). Furthermore, topographical distribution of immunoreactive mast cells (see Fig. 7) is suggestive of a not yet described interaction with cuticular tumor cells and their participation in duct formation.

Acknowledgement. This study was supported in part by the "BMFT-Projekt: Klinisch-orientierte Neurowissenschaften." The technical assistance of Ms. S. Feldrappe is highly appreciated.

References

Abenoza P, Ackerman AB (1990) Neoplasms with eccrine differentiation. Lea and Febiger, Philadelphia

Akiyoshi E, Nogita T, Yamaguchi R, Toyoda H, Kawashima M, Hidano A (1991) Eccrine porocarcinoma. Dermatologica 182:239–242

Beresford WA (1990) Direct transdifferentiation: can cells change their phenotype without dividing? Cell Differ Dev 29:81–93

Eckert F, Betke M, Schmoeckel C, Neuweiler, J, Schmid U (1992) Myoepithelial differentiation in benign sweat gland tumors. J Cutan Pathol 19:294–301
Eckert F, Schmid U, Hardmeier T, Altmannsberger M (1993) Cytokeratin expression in mucinous sweat gland carcinomas: an immunohistochemical analysis of four cases. Histopathology 21:161–165
Guelstein VI, Tchypysheva TA, Ernilova VD, Livinova LA, Troyanovsky SM, Bannikov G (1988) Monoclonal antibody mapping of keratins 8 and 17 and of vimentin in normal human mammary gland, benign tumours, dysplasias and breast cancer. Int J Cancer 42:147–153
Hashimoto K, Gross BG, Lever WF (1965) The ultrastructure of the skin of human embryos. I. The intraepidermal eccrine sweat duct. J Invest Dermatol 45:139–151
Hashimoto K, Gross BG, Lever WF (1966) The ultrastructure of the skin of human embryos. II. The formation of intradermal portion of the eccrine sweat duct and the secretory segment during the first half of embryonic life. J Invest Dermatol 46:513–529
Hashimoto K, Mehregan AH, Kumakiri M (1987) Tumors of skin appendages. Butterworth, Stoneham
Landa NG, Winkelmann RK (1991) Epidermotropic eccrine porocarcinoma. J Am Acad Dermatol 24:27–31
Lever WF, Schaumburg-Lever G (1990) Histopathology of the skin, 7th edn. Lippincott, Philadelphia
Massa M, Medenica M (1987) Cutaneous adnexal tumors and cysts: a review, part II. Tumors with apocrine and eccrine glandular differentiation and miscellaneous cutaneous cysts. Pathol Annu 22:225–276
McGuire LJ, Ng JPW, Lee JCK (1988) Coexpression of cytokeratin and vimentin. Appl Pathol 7:73–84
Mehregan AH, Hashimoto K, Rahbari H (1983) Eccrine adenocarcinoma. A clinicopathologic study of 35 cases. Arch Dermatol 119:104–111
Mita H, Takigawa M, Iwatsuki K, Todura Y, Inoue K, Yamada M (1989) An immunohistologic study on eccrine gland carcinoma. J Am Acad Dermatol 20: 693–696
Pinkus H, Mehregan AH (1963) Epidermotropic eccrine carcinoma. Arch Dermatol 88:597–606
Pinkus H, Rogin JR, Goldman P (1956) Eccrine Poroma. Tumors exhibiting features of the epidermal sweat duct unit. Arch Dermatol 74:511–521
Requena L, Sánchez M, Aguilar A, Ambrojo P, Sánchez Yus E (1990) Periungual porocarinoma. Dermatologica 180:177–180
Sikora LKJ, Pinto A, Demetrick DJ, Dixon WT, Urbanski SJ, Temple W, Jerry LM (1987) Characterization of a novel neuroglandular antigen (NGA) expressed on abnormal melanocytes. Int J Cancer 39:138–145
Shaw M, McKee PH, Lowe D, Black MM (1982) Malignant eccrine poroma: a study of twenty-seven cases. Br J Dermatol 107:675–680
Snow SN, Reizner GT (1992) Eccrine porocarcinoma of the face. J Am Acad Dermatol 27:306–311
Wick MR, Swanson PE (1991) Cutaneous adnexal tumors. A guide to pathologic conditions. ASCP Press, Chicago
Winkelmann RK, McLeod WA (1966) The dermal duct tumor. Arch Dermatol 94:50–55
Wollina U (1991) Human eccrine sweat gland. Expression of neuroglandular antigens and coexpression of intermediate filaments. Histol Histopathol 6:191–198
Wollina U (1993) Diversity of epithelial skin tumors: thoughts and comments on some basic principles. In: Hecker E, Jung EG, Marks F, Tilgen W (eds) Skin carcinogenesis in man and in experimental models. Springer, Berlin Heidelberg New York, pp 153–178 (Recent results in cancer research, vol 128)

Wollina U, Castelli E (1993) Immunohistochemistry of eccrine porocarcinoma. Oncology Rep 1:101–105

Wollina U, Henkel U, Schaarschmidt H, Knopf B, Hipler C (1991) Human eccrine sweat glands – a histochemical approach. Anat Anz 173:155–159

Wollina U, Rülke D, Schaarschmidt HH (1992a) Distribution of calmodulin-immunoreactivity (CaM-IR) and neuroglandular antigen among adnexal tumors of skin. Eur J Dermatol 2:435–439

Wollina U, Rülke D, Schaarschmidt HH (1992b) Dermal cylindroma. Expression of intermediate filaments, epithelial and neuroectodermal antigens. Histol Histopathol 7:575–582

Wollina U, Schaarschmidt H, Rülke D (1992c) Sweat gland tumors of skin: immunohistochemistry with common antibodies in the paraffin section. Int J Oncol 1:395–402

V. Treatment and Management

Excision of Primary Melanoma Should Allow Primary Closure of the Wound

N. Cascinelli and M. Santinami

Surgical Oncology B, National Cancer Institute, Via G. Venezian, 1, 20133 Milan, Italy

Abstract

There is no doubt about the fact that surgery is mandatory for primary melanoma. The problem in the recent past has been how wide and deep the excision of primary melanoma has to be. Results published from the World Health Organization (WHO) Melanoma Program have clearly demonstrated that a procedure involving up to 2-mm thickness and 1-cm margins is safe. Further trials dealing with melanoma thicker than 2 mm are being carried out, and preliminary results confirm that even in this case narrow excision is the correct procedure. At present we may assume that for stage I melanoma the excision of the primary tumor should in the majority of cases allow primary closure of the wound.

Introduction

Up to the 1960s and later, the conventional therapy for primary melanoma was wide excision (3- to 5-cm margin) plus plastic repair if needed. The reason for this width was to remove any neoplastic cells in the tissue surrounding the primary that may lead to local recurrences, in transit metastases, or distant metastases (Cochran 1971; Olsen 1966). When Breslow and Macht (1977) introduced their new histologic parameter in the 1970s, strictly correlated with prognosis, surgeons began to reconsider the problem of wide excision. There is no doubt that melanomas with a thickness of up to 0.76 mm do not require wide excision of any kind; in fact, all surgeons agree on this issue that 1 cm margin is sufficient. However, for thicker melanomas the surgical margins vary according to the ideas of different authors (Cascinelli et al. 1980; Milton et al. 1980; Day et al. 1982; Goldman and Byrd 1988; Balch et al. 1979) in relation to various histologic parameters. To create some degree of order in this field, at the end of the 1970s the

Recent Results in Cancer Research, Vol. 139

WHO Melanoma Program started a randomized clinical trial comparing wide versus narrow excision for melanomas up to 2 mm thick. After a narrow excision of 1 cm, the study was based on two arms: one requiring the traditional wide excision (3-cm margin from the surgical scar) and the other being the control group. The trial was completed on 1988, 612 patients having been entered into the study. Results published by Veronesi and Cascinelli (1991) demonstrated that for Breslow's thickness of up to 2 mm narrow excision is a safe procedure. In fact (Fig. 1), overall survival is similar in both arms, and local recurrences (Table 1) only appeared in four cases. The frequency of adverse events during follow-up was similar in the two groups when regional lymph node metastases, in-transit metastases, and metastatic spread to distant sites were taken into consideration. The histologic examination of the four local recurrences (all in the narrow excision arm) did not establish whether they were cases of local residual disease or a metastatic event. A subsequent analysis of the four cases, including time elapsed from primary treatment and the characteristics of primary, seems to support the view that local recurrences were unrelated to the width of excision of primary tumor.

At present, we can state that for primary melanomas up to 2 mm thick, narrow excision (1-cm margin) is the recommended procedure (Veronesi

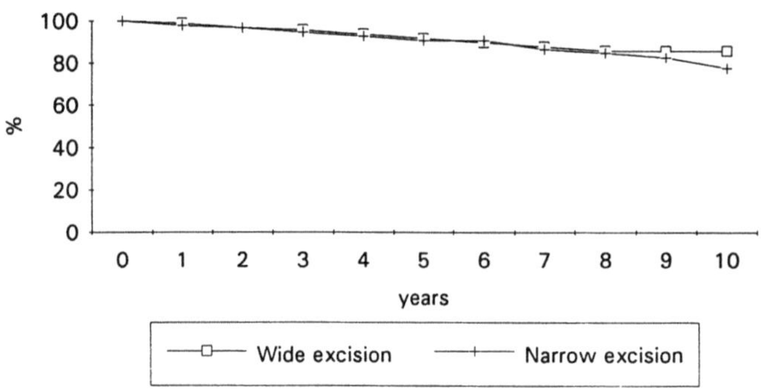

Fig. 1. Overall survival of stage I patients (n = 612; Veronesi 1991)

Table 1. Site of first relapse (Veronesi 1991)

Recurrences	Narrow excision	Wide excision	Total
Local recurrence	4	0	4
In-transit metastases	2	2	4
Regional node metastases	21	24	45
Distant metastases	17	14	31
Total	44	40	84

and Cascinelli 1991; Cosimi et al. 1984; Day et al. 1982; Ackerman and Scheiner 1983).

More recently, the Melanoma Intergroup started another randomized trial, the goal of which is to verify whether 2 cm or 4 cm is adequate for melanoma ranging from 1 to 4 mm: preliminary results of this study confirm that a 2-cm excision margin (in most instances compatible with primary closure of the wound) is safe in this group of patients. A reasonable policy for the surgical treatment of primary melanoma as a function of tumor thickness is given in Table 2.

Surgical Treatment

Surgical treatment of primary melanoma is an easy task; usually an elliptical incision is performed in the direction of lymphatic drainage, allowing skin closure in the majority of cases; another possibility, especially for melanoma located on the trunk, is to remove a square area with the primary in the center and to close the wound by rotating a contiguity flap. Nevertheless, it does not matter what type of surgical excision or plastic repair is used, as they do not influence survival or appearance of local recurrences. For cosmetic reasons we recommend the avoidance of skin graft as far as possible.

The other controversial point is the removal of the underlying fascia. On the basis of observations by Olsen (1964), many surgeons still continue to excise the deep fascia. However, Kenady (Kenady et al. 1982) showed that the removal of fascia is not relevant in term of survival of local recurrence. Even in our experience, the removal of fascia is useless, and for primary tumors in certain locations, such as the extremities, it may cause problems in closure and functionality (muscle hernia).

In view of this, the excision of primary melanoma in depth should be extended as far as the fascia, but does not require the removal of fascia.

Obviously, there are some particular areas in which excisions of melanoma require a different procedure, such as in the fingers , toes, face, or breast.

Table 2. Surgical treatment of primary melanoma

Primary	Margin (cm)
In situ	A few mm
<2 mm	1 cm
>2 mm[a]	2–3 cm
LLMM	1 cm

LLMM, Lentigo Maligna
[a] Results of the Melanoma Intergroup study still awaited.

Face

Obviously, excision in the face must be limited for cosmetic reason. So far, excision is usually limited to 1-cm margins, regardless of the Breslow's thickness. For melanoma on the ear, we recommend prolonging the triangular excision as far as the external auricular canal in order to facilitate closure.

Fingers and Toes

The goal of excision of primary tumors located on the fingers or toes is to reduce as much as possible the degree of amputation required in order to preserve functionality. Thus if the primary tumor is located on the nail bed, amputation at level of the interphalangeal joint is required. Metacarpophalangeal disarticulation is required if it is located on the other part of the finger. For melanoma located on the toes, metatarsophalangeal disarticulation is appropriate and does not cause any particular problems to the patient.

Breast

Even in the breast, the correct indication is an excision as performed in any other part of the skin surface. There is no need for total mastectomy, as used to be performed (Papachristou et al. 1979; Roses et al. 1979; Lee et al. 1977; Ariel and Caron 1972).

References

Ackerman AB, Scheiner AM (1983) How wide and deep is wide and deep enough? Hum Pathol 14:743
Ariel IM, Caron AS (1972) Diagnosis and treatment of malignant melanoma arising from the skin of the female breast. Am J Surg 124:284
Balch CM, Murad TM, Soong S-J, Ingalls AL, Richards PC, Maddox WA (1979) Tumour thickness as a guide to surgical management of stage I melanoma patients. Cancer 43:883
Breslow A, Macht SD (1977) Optimal size of resection margin for thin cutaneous melanoma. Surg Gynecol Obstet 143:973
Cascinelli N, Van der Esch EP, Breslow A, Morabito A, Bufalino R (1980) Stage I melanoma of the skin: the problem of resection margin. Eur J Cancer 16:1079
Cochran AJ (1971) Studies of the melanocytes of the epidermis adjacent to tumours. J Invest Dermatol 57:38
Cosimi AB, Sober AJ, Mihm MC, Fitzpatrick TB (1984) Conservative surgical management of superficially invasive cutaneous melanoma. Cancer 53:1256
Day CL Jr, Mihm MC, Sober AJ, Fitzpatrick TB, Malt RA (1982) Narrower margins for clinical stage I malignant melanoma. N Engl J Med 306:479

Goldman LI, Byrd R (1988) Narrowing resection margins for patient with low risk melanoma. Am J Surg 155:242
Kenady DE, Brown BW, McBride CM (1982) Excision of underlying fascia with primary malignant melanoma: effects on recurrence and survival rates. Surgery 92:615
Lee YN, Sparks FC, Morton DL (1977) Primary melanoma of the skin of the breast region. Ann Surg 185:17
Milton GW, Shaw HM, Farago GA, McCarthy WJ (1980) Tumour thickness and site and time of first recurrence in cutaneous malignant melanoma (stage I). Br J Surg 67:543
Olsen G (1964) Removal of fascia – cause of more frequent metastases of malignant melanomas of the skin to regional lymph nodes? Cancer 17:1159
Olsen G (1966) The malignant melanoma of the skin: new theories based on a study of 500 cases. Acta Chir Scand Suppl 365:1
Papachristou DN, Kinne DW, Rosen PP, Ashikari R, Fortner JG (1979) Cutaneous melanoma of the breast. Surgery 85:322
Roses DF, Harris MN, Stern JS, Gumport SL (1979) Cutaneous melanoma of the breast. Ann Surg 189:112
Veronesi U, Cascinelli N (1991) Narrow excision (1-cm margin). A safe procedure for thin cutaneous melanoma. Arch Surg 126:438

Role of Elective Lymph Node Dissection in Stage I Malignant Melanoma: Evaluation by Matched Pair Analysis

R. Rompel[1], C. Garbe[2], P. Büttner[2], K. Teichelmann[1], and J. Petres[1]

[1] Department of Dermatology, Municipal Clinics of Kassel, Kassel, Germany
[2] Department of Dermatology, Free University of Berlin, Berlin, Germany

Abstract

The role of elective lymph node dissection (ELND) in clinical stage I malignant melanoma continues to be controversial. We present a matched pair analysis of 375 patients treated in the Department of Dermatology in Kassel between 1979 and 1991 by wide local excision (WLE) plus ELND. Multivariate analysis revealed tumor thickness, level of invasion, age, sex, and localization as independent prognostic factors, and 375 patients treated by WLE alone were matched as controls to the patients treated by ELND and WLE. There was no significant benefit from WLE plus ELND compared to WLE alone in the total group as shown by the 5-year survival rates (87.3% versus 86.4%) and 10-year survival rates (80.1% versus 77.82%). Increased survival rates were noted for tumor thicknesses 1.51–4.0 mm for the WLE plus ELND group, as shown by the 10-year survival rates of 73.1% versus 60.3%. However, these data were not significant ($p = 0.14$). Disease-free survival rates were significantly higher in the group treated by additional ELND for all tumor thicknesses ($p < 0.05$) and even more in intermediate tumor thicknesses of 1.51–4.0 mm ($p < 0.001$). A significant benefit of elective lymph node dissection was detected for malignant melanoma of the trunk (all tumor thicknesses), as shown by the 5-year survival rates of 92.0% versus 79.7% and 10-year survival rates of 80.4% versus 45.16% ($p < 0.05$). Malignant melanoma of the extremities revealed no significant differences in survival rates. We conclude that there is a certain benefit from ELND in clinical stage I malignant melanoma for tumor thicknesses of 1.51–4.00 mm. Especially in malignant melanoma of the trunk, WLE plus ELND was more beneficious than WLE alone.

Recent Results in Cancer Research, Vol. 139

Introduction

The role of elective lymph node dissection (ELND) in stage I malignant melanoma has been discussed quite controversially in recent decades. The rational background for the ELND is based on the hypothesis of a stepwise spread from the primary to the regional nodes and then to distant sites, which is true for the majority of cases, but of course not for all. In clinical stage I melanoma, the ELND is intended to eliminate possible micrometastases of the regional lymph nodes.

Several retrospective studies on large patient collectives have shown prognostic improval concerning disease-free survival and overall survival time. Most of these studies revealed significant prognostic improvements for intermediate tumor thicknesses (Fortner et al. 1977; Balch 1980; Milton et al. 1982; Balch et al. 1982; Reintgen et al. 1983; Shaw et al. 1987; McCarthy et al. 1985, 1988; Balch 1988; Balch et al. 1992; Drepper et al. 1993). This had been explained by the low metastatic risk in small thicknesses and, on the other hand, the increased risk of distant metastases in greater tumor thicknesses, which overrides the effect of ELND. Opponents of ELND refer mainly to the two prospective studies carried out by WHO (Veronesi et al. 1977, 1982) and the Mayo Clinic (Sim et al. 1978, 1986); however, even these studies have not withstood all criticism. Further retrospective studies on relatively small patient collectives also did not demonstrate a significant benefit of ELND (Elder et al. 1985; Karakousis et al. 1987; Binder et al. 1990).

We present data of a matched pair analysis of 375 patients treated by wide local excision (WLE) plus ELND (Department of Dermatology, Municipal Clinics, Kassel, Germany) and 375 patients treated by wide local excision alone (data from the Central Malignant Melanoma Registry of the German Dermatological Society).

Patients and Methods

Between 1979 and 1991, a total of 1269 patients were treated at the Department of Dermatology, Municipal Clinics of Kassel, Germany. Of these, a series of 375 patients with clinical stage I malignant melanoma of the trunk or extremities was treated by WLE (≥3.0 cm) and ELND, taking into consideration medium or high risk for local or distant metastasis. Inclusion criteria for the ELND were: Breslow thickness of 0.75 mm or more, and/or Clark level of III or more, and/or ulceration. Inclusion criteria were the same throughout the treatment period.

The operative technique for ELND was the same throughout the study, and the operations were performed by only four experienced dermatosurgeons at the Department of Dermatology in Kassel. All surgical procedures strived for maximal radicality according to the strategies and techniques described by Balch and by Karakousis et al., respectively (Balch 1990; Karakousis et al. 1986, 1989). Patients with malignant melanoma located on the trunk underwent ^{99}Tc lymphoscintigraphy for detection of the lymphatic drainage. In the case of bilateral and/or axilloinguinal drainage, the concerning lymphatic regions were dissected.

Disease-free and overall survival rates of the 375 patients treated by WLE and ELND were compared to those of a pool of 1393 patients with stage I malignant melanoma documented by the Central Malignant Melanoma Registry of the German Dermatologic Society. These patients had been treated by WLE only.

In both groups a standardized follow-up in all patients was performed at intervals of 3 months during the first 5 years and at intervals of 6 months between the sixth and tenth year. Complete tumor staging (chest X-ray, abdominal sonography, sceletal scintigraphy, cranial computed tomography) was performed at least once every year.

Data analysis was performed in two steps: first, the multivariate Cox hazard analysis was performed to identify the major independent prognostic factors within the entire collective, including all patients of both treatment groups. This analysis was performed regarding disease-free and overall survival rates. Second, a matched pair comparison between 375 cases treated by WLE plus ELND and 375 patients treated by WLE alone was performed and univariate disease-free survival and overall survival, respectively, were calculated by means of the actuars method (Cutler and Ederer 1958). Matching was done for the major independent prognostic factors such as tumor thickness (≤0.75 mm, 0.75–1.50 mm, 1.50–4.00 mm, >4.00 mm), level of invasion (II, III, IV, V), age (≤40 years, >40 years), sex, and localization (trunk, extremities). The selection of control cases was performed by a random computer program on the basis of dBASE IV.

Results

The results of the multivariate analysis are shown in Tables 1–3. Age, sex, Breslow thickness, Clark level, tumor type, and localization were confirmed as major independent prognostic factors. In addition, ELND was noted as a significant prognostic parameter for the disease-free interval, while it was not significant for the overall survival time in the entire collective.

Following the matching, patient characteristics and prognostic factors were virtually the same in both groups, as shown in Table 4. The chi-square test and *t* test, respectively, revealed no significant differences between the two groups, except for ulceration, which was higher in the WLE plus ELND group. the median age for patients treated by WLE plus ELND was 53 years (mean, 51.2; standard deviation, SD, 14.1). The matched control group treated by WLE alone had a median age of 52 years (mean, 51.6; SD, 14.6). Tumor thickness as the major prognostic factor was com-

Table 1. Multivariate Cox hazard analysis; independent prognostic factors for disease-free survival

Factor	Coefficient	*p* Value	RR	95% CI
Age				
>40 vs. ≤40 years	0.436	<0.05	1.6	1.1, 2.2
Sex				
Male vs. female	0.471	<0.001	1.6	1.2, 2.1
Breslow thickness				
>0.75 vs. ≤0.75 mm	1.183	<0.001	3.3	1.7, 6.2
>1.50 vs. 0.76–1.50 mm	0.840	<0.001	2.3	1.6, 3.4
>4.00 vs. 1.51–4.00 mm	0.627	<0.001	1.9	1.4, 2.6
Clark level				
≥III vs. II	1.707	<0.01	5.5	1.7, 18.5
≥IV vs. III	0.405	<0.05	1.5	1.1, 2.1
Tumor type				
ALM vs. others	0.551	<0.05	1.7	1.1, 2.7
Localization				
Trunk vs. extremities	0.298	<0.05	1.4	1.0, 1.8
ELND				
WLE vs. WLE + ELND	0.473	<0.01	1.6	1.2, 2.2

RR, relative risk; CI, confidence interval; ALM, acral lentiginous melanoma; WLE, wide local excision; ELND, elective lymph node dissection.

Table 2. Multivariate Cox hazard analysis; independent prognostic factors for overall survival

Factor	Coefficient	*p* Value	RR	95% CI
Sex				
Male vs. female	0.520	<0.01	1.7	1.2, 2.4
Breslow thickness				
>0.75 vs. ≥0.75 mm	0.724	<0.05	2.1	1.0, 4.2
>1.50 vs. 0.76–1.50 mm	1.028	<0.001	2.8	1.9, 4.2
>4.00 vs. 1.51–4.00 mm	0.960	<0.001	2.6	1.8, 3.9
Clark level				
≥III vs. II	2.654	<0.05	14.2	1.9, 106.6
Tumor type				
ALM vs. others	0.776	<0.01	2.2	1.3, 3.8
Localization				
Trunk vs. extremities	0.298	<0.05	1.4	1.0, 1.8
ELND				
WLE vs. WLE + ELND		n.s.		

RR, relative risk; CI, confidence interval; ALM, acral lentiginous melanoma; WLE, wide local excision; ELND, elective lymph node dissection.

Table 3. Multivariate Cox hazard analysis, influence of ELND on overall survival (adjusted to all prognostic factors)

Factor	Coefficient	*p* Value	RR	95% CI
Age				
>40 vs. ≤40 years	0.2339	n.s.	1.3	0.8, 1.9
Sex				
Male vs. female	0.523	<0.01	1.7	1.2, 2.4
Breslow thickness				
>0.75 vs. ≤0.75 mm	0.657	n.s.	1.9	1.0, 3.9
>1.50 vs. 0.76–1.50 mm	1.426	<0.001	4.2	2.0, 8.7
>4.00 vs. 1.51–4.00 mm	2.364	<0.001	10.6	4.7, 23.9
Clark level				
≥III vs. II	2.600	<0.05	13.5	1.8, 101.9
≥IV vs. III	2.948	<0.05	19.1	2.4, 149.0
≥V vs. IV	2.630	<0.05	13.9	1.6, 120.9
Tumor type				
NM vs. SSM	0.202	n.s.	1.2	0.9, 1.8
LMM vs. SSM	0.368	n.s.	1.5	0.8, 2.6
ALM vs. SSM	0.872	<0.01	2.4	1.3, 2.4
Localization				
Trunk vs. extremities	0.542	<0.01	1.7	1.2, 2.5
ELND				
WLE vs. WLE + ELND	0.005	n.s.	1.0	0.7, 1.4

ELND, elective lymph node dissection; RR, relative risk; CI, confidence interval; WLE, wide local excision; NM, nodular melanoma; SSM, superficially spreading melanoma; LMM, lentigo malignant melanoma, ALM, acral lentiginous melanoma; n.s., not significant.

parable, as shown by the median tumor thickness of 1.20 mm for the WLE plus ELND group (mean, 1.96 mm; SD, 2.56 mm) and 1.15 mm for the WLE group (mean, 1.76 mm; SD, 1.68 mm).

Concerning the overall survival times in the whole group, there was no significant benefit from WLE plus ELND compared to WLE, as demonstrated by the 5-year survival rates of 87.3% versus 86.4% and 10-year survival rates of 80.1% versus 77.8% (log-rank test: $p = 0.72$, not significant; Fig. 1). When further divided into four classes of tumor thicknesses, increased survival rates were noted for intermediate tumor thicknesses of 1.51–4.0 mm for the WLE plus ELND group, as shown by 5-year survival rates of 85.3% versus 76.7% and 10-year survival rates of 73.1% versus 60.3%. However, these data were not significant (log-rank test: $p = 0.14$, not significant; Fig. 2c). As depicted in Fig. 2a and b, the subgroups with lower tumor thicknesses (≤0.75 mm and 0.76–1.50 mm) showed no significant differences in survival rates (log-rank test: $p = 0.52$ and $p = 0.15$, respectively). In cases of high tumor thicknesses (≥4.00 mm), ELND seemed to be disadvantageous (Fig. 2d); however, only a small number of patients

Table 4. Patient characteristics and prognostic criteria in the two treatment groups

	WLE + ELND (n = 375; %)	WLE only (n = 375; %)	p Value (n.s.: $p > 0.05$)
Sex			
Female	58.4	58.4	
Male	41.6	41.6	n.s.
Age (years)			
<41	23.2	23.2	
41–60	48.3	47.5	n.s.
>60	28.5	29.3	
Localization			
Breast	4.3	5.6	
Back	14.9	16.3	
Abdomen	4.0	1.6	
Nates	1.1	0.8	
Upper arm	22.4	13.1	
Forearm	6.4	9.3	n.s.
Hand	1.3	2.1	
Thigh	10.1	11.7	
Lower leg	29.6	30.9	
Foot	5.9	8.5	
Tumor thickness (mm)			
<0.76	29.3	29.3	
0.76–1.50	29.1	29.1	
1.51–4.00	34.4	34.4	n.s.
>4.00	7.2	7.2	
Clark level			
II	5.1	5.1	
III	49.6	49.6	
IV	40.5	43.7	n.s.
V	4.8	1.6	
Type of Tumor			
SSM	67.5	60.0	
NM	22.7	20.8	
LMM	1.1	8.5	n.s.
ALM	5.1	4.5	
Others	3.7	6.1	
Ulceration			
Yes	20.3	5.6	
No	79.7	94.4	$p < 10^{-4}$

WLE, wide local excision; ELND, elective lymph node dissection; NM, nodular melanoma; SSM, superficially spreading melanoma; LMM, lentigo malignant melanoma; ALM, acral lentiginous melanoma; n.s., not significant.

belonged to this subgroup, and these data were not significant (log-rank test: $p = 0.23$, $n = 27$ per group).

When subdivided for the localization of the primary, ELND showed a significant improval for malignant melanoma of the trunk, as shown by the 5-year survival rates of 92.0% versus 79.7% and 10-year survival rates of

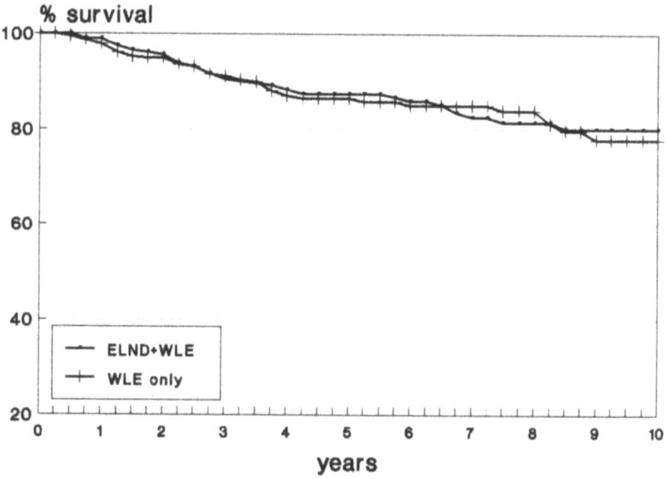

Fig. 1. Univariate comparison of survival time in the total of the two groups of each 375 patients ($n = 750$); $p = 0.72$, not significant (log-rank test). *ELND*, elective lymph node dissection; *WLE*, wide local excision

80.4% versus 45.2% (log-rank text: $p < 0.05$; Fig. 3a). Malignant melanoma of the extremities revealed no significant differences in survival rates (log-rank test: $p = 0.36$; Fig. 3b).

Regarding the disease-free survival, there were higher rates of 83.0% versus 79.7% after 5 years and of 80.5% versus 70.7% after 10 years in the total group of patients treated by additional ELND (log-rank test: $p < 0.05$; Fig. 4a). In intermediate tumor thicknesses (1.51–4.0 mm), there was an even highly significant benefit from ELND concerning disease-free survival ($p < 0.001$; Fig. 4b).

Discussion

The results of our matched pair study confirm the results of several investigators who demonstrated a positive influence of ELND on disease-free survival and/or overall survival for patients with malignant melanoma of intermediate Breslow thickness. There were no significant differences regarding overall survival time of WLE plus ELND compared to WLE only. As subdivided into classes of different Breslow thicknesses, markedly higher 5- and 10-year survival rates were noted for the WLE plus ELND group in intermediate tumor thicknesses (1.51–4.00 mm). In tumor thicknesses of 4.00 mm or more, a negative influence seemed to result from additional ELND. However, the findings were not statistically significant. In patients with malignant melanoma of the trunk treated by WLE plus ELND, a significant improvement in survival time was demonstrated, while there were

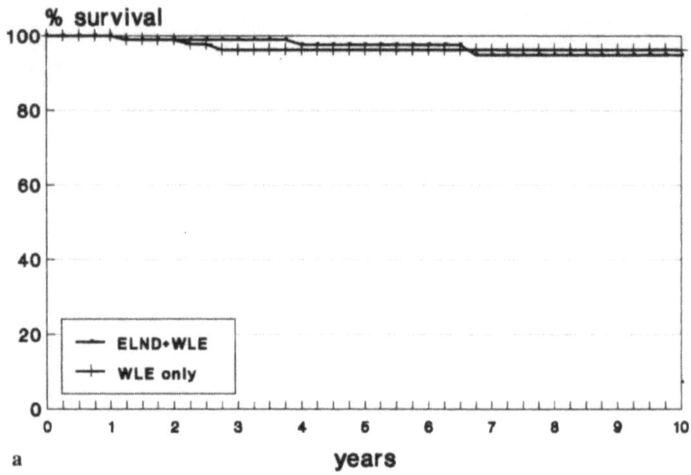

a

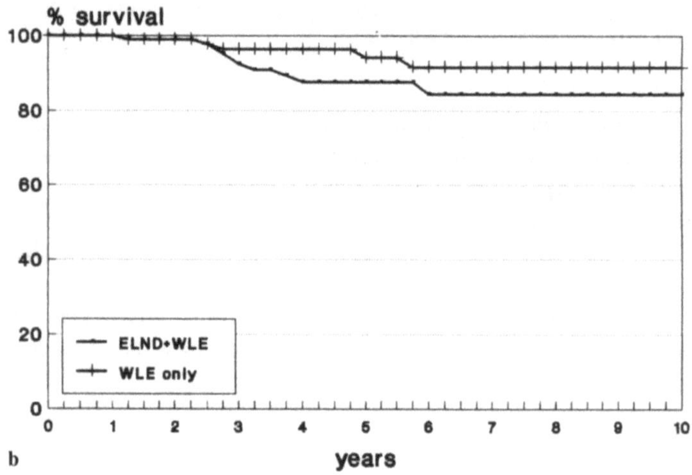

b

Fig. 2a–d. Survival time for Breslow's thickness less than 0.75 mm (n = 220), p = 0.52, not significant (**a**), 0.76–1.50 mm (n = 218), p = 0.15, not significant (**b**), 1.51–4.00 mm (n = 258), p = 0.14, not significant (**c**), and greater than 4.00 mm (n = 54), p = 0.23, not significant (**d**). *ELND*, elective lymph node dissection; *WLE*, wide local excision

no marked differences in survival rates of both treatment groups in cases of melanoma located on the extremities. Concerning disease-free survival time, a significant benefit from additional ELND was shown for the total group and an even highly significant effect for intermediate tumor thicknesses. Multivariate analysis confirmed the independent positive influence of ELND on disease-free interval. However, concerning overall survival, a significant benefit from ELND was not demonstrated in the entire collective.

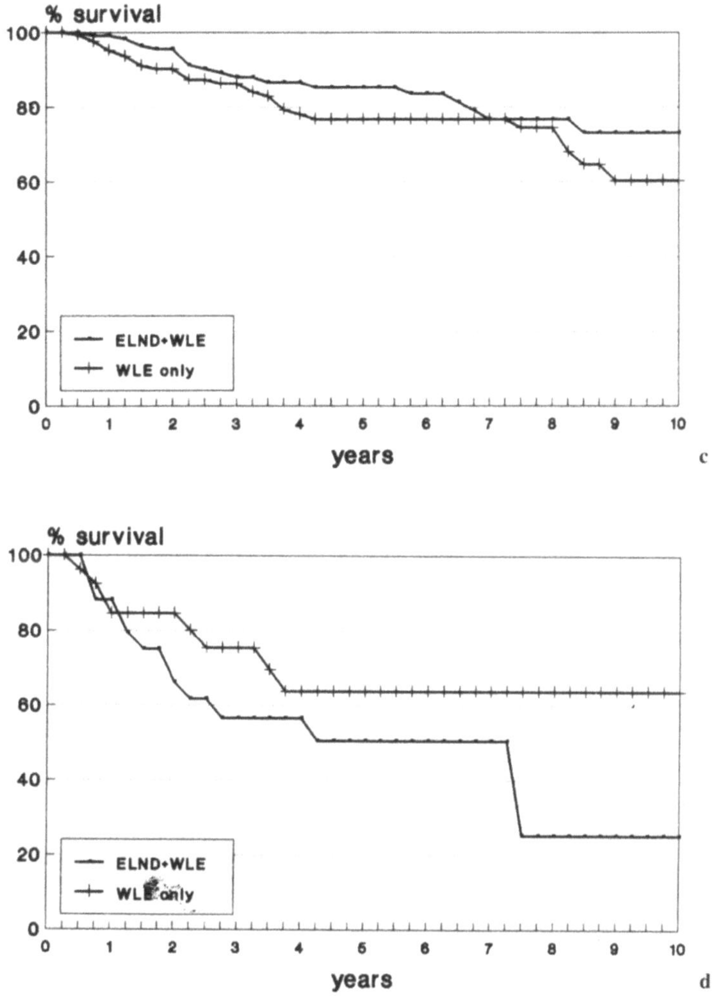

Fig. 2c,d

Several retrospective, nonrandomized studies have been undertaken showing significant benefits, or at least trends towards a better prognosis, from ELND for patients with intermediate Breslow thickness (Fortner et al. 1977; Balch 1980; Milton et al. 1982; Balch et al. 1982; Reintgen et al. 1983; Shaw et al. 1987; McCarthy et al. 1985, 1988; Balch 1988; Drepper et al. 1993). ELND done at an early stage is thought to provide a definitive surgical treatment with a maximum extent of elimination of tumor tissue. On the other hand, delayed dissection of regional lymph nodes bears the risk of increasing tumor masses, which itself are a new starting point for tumor spread (Balch 1988; Cochran et al. 1992).

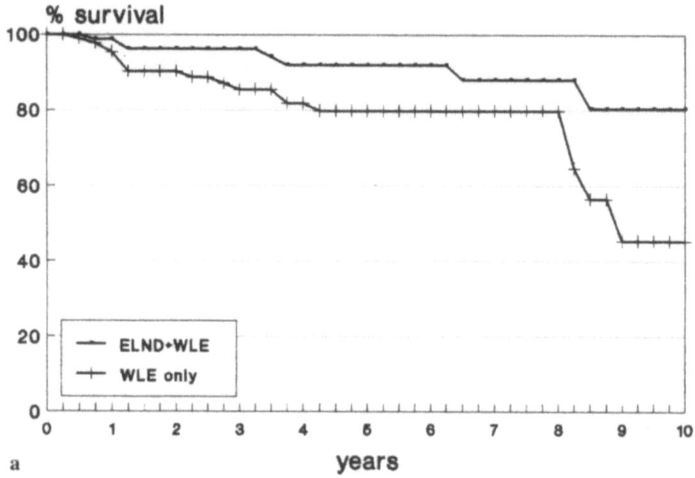

a

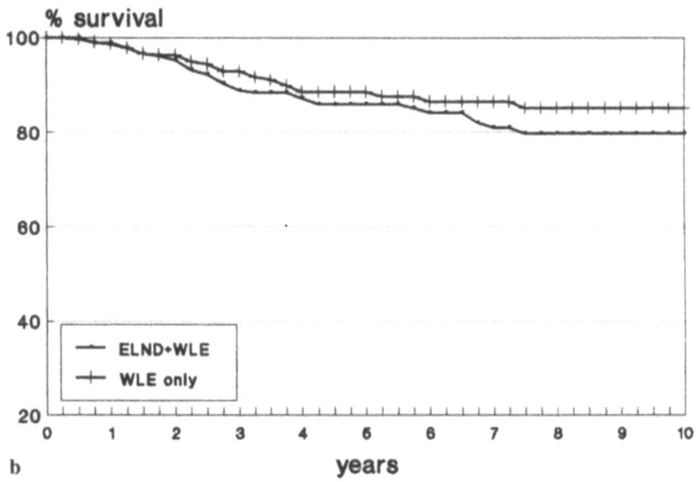

b

Fig. 3a,b. Survival time for all patients with malignant melanoma located on the trunk (n = 182), $p < 0.05$ (**a**) and on the extremities (n = 568), $p = 0.36$, not significant (**b**). *ELND*, elective lymph node dissection; *WLE*, wide local excision

The two major prospective randomized studies, one from the WHO Melanoma Group and the other from Mayo Clinic, have shown no significant benefit from ELND (Sim et al. 1978, 1986; Veronesi et al. 1977, 1982). However, the study by the Mayo Clinic included only a small number of patients with melanoma of intermediate Breslow thickness. Therefore, the value of ELND cannot be judged from these data. The study by the WHO was criticized for the lack of optimal stratification according to the major prognostic factors and deficiencies in standardization of histological and

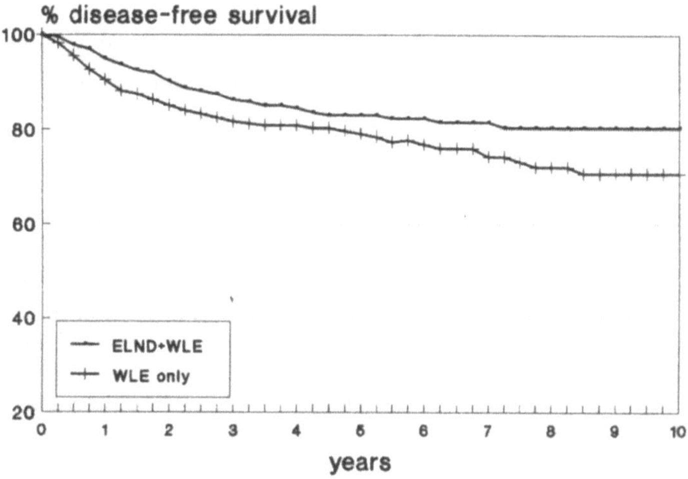

a

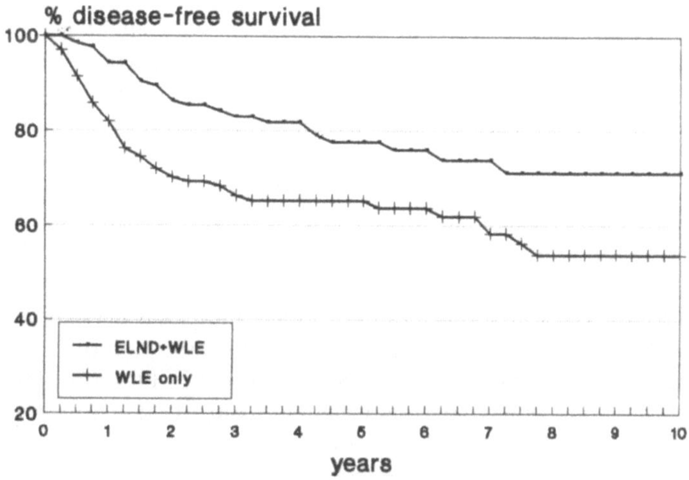

b

Fig. 4a,b. Disease-free survival. **a** All tumor thicknesses ($n = 750$), $p < 0.05$. **b** Breslow's thickness 1.51–4.00 mm ($n = 258$), $p < 0.001$. *ELND*, elective lymph node dissection; *WLE*, wide local excision

clinical staging and in the performance of surgical treatment (Balch 1988; McCarthy et al. 1992; Scott and McKay 1993). Any multicenter study will be impaired by differences in the quality, i.e. the radicality of the lymph node dissection, while a large number of surgeons with different levels of experience will have carried out the operations. The technique for ELND in malignant melanoma must be of a higher radicality than in breast cancer, while in the latter the procedure has more or less the aim of completing the primary staging before adjusting adjuvant chemotherapy (Balch 1990; Ross and Balch 1992). The varying rates for local recurrences in the regional lymph nodes in malignant melanoma following ELND or TLND give some idea about the variability in the surgical techniques and experience of different surgeons at different centers (Bowsher et al. 1986; Balch 1990; Shaw and Rumball 1990).

The regional lymph nodes are most frequently the first site of metastasis in the natural course of malignant melanoma (Little and Davis 1978; Balch 1980; O'Rourke and Louis 1982). In the study of the WHO, 56% of the intermediate thickness group with clinical stage I malignant melanoma treated initially by wide excision alone later developed metastasis to the lymph nodes (Veronesi et al. 1977). This high percentage of patients will undergo therapeutic lymph node dissection, which carries a very much higher risk than initial ELND (Ingvar et al. 1984; Shaw and Rumball 1990). On the other hand, the majority of patients that undergo ELND do not have any occult metastasis of the regional lymph nodes, and the benefit of ELND in these patients is doubtful. Therefore, the major task in evaluating the role of ELND is to find out which patients most benefit from the procedure and to exclude those patients who might not benefit from the procedure, thus sparing them the risk of the operation. Breslow thickness as the most important prognostic parameter in primary malignant melanoma is thought to indicate the patients who might have most benefit from ELND (Balch et al. 1979). In those studies that showed positive influences on disease-free survival and overall survival time, intermediate Breslow thicknesses in particular showed significant benefit (Balch et al. 1979; Balch et al. 1982; Milton et al. 1982; Shaw et al. 1987; McCarthy et al. 1985, 1988; Balch 1988; Drepper et al. 1993). In the case of thick cutaneous melanoma, i.e. Breslow thickness of 4.00 mm or more, there was no significant benefit from ELND (Crowley and Seigler 1990). The localization of the primary seems to be another important factor. Some reports in literature favored melanoma of the trunk as having greater benefit from ELND (Milton et al. 1982; Ariel 1982). A report on BANS (upper back, posterior arm, posterior neck, posterior scalp) melanoma revealed a tendency of better prognosis for the ELND group, although this was not significant (Auguste et al. 1991).

On the basis of our results, we recommend ELND for intermediate Breslow thicknesses (1.51–4.00 mm). In addition, the total group of malignant melanoma of the trunk has shown a significant improvement in survival by ELND. This group included a large proportion of patients with melanoma located on the back, which is regarded as a high-risk localization. Therefore, we recommend that especially melanoma in high-risk localizations should be considered for ELND.

References

Ariel IM (1982) Malignant melanoma of the trunk: a retrospective review of 1128 patients. Cancer 49:1070–1078
Auguste LJ, Belluco C, Peralo J (1991) Surgical management of BANS malignant melanoma. Surgery 110:598–603
Balch CM (1980) Surgical management of regional lymph nodes in cutaneous melanoma. J Am Acad Dermatol 3:511–524
Balch CM (1988) The role of elective lymph node dissection in melanoma: rationale, results, and controversies. J Clin Oncol 6:163–172
Balch CM (1990) Axillary lymph node dissection: differences in goals and techniques when treating melanoma and breast cancer. Surgery 108:118–119
Balch CM, Murad T, Soong S et al (1979) Tumour thickness as a guide to surgical management of clinical stage I melanoma patients. Cancer 43:883–888
Balch CM, Soong SJ, Milton GW et al (1982) A comparison of prognostic factors and surgical results in 1786 patients with localized (stage I) melanoma treated in Alabama, USA, and New South Wales, Australia. Ann Surg 196:677–684
Balch CM, Soong S-J, Shaw HM et al (1992) An analysis of prognostic factors in 8500 patients with cutaneous melanoma. In: Balch CM, Houghton AN, Milton GW, Sober AJ, Soong S-J (eds) Cutaneous melanoma, 2nd edn. Lippincott, Philadelphia, pp 165–187
Binder M, Pehamberger H, Steiner A et al (1990) Elective regional lymph node dissection in malignant melanoma. Eur J Cancer 26:871–873
Bowsher WG, Taylor BA, Hughes LE (1986) Morbidity, mortality and local recurrence following regional node dissection for melanoma. Br J Surg 73:906–908
Cochran AJ, Wen DR, Morton DL (1992) Management of the regional lymph nodes in patients with cutaneous malignant melanoma. World J Surg 16:214–221
Crowley NJ, Seigler HF (1990) The role of elective lymph node dissection in the management of patients with thick cutaneous melanoma. Cancer 66:2522–2527
Cutler SJ, Ederer F (1958) Maximum utilization of the life table method in analyzing survival. J Chron Dis 8(6):87–94
Drepper H, Köhler CO, Bastian B et al (1993) Benefit of elective lymph node dissection in subgroups of melanoma patients. Results of a multicenter study of 3616 patients. Cancer 72:741–749
Elder DE, Guerry D, van Horn M et al (1985) The role of lymph node dissection for clinical stage I malignant melanoma of intermediate thickness (1.51–3.99 mm). Cancer 56:413–418
Fortner JH, Woodruff J, Schottenfeld D et al (1977) Biostatistical basis for elective lymph node dissection for malignant melanoma. Ann Surg 186:101–103
Ingvar C, Erichsen C, Jonsson PE (1984) Morbidity following prophylactic and therapeutic lymph node dissection for melanoma: a comparison. Tumori 70:529–533
Karakousis CP, Emrich LJ, Rao U (1986) Groin dissection in malignant melanoma. Am J Surg 152:491–495
Karakousis CP, Kachrimanidis S, Rao U et al (1987) Changes in survival with clinical stage I malignant mealnoma. J Surg Oncol 34:155–159
Karakousis CP, Hena MA, Emrich LJ et al (1989) Axillary node dissection in malignant melanoma: results and complications. Surgery 108:10–17
Little JH, Davis NC (1987) Secondary malignant melanoma in lymph nodes: incidence, time of occurrence, and mortality. Aust N Z J Surg 48:9–13
McCarthy WH, Shaw HM, Milton GW (1985) Efficacy of elective lymph node dissection in 2347 patients with clinical stage I malignant melanoma. Surg Gynecol Obstet 161:575–580

McCarthy WH, Shaw HM, Thompson JF et al (1988) Time and frequency of recurrence of cutaneous stage I malignant melanoma with guidelines for follow-up study. Surg Gynecol Obstet 166:497–502

McCarthy WH, Shaw HM, Cascinelli N et al (1992) Elective lymph node dissection for melanoma: two perspectives. World J Surg 16:203–213

Milton GW, Shaw HM, McCarthy WH, et al (1982) Prophylactic lymph node dissection in clinical stage I cutaneous malignant melanoma: results of surgical treatment in 1319 patients. Br J Surg 69:108–111

O'Rourke MG, Louis A (1982) Metastases in malignant melanoma. Aust N Z J Surg 52:154–157

Reintgen DS, Cox EB, McCarty KS Jr et al (1983) Efficacy of elective lymph node dissection in patients with intermediate thickness primary melanoma. Ann Surg 198:379–385

Ross MI, Balch CM (1992) General principles of regional lymphadenectomy. In: Balch CM, Houghton AN, Milton GW, Sober AJ, Soong S-J (eds) Cutaneous melanoma, 2nd edn. Lippincott, Philadelphia, pp 339–344

Scott RN, McKay AJ (1993) Elective lymph node dissection in the management of malignant melanoma. Br J Surg 80:284–288

Shaw HM, McCarthy WH, McCarthy SW et al (1987) Thin malignant melanomas and recurrence potential. Arch Surg 122:1147–1150

Shaw JH, Rumball EM (1990) Complications and local recurrence following lymphadenectomy. Br J Surg 77:760–764

Sim FH, Taylor WF, Ivins JC et al (1978) A prospective randomized study of the efficacy of routine elective lymphadenectomy in management of malignant melanoma: preliminary results. Cancer 4:948–951

Sim FH, Taylor WF, Pritchard DJ et al (1986) Lymphadenectomy in the management of stage I malignant melanoma: a prospective randomized study. Mayo Clin Proc 61:697–705

Veronesi U, Adamus J, Bandiera DC et al (1977) Inefficacy of immediate node dissection in stage I melanoma of the limbs. N Engl J Med 297:627–630

Veronesi U, Adamus J, Bandiera DC et al (1982) Delayed regional lymph node dissection in stage I melanoma of the skin of the lower extremities. Cancer 49:2420–2430

Clinical Activity of a Polyvalent Melanoma Antigen Vaccine

J.-C. Bystryn

Ronald O. Perelman Department of Dermatology, Melanoma Program,
Kaplan Comprehensive Cancer Center, New York University School of Medicine,
560 First Avenue, New York, NY 10016, USA

Abstract

We have developed a partially purified, polyvalent melanoma vaccine from surface material shed into culture medium by a pool of selected melanoma cells. The vaccine contains a broad spectrum of melanoma antigens to circumvent the antigenic heterogeneity of melanoma and to obviate the need to identify individual antigens that mediate tumor-protective immunity.

Vaccine treatment augments antimelanoma humoral and/or cellular immunity in over 50% of patients and can increase immunity to a patient's own melanoma. Vaccine-induced antibodies are directed at one or more surface antigens with molecular masses of 210, 150, 110, 75, or 38 kDa. The 210- and 110-kDa antigens are melanoma associated, as they were expressed by four of five human melanoma cell lines, but by only two of 12 control cell lines, and are unrelated to previously described melanoma antigens.

The disease-free (DF) and overall survival (OS) of vaccine-treated patients with surgically resected stage II (regional) disease is 50% longer than that of historical controls. Survival is particularly prolonged in patients who develop an immune response. Median DF survival is 4.7 years longer and OS 3.7 years longer in patients with a strong, as opposed to no, cellular immune response to vaccine treatment ($p = <0.02$). Similarly, median DF survival of patients with vaccine-induced melanoma antibodies is significantly longer than that of nonresponders (65 months vs. 17 months, respectively), as is overall survival ($p = 0.01$). These differences in outcome are unrelated to disease severity or to the overall immunological competence of the patients, suggesting they result from vaccine treatment.

Thus melanoma vaccine treatment is safe, capable of stimulating antimelanoma immunity in many patients, and appears to be clinically effective in delaying the progression of this cancer in some individuals.

Recent Results in Cancer Research, Vol. 139

Introduction

Active, specific immunotherapy of malignant melanoma with melanoma vaccines is now an accepted, albeit still experimental, method of treating malignant melanoma. The rationale for using vaccines to treat melanoma is based on the fact that melanoma cells differ from normal adult pigment cells, that these differences can be recognized by immunocompetent cells and stimulate antimelanoma immune responses, and that the resulting immune responses can destroy melanoma cells in vitro. Several observations support this hypothesis. Two are particularly compelling. Spontaneous destruction of melanoma cells occurs in 15%–20% of primary lesions. This dramatic event indicates that host-protective mechanisms which can selectively destroy melanoma cells are present in man. Vaccine immunotherapy with crude or partially purified melanoma vaccines can prevent tumor growth in 50%–100% of mice immunized to otherwise lethal doses of melanoma cells (Bystryn 1978). The protection is specific, indicating it is mediated by immune mechanisms. This demonstrates directly that melanoma vaccines can effectively increase resistance to this cancer. The challenge is to devise vaccine design strategies that will induce similar immunoprotective responses in man.

Desired Properties of Cancer Vaccines

The essential requirements for cancer vaccines to be effective is that they contain tumor antigens that can stimulate tumor-protective immune responses in man and that at least some of these antigens are expressed by the tumor to be treated. Unfortunately, the melanoma antigens which induce tumor-*protective* immunity in man are not known, and because of the heterogenous expression of tumor antigens on different melanomas, the actual antigens expressed by the tumor to be treated is also not known. Melanoma vaccines should fulfill a number of other important requirements. They should be safe to use, produced in a reproducible manner, their essential properties characterized, and they should be simple to use to retain the cost-effectiveness of this method of therapy.

Rationale for Preparing a Polyvalent Vaccine from Shed Antigens

The strategy we have selected to design a polyvalent melanoma antigen vaccine addresses the two most essential requirements of cancer vaccines – their need to include antigens that: 1) can stimulate protective immunity and 2) circumvent the antigenic heterogeneity of melanoma. This design strategy seeks to retain the advantages of constructing cancer vaccines from whole tumor cells or from pure tumor antigens, while minimizing the problems associated with each of these methods (Bystryn 1993).

The key element in this strategy is to prepare the vaccine from material shed by viable tumor cells into culture medium. Tumor cells rapidly release a broad range of molecules expressed on their external surface, including tumor antigens (Bystryn et al. 1981). This process, which is called shedding, is of interest because cell surface material is released much more rapidly than the bulk of unrelated cellular material which is in the cytoplasm or the nucleus of the cells. Consequently, shed material is highly enriched in cell surface macromolecules and antigens and provides a simple method of obtaining a broad range of cell surface tumor antigens in a fairly purified form.

The major advantages of this method of vaccine production are twofold. First, it results in a formulation that contains a broad range of antigens expressed on the surface of melanoma cells. The polyvalent nature of the vaccine increases its chance of containing immunogenic antigens that stimulate tumor protective immunity and, by so doing, obviates the need to identify and purify the individual antigens that induce these responses. It also makes it more likely that the vaccine will contain antigens present on the tumor to be treated, circumventing antigenic heterogeneity. Furthermore, the presence of multiple antigens will stimulate different antitumor immune responses, increasing the chances of tumor destruction and clinical effectiveness. The range of antigens in the vaccine is further increased by preparing it from a pool of melanoma cells, selected because they express different patterns of tumor antigens. Second, the shed tumor antigens are partially purified, as they are separated from the bulk of the cellular material, which is poorly shed. This simplifies the characterization of the vaccine, reduces the possibility of toxicity, and promotes effectiveness by decreasing the presence of possible suppressive factors in the vaccine and of antigenic competition by irrelevant antigens. Other advantages of vaccine prepared in this fashion are summarized in Table 1.

The vaccine is prepared from material shed into culture medium in 3 h by a pool of four melanoma cell lines (Bystryn et al. 1986). The cells were selected because each expresses a different pattern of cell surface melanoma-associated antigens. The cells have been adapted to long-term growth in serum-free medium, to exclude from the vaccine highly immunogenic fetal calf serum proteins, which confuse the analysis of immune responses to vaccine treatment. The shed antigens are further purified by detergent treatment and ultracentrifugation to deplete HLA antigens. The vaccine contains xenogeneic proteins, which are thought to potentiate vaccine immunogenicity through xenogenization. The xenogeneic proteins do not interfere with assays of vaccine-induced antimelanoma immune responses, since all assays are conducted using human melanoma cells as targets. Seed and working cell banks have been established to ensure reproducible preparation of vaccine.

Table 1. Important features of polyvalent melanoma antigen vaccine

- Contains multiple melanoma antigens
  - More likely to contain immunogenic antigens and antigens expressed by patient's own tumor
  - More likely to circumvent antigenic heterogeneity of tumors
- Enriched in surface antigens
  - More relevant for immunotherapy
- Partially purified
  - Minimizes contamination by cytoplasmic and nuclear material
  - Reduces potential toxicity
  - Simplifies characterization of vaccine
  - Reduces presence of possible suppressive factors
  - Reduces antigenic competition by irrelevant antigens
- Prepared from cultured cells
  - Permits preparation of generic vaccine
  - Permits treatment of patients with no available tumor tissue
  - Permits treatment of early disease and prophylaxis
- Cells adapted to long-term growth in serum-free medium
  - Prevents sensitization to fetal calf serum proteins
  - Simplifies assays of vaccine induced antitumor immune responses

Side Effects of Vaccine Treatment

Over 375 patients with predominantly stage III (AJCC classification, regional disease) malignant melanoma have been repeatedly immunized six to 20 times with 20–40 μg vaccine for up to 5 years. There has been no acute or chronic toxicity other than transient urticaria at the site of injection (Bystryn et al. 1988, 1992), apart for one patient who developed a mild febrile episode following each vaccine immunization. The lack of toxicity makes the vaccine particularly attractive as an adjuvant treatment for surgically resected, high-risk melanoma.

Vaccine Immunogenicity

The vaccine is immunogenic in man. It can stimulate antibody and/or cellular immune response to melanoma in approximately 50% of patients, as described below (Bystryn et al. 1988, 1989, 1992). These responses have the functional capacity to kill melanoma cells in vitro (Cui et al. 1992; Adler et al. 1990) and are directed, at least in part, to melanoma-associated antigens and to antigens expressed by autologous melanoma in vivo (Oratz et al. 1989). Some of these antigens have been identified at the molecular level (Bystryn 1992) and appear to be good candidates to construct second-generation vaccines from purified antigens.

Stimulation of Antimelanoma Antibody Responses by Vaccine Treatment

The antibody response to vaccine treatment has been measured by an immunoprecipitation sodium dodecyl sulfate polyacrylamide gel electrophoresis (SDS-PAGE) analysis assay, which measures antibodies to individual melanoma cell surface antigens, and by complement-dependent cytolysis, which measures the functional ability of antibodies to kill melanoma cells. Both assays detect antibodies to surface antigens – the ones most likely to be biologically relevant.

With the immunoprecipitation assay, vaccine-induced antibody responses are detected by comparing the pattern of antigens bound by pre- and postimmunization sera in the same patient, as illustrated in Fig 1. Vaccine treatment was found to stimulate antibody responses to melanoma in 16 (61%) of 26 sequential patients (Bystryn 1992). The antibodies were directed against one or more antigens with approximate molecular masses of 210, 150, 110, 75, or 38 kDa. Antibodies were directed most often the 210- and 110-kDa antigens. These two antigens appear to be melanoma associated, as they were expressed by four of five human melanoma cells, but by only two of 11 unrelated control cells (Bystryn 1992). These antigens are unrelated to HLA class I or II molecules or to antigens defined by a large panel of murine monoclonal antibodies to currently known melanoma associated antigens. The latter observation indicates that the melanoma antigens which are immunogenic in man differ from those which are immunogenic in mice.

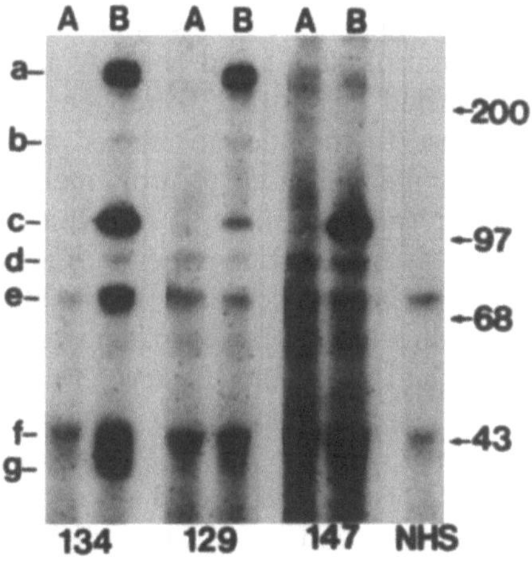

Fig. 1. Antibody response to melanoma vaccine immunization. Pattern of radioiodinated melanoma (SF SK-Mel 28) antigens precipitated by pre- (*lane A*) and post- (*lane B*) vaccine treatment sera in three patients. Note that vaccine immunization induced antibody responses to one or more antigens with approximate molecular masses of 200+, 150, 110, 75, or 38 kDa. *NHS*, pattern of antigens prescribed by a control normal human sera

The functional ability of vaccine-induced antibodies to kill melanoma cells was measured by complement-dependent cytolysis. Cytolytic antibodies to melanoma were present prior to vaccine treatment in one (4%) of 27 patients with AJCC stage III melanoma and in 21 (77%) of the patients 1 week after four vaccine immunizations (Cui et al. 1992). These antibodies were selectively directed against melanoma, as a panel of five sera with strong cytolytic activity against melanoma did not kill two control cell lines.

In more recent studies using a western immunoblot assay, we have found that vaccine-induced antibodies can react to antigens expressed in fresh melanoma tissue and antigens that are expressed in vivo in the patient's own tumor.

Stimulation of Cellular Immune Responses by Vaccine Treatment

This has been measured in vivo by delayed-type hypersensitivity (DTH) response to skin tests to vaccine and in vitro by assays of T cell-mediated cytolysis and of precursor cytolytic T cells.

A DTH response to the vaccine is induced in a variable number of patients, depending on the immunization procedure used. The most immunogenic regimen of those evaluated to date uses alum as an adjuvant and stimulated strong DTH responses in 54% of 24 patients (Bystryn et al. 1989). The DTH response appears to be selectively directed to melanoma. Patients with a DTH response to the vaccine do not react to an equal amount of a control vaccine prepared from pooled allogeneic lymphocytes (Bystryn et al. 1992). Since pooled lymphocytes are a rich source of a broad spectrum of class I and II HLA antigens, it is unlikely the DTH response is directed against HLA antigens. Only one of 24 patients with a DTH response to the vaccine reacted to skin tests with concentrated complete culture medium used to grow melanoma cells, making it unlikely that the DTH response is directed at a culture medium contaminant (Bystryn et al. 1992). By skin testing patients to individual vaccines, each prepared from a single melanoma cell line, we established that the DTH response was in all cases directed at least in part at one of the human melanoma cells used to construct the vaccine (Bystryn et al. 1992).

Vaccine treatment also stimulates both specific and nonspecific cell-mediated cytolytic immune responses. Peripheral blood lymphocytes from 18 patients were collected prior to and following two to six vaccine immunizations and tested for cytolytic activity against melanoma and nonmelanoma targets by a ^{51}Cr release assay. Lytic activity (defined as more than 15 lytic units) to melanoma cells was present in two of 18 (11%) patients prior to and in 16 (89%) following vaccine treatment (Adler et al. 1990). Augmentation of antimelanoma cytolytic responses (defined as more than 50% increase in lytic activity over baseline measurement in the same patient) was detected in 28%–100% of patients, depending on the melanoma cells used as target. Specificity analysis of the response showed that in some patients it was directed selectively to melanoma, while in others it was directed nonspecifically to both melanoma and unrelated tumor control cells. Vaccine treatment has little effect on NK or LAK cells. Cytotoxicity to melanoma was not blocked by monoclonal antibody to class I or to class II HLA, indicating it was not directed to transplantation alloantigens.

Detection of vaccine-induced antimelanoma cellular responses is enhanced by using an in vitro sensitization (IVS) assay, which measures precursor cytolytic T cells (pCTL). Using this assay, pCTL were detected in 83% (15 out of 18) vaccine-treated compared to none of 13 untreated patients and none of five normal donors. The magnitude of antimelanoma lytic responses in vaccine-treated patients was ignificantly higher when measured by IVS than by direct cytolytic assay (mean cytolysis of 46.4% versus 9.9%, respectively), $p < 0.001$. The enhanced IVS cytolytic responses were mediated by $CD3^+$ T cells, which were of mixed phenotype: $CD4^+/CD^-$ and/or $CD8^+/CD56^+$ or $CD56^-$.

An important requirement for cancer vaccines is that they stimulate immune responses to antigens expressed by the patient's own tumor in vivo. To address this question we studied the density and distribution of cellular infiltrates (TIL cells) in subcutaneous melanoma nodules removed from vaccine-treated patients (Oratz et al. 1989). This provides an indication of host immunity to autologous tumor in vivo. Normally there is only a slight infiltrate of TIL in melanoma nodules, indicating that patients have minimal immune responses to their own tumor. By contrast, there is a dense infiltrate in most tumor nodules removed from vaccine-treated patients. Overall, a dense (>15 cells/high power field) infiltrate of TIL was present in 91% of subcutaneous melanoma nodules removed from 11 vaccine-treated patients compared to 41% of 22 similar nodules removed from control patients, $p < 0.02$. In addition, the TIL in most vaccine-treated patients infiltrate into the tumor nodules, while in untreated patients they are found mainly at the periphery. In most (eight of nine tumor nodules studied), the predominant (80%–90%) effector cell population infiltrating the tumor is $CD3^+/CD4^+$.

Phase II clinical trials have been conducted to explore different approaches to potentiate vaccine immunogenicity (different dose schedule, vaccine aggregation, pretreatment with low-dose cyclophosphamide, use of novel adjuvants such as Detox). The most effective regimen used so far was using alum as an adjuvant, which induced DTH responses to the vaccine in 54% of 24 patients (Bystryn et al. 1989). Pretreatment with a low dose of cyclophosphamide ($300\,mg/m^2$ 3 days prior to each immunization; Oratz et al. 1991) or the use of the adjuvant Detox (Schultz et al. 1992) did not further potentiate vaccine immunogenicity or clinical effectiveness.

These results indicate that vaccine treatment increases immunity to melanoma in many patients.

Clinical Effectiveness of Vaccine Treatment

Two sets of observations suggest, but do not prove, that vaccine treatment is clinically effective:

1. The median disease-free (DF) and overall survival of vaccine-treated patients are both increased by more than 50% over that of similar historical control patients (Bystryn et al. 1991, 1992). The median DF survival of the first 94 vaccine-treated patients with AJCC stage III surgically resected melanoma was 30 months versus 18 months for similar, non-vaccine treated, historical controls (Balch et al. 1985; Veronesi et al. 1982; Berdeaux et al. 1989; Table 2), and overall 5-year survival was 50% compared to 33 (Table 3).
2. The recurrence of melanoma is particularly delayed in those patients who develop strong immune responses to vaccine treatment, as described below.

Table 2. Disease-free survival in regional (AJCC stage III) melanoma

Study	Patients (n)	Median disease-free survival (months)
Bach 1978	?	16
Veronesi 1982	761	18
Sterchi 1985	24	8–19
Berdeaux 1989	137	19
Historical average	922	18
Bystryn	94	30

Table 3. Overall survival in regional (AJCC stage III) melanoma

Study	Patients (n)	Overall survival (%)	
		3 Years	5 Years
Milan	45	31	27
Sydney	366	48	37
Erlangen	185	41	33
UCLA	150	46	37
Boston	33	52	30
Alabama	119	46	28
Brisbane	64	32	27
Hersey 1992	206	47	35
Morton 1992	126	–	18
Historical average	1294	43	30
Bystryn 1992	94	62	50

The presence and magnitude of vaccine-induced cellular immune responses to melanoma was determined by comparing DTH response to vaccine prior to vaccine treatment and at the fourth vaccine immunization in the same patient. The analysis was conducted in 94 evaluable sequential patients with surgically resected regional disease (AJCC stage III melanoma; Bystryn et al. 1991, 1992). Median DF survival was 4.7 years longer and overall survival 3.7 years longer in the patients with a strong vaccine-induced DTH response than in nonresponders (Table 4). Three years after onset of treatment, 70% patients with a strong DTH response, but only 31% of nonresponders, were still disease free. By Cox proportional hazard analysis, the relation between the strength of the DTH response and increased DF survival was significant ($p = 0.02$) and independent of differences in disease severity (thickness or level of primary lesion, age, sex, number of involved regional nodes, nodes clinically positive at presentation) or of the immunological competence of the patients (as evaluated by responses to recall antigens or ability to be sensitized to a new control antigen, DNCB).

A correlation also exists between vaccine-induced antimelanoma antibodies and improved survival (Table 5). Antibodies to melanoma were measured (by immunoprecipitation) at baseline and following the fourth immunization in a group of 81 patients with surgically resected AJCC stage III melanoma. The median DF survival of patients with vaccine-induced antibody responses was 47 months compared to 19 months for nonresponders, and overall survival was 62 months compared to 46 months, respectively ($p = 0.01$). Again, there was no significant difference in disease severity or immunological competence between the two groups.

These results indicate that antibody and cellular immune responses to vaccine treatment are immunological markers of vaccine activity which

Table 4. Relation between delayed-type hypersensitivity (DTH) response to melanoma vaccine immunization and survival in AJCC stage III melanoma

Increase in (DTH) response[a]	No. of patients[b] ($n = 94$)	Median survival (months)	
		Disease-free[c]	Overall[d]
0	41	15	44
1–14	24	24	57
≥15	29	>72	>89

[a] Increase (in mm) in induration over baseline.
[b] All with postsurgical stage II melanoma.
[c] Median survival from surgical treatment of stage II disease to recurrence.
[d] Median from surgical treatment of stage II disease to death.

Table 5. Relation between antibody response to vaccine and survival

Antibody response[a]	Percentage of patients ($n = 82$)	Median disease-free survival (months)	5-year survival (%)
Present	39	65	71
Absent	61	17*	44**

[a] By immunoprecipitation sodium dodecyl sulfate polyacrylamide gel electrophoresis (SDS-PAGE) analysis.
*$p = 0.01$.
**$p = 0.001$.

are predictive of an improved clinical outcome. As the improved clinical outcome is independent of disease severity or of the immunological competence of the patients, the clinical benefits appear to be a result of vaccine treatment.

Mechanism of Melanoma Vaccine Clinical Effectiveness

The immunological mechanisms by which melanoma vaccines mediate their clinical benefits remain unclear. Several studies indicate significant correlations between the stimulation of cellular, antimelanoma, immune responses by vaccine treatment and improved clinical outcome, suggesting that T cell immunity is an important factor. The role of antibody responses is less clear, as some studies show correlations between vaccine-induced antibody responses and improved clinical outcome and others do not. Given that melanoma vaccine treatment can stimulate different types of immune responses and that it is feasible to modulate these responses in desired directions, a central question regarding vaccine therapy of melanoma is the identity of melanoma vaccine-induced antitumor immune responses, which are effective in mediating the therapeutic effects of the vaccine. Our results indicating that antibody and cellular (DTH) responses to vaccine treatment are each independently associated with an improved outcome suggest that both types of responses can mediate tumor-protective immunity. The best outcome was seen in patients who had both antibody and strong DTH responses to vaccine treatment, suggesting the beneficial effects associated with these different responses may be additive. The implications of these observations is that tumor vaccine design and immunization strategies should be aimed at magnifying both cellular and antibody responses to vaccine treatment, since both responses appear to provide tumor protective effects.

Prevention of Melanoma with Vaccines

A unique and potentially the most significant application of melanoma vaccines is their use to prevent this cancer in normal individuals. Several observations suggest this may ultimately be feasible. It is well established that melanoma vaccines can prevent this cancer in animals (Bystryn 1978, 1990; Bystryn et al. 1981, 1986). It is also clear, in animals, that vaccine treatment is more effective in preventing melanoma than in treating the disease once it is established. As noted by our results and those of other investigators described elsewhere in this volume, melanoma vaccines appear to be clinically effective in patients with established melanoma. Consequently, the logic of the animals studies suggest it should be feasible for vaccines to prevent melanoma in man and that in fact this might prove to be easier than treating patients who already have the disease.

Acknowledgment. This work was supported in part by USPHS Research Grant Nos. RO1 AM 27663-09, CA53468, P30CA16087, and AR39749, and by grants from the Rose M. Badgeley Trust, the Pardee Foundation, the Share foundation, and the NIH Skin Disease Research Center 5P30AR39749.

References

Adler A, Oratz R, Liebes L, Bystryn J-C (1990) Effect of allogeneic melanoma vaccine on the in vitro cellular immune response. Proc Am Assoc Cancer Res 31:252

Balch CM, Soong S-J, Shaw HM (1985) A comparison of world-wide melanoma data. In: Shaw HM, Seng-Jaw S (eds) Cutaneous melanoma. Lippincott, Philadelphia, pp 507–518

Berdeaux DH, Meyskens FL Jr, Parks B et al (1989) Cutaneous malignant melanoma. II. The natural history and prognostic factors influencing the development of stage II disease. Cancer 63:1430–1436

Bystryn J-C (1978) Antibody response and tumor growth in syngeneic mice immunized to partially purified B16 melanoma associated antigens. J Immunol 120:96–101

Bystryn J-C (1990) Tumor vaccines. Cancer Metastasis Rev 9:81–91

Bystryn J-C (1992) Identification of immunogenic human melanoma antigens in a polyvalent melanoma vaccine. Cancer Res 52:5948–5953

Bystryn J-C (1993) Immunogenicity and clinical activity of a polyvalent melanoma antigen vaccine prepared from shed antigens. In: Bystryn J-C, Ferrone S, Livingston P (eds) Specific immunotherapy of cancer with vaccines. Ann NY Acad Sci 690:190–203

Bystryn J-C, Tedholm CA, Heaney-Kieras J (1981) Release of surface macromolecules by human melanoma and normal cells. Cancer Res 41:910–914

Bystryn J-C, Jacobsen S, Harris MN, Roses DF, Speyer JL, Levin M (1986) Preparation and characterization of a polyvalent human melanoma antigen vaccine. J Biol Response Mod 5:221–224

Bystryn J-C, Oratz R, Harris MN, Roses DF, Golomb FM, Speyer JL (1988) Immunogenicity of a polyvalent melanoma antigen vaccine in man. Cancer 61:1065–1070

Bystryn J-C, Dugan M, Oratz R, Speyer J, Harris MN, Roses DF (1989) Vaccine immunotherapy of human malignant melanoma: relationship between method of immunization, immunogenicity, and tumor progression. In: Fred Fox C (ed) Human tumor antigens and specific tumor therapy. Liss, New York, pp 307–315

Bystryn J-C, Oratz R, Roses DF, Harris MN, Henn M, Lew R (1991) Improved survival of melanoma patients with delayed type hypersensitivity response to melanoma vaccine immunization. Clin Res 39:503A

Bystryn J-C, Oratz R, Henn M, Adler A, Harris MN, Roses DF (1992) Relationship between immune response to melanoma vaccine and clinical outcome in stage II malignant melanoma. Cancer 69:1157–1164

Cui J, Oratz R, Harris M, Roses D, Henn M, Bystryn J-C (1992) Induction of cytolytic melanoma antibodies by immunization to a polyvalent melanoma antigen vaccine. Proc Am Assoc Cancer Res 32:256

Oratz R, Cockerall C, Speyer J, Harris MN, Roses DF, Bystryn J-C (1989) Induction of tumor-infiltrating lymphocytes in malignant melanoma metastasis by immunization to melanoma antigen vaccine. J Biol Response Mod 8:355–358

Oratz R, Dugan M, Roses DF, Harris MN, Speyer JL, Hochster H, Weissman J, Henn M, Bystryn J-C (1991) Lack of effect of cyclophosphamide on the immunogenicity of a melanoma antigen vaccine. Cancer Res 51:3643–3647

Schultz N, Oratz R, Chen D, Bystryn J-C (1992) Effect of DETOX on the immunogenicity of a polyvalent melanoma antigen vaccine in man. Proc Am Soc Clin Oncol 11:1180

Veronesi U, Adamus J, Aubert C et al (1982) A randomized trial of adjuvant chemotherapy and immunotherapy in cutaneous melanoma. N Engl J Med 307: 913–916

Perspectives of Cytokine Treatment in Malignant Skin Tumors

C. Garbe

University Department of Dermatology, Medical Center Steglitz,
The Free University of Berlin, Hindenburgdamm 30, 12200 Berlin, Germany

Abstract

Cytokines have been tested in the treatment of different skin cancers during the last decade, and treatment schedules have been established or proposed for several malignant skin tumors. Preferentially, the interferons and interleukin-2 were found to be effective in treating skin cancers. Interferons alpha and beta have been approved for the treatment of human immunodeficiency virus (HIV)-associated Kaposi's sarcoma, cutaneous T cell lymphoma, and malignant melanoma in several countries. Interferon alpha was found to be most effective in cutaneous T cell lymphoma with 40%–60% overall responses. When combining interferon alpha with psoralens and ultraviolet A (PUVA) or with retinoids, even higher response rates up to 60%–90% were reported, and long-term remissions have been described. A considerable activity of interferon alpha was found in HIV-associated Kaposi's sarcoma with response rates of 30%–50%. The effectiveness of Kaposi's sarcoma's treatment was further improved by combining interferon alpha and zidovudine. Responses to interferon alpha in metastatic malignant melanoma are rather seldom (10%–15%), but a stabilization of the disease with prolonged survival was reported after interferon alpha treatment. Additionally, interleukin-2 was found to be active in metastatic melanoma, with overall response rates of about 20%, and both biological agents were found to have an additive efficacy in combination. Several combined regimens of interferon alpha, interleukin-2, and polychemotherapy have been described in metastatic melanoma, and overall response rates higher than 50% were found with these combined treatment modalities. Interferon alpha and beta were also intralesionally injected into basal cell carcinomas and other epithelial skin cancers, and complete responses were found in more than 80% of tumors treated. Local applications of interferons and interleukin-2 were likewise found to be effective in the treatment of cutaneous melanoma metastases and cutaneous manifestations of Kaposi's

Recent Results in Cancer Research, Vol. 139

sarcoma. Cytokines and their combination with other treatment modalities has greatly enriched the treatment facilities in malignant skin tumors during recent years, and additional new cytokines will be introduced in skin cancer treatment in near future.

Introduction

The effects of several cytokines in skin cancer have been investigated extensively during the last decade. The use of cytokines enriched the therapeutic approaches to skin cancer treatment and new strategies were added to classic therapies. Cytokines are defined as low molecular weight proteins predominantly released by cells of the immune system. They specifically bind with great affinity to target cell receptors and regulate their proliferation, differentiation, and functional activation. In contrast to endocrine hormones, they are produced by cells of different tissue origin rather than by specialized glands. They are often not detectable in the serum and they preferentially act on target cells in a paracrine or autocrine manner. Cytokines are known to play an important role in regulating host antitumor defence mechanisms.

Antitumor effects are mediated by different actions of cytokines. Several cytokines display direct antiproliferative effects on different tumor cells in vitro and in vivo. This kind of cytostatic effects has been preferentially described for the interferons (Garbe and Krasagakis 1993). Interestingly, interferons seem to selectively inhibit the growth of tumor cells, but not of normal cells of the same tissue or region. A selective growth inhibition by interferons was described for basal cell carcinoma cells in contrast to normal keratinocytes (Brysk et al. 1992), and we similarly found potent growth inhibition of melanoma cells, but not for normal human melanocytes (Krasagakis et al. 1991). Additionally, cytokines modulate the cell surface antigen expression of tumor cells. Enhancement of HLA class I and II antigens was observed after incubation of melanoma cells with interferons and other cytokines, and also other surface molecules involved in immunological recognition such as the intercellular adhesion molecule 1 (ICAM-1) were affected by different cytokines (Garbe et al. 1990). Cytokines also act via the host's immune response. Several cytokines stimulate the proliferation and functional activation of different lymphocyte subtypes and monocytes. The antitumor effect of certain cytokines such as interleukin-2 (IL-2) is predominantly mediated by stimulation of the cellular immune response against the tumor.

In recent years, cytokine treatments have been established or proposed for several malignant skin tumors. Type-I interferons (alpha and beta) have been approved in different countries for the treatment of cutaneous T cell lymphoma, human immunodeficiency virus (HIV)-associated Kaposi's sarcoma, and for malignant melanoma. Additionally, the local injection of cytokines into skin tumors seems to be effective in different tumor types. The inclusions of cytokines into therapeutic strategies proved, therefore, to be a major step forward in treatment of disseminated or advanced skin cancer during the last decade.

The following review is based to a great part on literature. It is also based on extensive personal experience in treating large collectives of skin cancer patients with different treatment modalities including chemotherapy, immunotherapy, surgery, and radiation. The purpose of this paper is to summarize the present status of skin cancer treatment with special attention to the role of cytokines within the advanced concepts.

Cutaneous T Cell Lymphoma

The efficacy of interferon alpha treatment in cutaneous T cell lymphoma (mucosis fungoides) was first described in the mid-1980s. The long-term benefit of patients treated with interferon alpha was striking and the activity of intralesional application was recognized (Bunn et al. 1984). Response rates of cutaneous T cell lymphoma after treatment with interferon alpha were 40% or higher in early stages with 10%–15% complete responses. Toxicity was found to be rather mild in comparison to chemotherapeutic regimens (Bunn et al. 1986; Foon et al. 1987). Further trials revealed that even intermediate doses of interferon alpha were sufficient to achieve objective remissions and that discontinuation of treatment led to immediate relapses (Simoni et al. 1987; Tura et al. 1987; Olsen et al. 1989; Nicolas et al. 1989; Vegna et al. 1990; Table 1). Dose escalation of interferon alpha did not improve objective response rates (Kohn et al. 1990). More than 90% of responses were reported after combination of photochemotherapy with psoralens and ultraviolet A light (PUVA) and with interferon alpha (Roenigk et al. 1990; Kuzel et al. 1990; Otte et al. 1992). Interestingly, the addition of PUVA to interferon alpha therapy in cutaneous T cell lymphoma supresses the formation of anti-interferon alpha antibodies (Kuzel et al. 1992). Additionally, a combination of interferon alpha with retinoids yielded promising therapeutic results (Thestup Pedersen et al. 1988; Zachariae et al. 1990; Altomare et al. 1993).

It is still a matter of debate whether the treatment of cutaneous T cell lymphoma should be with interferon alpha as monotherapy or as combined therapy initially. With interferon alpha monotherapy, up to 70% remission rates have been reported (Vegna et al. 1990; Ross et al. 1993). Neither the doses nor the routes of administration showed a significant influence on the clinical responses to interferon alpha treatment in different studies (Ross et al. 1993). In future, patients with good chances for clinical response to interferon alpha may possibly be detected by immunohistological investigations. Patients with cutaneous T cell lymphoma normally lose the expression of an antigen on normal basal cell keratinocytes, which is recognized by

Table 1. Therapeutic results of interferon-α (IFN-α) treatment and combined treatment modalities in cutaneous T cell lymphoma

	Number	CR + PR (%)
50 × 10(6) U IFN-α_{2a}/m^2 3 days/week Bunn et al. 1984, 1986	20	10 + 35
18 × 10(6) U IFN-α_{2a} 3 days/week Simoni et al. 1987	12	42 + 50
3–18 × 10(6) U IFN-α_{2a} 3 days/week Tura et al. 1987	15	20 + 60
3–36 × 10(6) U IFN-α_{2a} 3 days/week Olsen et al. 1989	22	14 + 45
18 × 10(6) U IFN-α_{2a} 3 days/week Nicolas et al. 1989	6	17 + 50
10–50 × 10(6) IFN-α_{2a}/m^2 days 1–5 every 3 weeks Kohn et al. 1990	24	4 + 25
3–18 × 10(6) U IFN-α_{2a} 3 days/week Vegna et al. 1990	23	35 + 39
6–30 × 10(6) U IFN-α_{2a} 3 days/week + PUVA Roenigk et al. 1990; Kuzel et al. 1990	15	80 + 13
3–9 × 10(6) U IFN-α_{2a} 3 days/week + PUVA Otte et al. 1992	11	45 + 55
6–36 × 10(6) U IFN-α_{2a} 3 days/week + 0.7 mg Entretinate/kg Thestrup Pedersen et al. 1988; Zachariae et al. 1990	11	18 + 45
IFN-α_{2b} (low dose) + Etretinate Altomare et al. 1993	13	54 + 23

CR, complete response; PR, partial response (>50%); PUVA, psoralens and ultraviolet A light.

monoclonal antibody MY7. The expression of this antigen can be reinduced under interferon alpha therapy. Patients with successful reinduction of this antigen mostly seem to respond to interferon alpha treatment (Dreno et al. 1992; Celerier et al. 1993). In addition, immunophenotyping of T cells in cutaneous T cell lymphoma may aid in distinguishing patients with poor responses to interferon alpha from those with favorable chances for response. Deletions of T cell CD7 and CD5 antigens were associated with poor response to interferon treatment (Springer et al. 1993).

In early stages of cutaneous T cell lymphoma, monotherapy may be adequate treatment. If treatment was started with photochemotherapy, PUVA refractory patients often respond to the combined treatment with PUVA and interferon alpha (Otte et al. 1992; Mostow et al. 1993). In later stages of cutaneous T cell lymphoma, combined treatment modalities may be used initially to optimize the chances for response. The combination of interferon alpha and retinoids should be further evaluated. This combination allows the use of lower doses of interferon alpha and thereby the reduction of side effects of interferon alpha (Dreno et al. 1993; Altomare et al. 1993). This may be particularly valuable in patients with severe toxity of interferon alpha.

Kaposi's Sarcoma

The activity of interferon alpha in Kaposi's sarcoma was already recognized at the beginning of the 1980s (Krown et al. 1983). In the first series treated with interferon alpha, 33%–67% responses in patients with HIV-associated Kaposi's sarcoma were reported (Groopman et al. 1984; Volberding et al. 1984; Rios et al. 1985). Subsequent series revealed objective response rates between 27% and 38% (Gelmann et al. 1985; Abrams and Volberding 1986; Krown et al. 1986; Real et al. 1986; Fischl et al. 1986; Volberding et al. 1987; Kern et al. 1987; Rozenbaum et al. 1990; Plettenberg et al. 1990; Table 2). Response rates were related to the doses applied, and higher doses produced increasing responses (Real et al. 1986). Subsequent trials found response rates less related to the doses given, but rather to the immune status of the patient (Volberding et al. 1987). Patients with a much reduced immune situation responded less often than those with higher total lymphocyte and $CD4^{+}$ T lymphocyte counts and absence of prior opportunistic infection (Gelmann et al. 1985). Patients with endogeneous interferon alpha blood levels responded less well than those without detectable interferon alpha in the peripheral blood (Gelmann et al. 1985; Sawyer et al. 1990). Interestingly, among the responders there were patients with long-term responses of 2–5 years (Schaart et al. 1991).

In order to improve the therapeutic results in Kaposi's sarcoma, combined interferon alpha and zidovudine therapy was introduced into the treatment of HIV-associated Kaposi's sarcoma. It turned out that intermediate doses of interferon alpha (9–18 million U/day) and low doses of zidovudine (up to 600 mg/day) were relatively well tolerated and simultaneously associated with disease improvement, including survival benefits (Fischl 1991). This combined regimen revealed greater efficacy than interferon alpha monotherapy and response rates between 40% and 50% were described (Kovacs et al. 1989; Krown et al. 1990; Stadler et al. 1990; Fischl et al. 1991; Baumann et al. 1991; Scadden et al. 1991b; Table 3). As the toxicity of this combined regimen consists mainly in myelosuppression, several authors proposed adding colony-stimulating factors (CSF) to this regimen in order to prevent neutropenia. The addition of granulocyte-macrophage CSF (GM-CSF) was not associated with increased toxicity and did not affect the antitumor activity of combined zidovudine and interferon alpha therapy (Scadden et al. 1991a,b). Low-dose GM-CSF readily ameliorated neutropenia associated with zidovudine and interferon alpha therapy and made it

Table 2. Therapeutic results of interferon-α (IFN-α) treatment in human immunodeficiency virus (HIV)-associated Kaposi's sarcoma

	Number	CR + PR (%)
1–50 × 10(6) U IFN-α_{2b}/m^2 5 days/week Groopman et al. 1984	24	8 + 25
1 × 10(6) U IFN-α_{2b}/m^2 every other week	9	22 + 11
5 × 10(6) U IFN-α_{2b}/m^2 5 days/week Volberding et al. 1984	20	10 + 30
20 × 10(6) U IFN-α_{N1}/m^2 per day Rios et al. 1985	12	33 + 33
7.5–2.5 × 10(6) U IFN-α_{N1}/m^2 per day Gelmann et al. 1985	30	10
30–50 × 10(6) U IFN-α_{2b}/m^2 3–7 days/week Abrams and Volberding 1986	50	32
3 × 10(6) U IFN-α_{2a}/m^2 per day	35	0 + 3
3–36 × 10(6) U IFN-α_{2a}/m^2 per day	34	9 + 6
36 × 10(6) U IFN-α_{2a}/m^2 per day Real et al. 1986	27	30 + 19
20 + 10(6) U IFN-α_{N1}/m^2 per day Fischl et al. 1986	20	15 + 45
1;30;50 × 10(6) U IFN-α_{2b}/m^2 per day Volberding et al. 1987	114	33; 28; 45
18–36 × 10(6) U IFNα_{2a} 3–7 days/week Kern et al. 1987	20	30
18–36 × 10(6) U IFN-α_{2a} per day Rozenbaum et al. 1990	120	35 + 8
18 × 10(6) U IFN-α_{2a}/m^2 3–7 days/week Plettenberg et al. 1990	41	12 + 17

CR, complete response; PR, partial response (>50%).

possible to apply the combined treatment regimen without major dose reductions (Davey et al. 1991). Granulocyte CSF (G-CSF) has been evaluated with similar results (Schröder et al. 1992).

Other biologic agents, including interferons beta and gamma, tumor necrosis factor, and interleukin-2, have also been tested, though to a lesser extent, in patients with Kaposi's sarcoma. Although systemically administered interferon beta has lead to objective responses in some cases, the role of this biologic agent has not been defined completely yet (Brockmeyer et al. 1989; Miles et al. 1990). Preliminary trials of interferon gamma in Kaposi's sarcoma have failed to demonstrate significant activity, and only few responses have been described in several trials (Krigel et al. 1985; Ganser et al. 1986; Lane et al. 1989; Heagy et al. 1990; Table 4). Additionally, the use of interleukin-2 in combination with type-I interferon led to an exazerbation of Kaposi's sarcoma in a small series of patients (Krigel et al. 1989).

Table 3. Therapeutic results of combined treatments with interferon-α (IFN-α) and zidovudine in human immunodeficiency virus (HIV)-associated Kaposi's sarcoma

	Number	CR + PR (%)
5–20 × 10(6) U IFN-α_{2b}/m^2 per day + 300–1500 mg zidovudine per day Kovacs et al. 1989	22	50
4.5–18 × 10(6) U IFN-α_{2a}/m^2 per day + 600–1200 mg zidovudine per day Krown et al. 1990	43	46
18 × 10(6) U IFN-α_{2a}/m^2 3 days/week + 800–1200 mg zidovudine per day Stadler et al. 1990	15	27 + 20
9–27 × 10(6) U IFN-α_{2a}/m^2 per day + 600–1200 mg zidovudine per day Fischl et al. 1991	56	47
10 × 10(6) U IFN-α_{N1}/m^2 per day + 500 mg zidovudine per day Baumann et al. 1991	15	7 + 7
9 × 10(6) U IFN-α_{2a}/m^2 per day + 1200 mg zidovudine per day + GM-CSF in neutropenia Scadden et al. 1991	29 (80% poor-prognosis patients)	50

CR, complete response; PR, partial response (>50%); GM-CSF, granulocyte-macrophage colony-stimulating factor.

Table 4. Therapeutic results of interferon-β (IFN-β) and IFN-γ treatments in human immunodeficiency virus (HIV)-associated Kaposi's sarcoma

	Number	CR + PR (%)
90–180 × 10(6) U IFN-β_{ser}/m^2 5 days/week Miles et al. 1990	38 (Poor-prognosis patients)	16
0.5 × 10(6) U IFN-γ per day Krigel et al. 1985	7	0
4 × 10(6) U IFN-γ per day Ganser et al. 1986	4	0
0.001–1 mg IFN-γ/m^2 per day Lane et al. 1989	16	0
0.03–3 mg IFN-γ/m^2 per day Heagy et al. 1990	17	6 + 12

CR, complete response; PR, partial response (>50%).

Interferon alpha therapy is particularly indicated in cutaneous and mucocutaneous Kaposi's sarcoma in patients with CD4 T lymphocyte counts greater than 100–200/μl. Response rates are increased by combining interferon alpha with zidovudine. As soon as visceral involvement of Kaposi's sarcoma occurs, treatment with interferon alpha is less effective according to our experience and treatment with combined cytostatic regimens should be considered. The role of biologic agents other than interferon alpha in the treatment of Kaposi's sarcoma is still to be defined.

Malignant Melanoma

Presently, no standard treatment for disseminated malignant melanoma exists. Distant metastasis of malignant melanoma is associated with a poor prognosis and patients normally die within 4–6 months. Combined cytotoxic drug regimens lead to responses in only 25%–35% of patients with disseminated melanoma, and it still remins unclear whether survival time can be prolonged by these drugs. Against this background, the establishment of cytokine therapies in malignant melanoma became attractive and numerous cytokines have since been tested in malignant melanoma in vitro and in vivo.

Interferons were the first cytokines to be introduced into melanoma therapy. All interferons (alpha, beta, gamma) exhibit direct antiproliferative effects on melanoma cells in vitro, with interferon beta revealing the highest antiproliferative potency (Garbe et al. 1990). Among the type-I interferons (alpha, beta), the order of their antiproliferative potency is related to the order of their binding affinity to type-I interferon receptor (Johns et al. 1992). It is still unclear whether the increased antitumor activity of interferon beta also corresponds to a better efficacy in melanoma treatment in vivo. Intralesional application of interferon beta into cutaneous melanoma metastasis resulted in partial or complete remissions in 50% of metastases treated. However, no systemic antitumor effects were observed in any of these cases (Fierlbeck et al. 1992). Possibly, high tissue binding of interferon beta leads to reduced systemic availability of this substance when applied subcutaneously. Additionally, subcutaneous interferon beta induces an antibody response in a high percentage of patients with the potential to neutralize the agent (Dummer et al. 1991; Fierlbeck et al. 1992).

Several cytokines display direct antiproliferative effects on melanoma cells in vitro. Among these are interferons alpha, beta, and gamma, tumor necrosis factor alpha, IL-1α, IL-1β, IL-4, and transforming growth factor beta. Indirect antitumor effects via the host's immune response are augmented by IL-2, -6, and -12 (Garbe and Krasagakis 1993; Brunda et al. 1993).

Cytokines, however, do not uniformly display antitumor activity, but may also promote tumor growth and the metastatic potential of tumor cells. We found that interferon gamma enhanced the expression of several tumor antigens which are upregulated during tumor progression and metastasis. This is true for the ICAM-1 molecule, the adhesion molecule VLA-2, and HLA class 2 antigens (Garbe et al. 1990). The metastatic potential of tumor cells was found to be enhanced by tumor necrosis factor alpha and by interferon gamma in experimental models (Lollini et al. 1990). Additional clinical evidence resulted from an adjuvant study in high-risk stage I and II cutaneous malignant melanoma with interferon gamma, which was prematurely discontinued due to the impaired of prognosis the group treated with interferon gamma (Meyskens et al. 1990). These results provide evidence that interferon gamma is a tumor-promoting substance rather than an anticancer agent in malignant melanoma.

Interferon alpha as a single substance has a moderate activity in metastatic melanoma. Objective responses were reported in an average of 10%–15% of patients treated when analyzing several series reported in the literature in common (Stadler and Garbe 1991). The number of objective responses is probably not the best criterium to judge the antitumor activity of interferon alpha in metastatic melanoma. With intermediate doses of interferon alpha, disease stabilization and a prolonged survival of patients was also found in metastatic melanoma (Pyrhonen et al. 1992b). These effects of interferon alpha have also been observed by the author, and additional studies should be performed to better clarify these inhibiting effects of disease progression.

Interferons were also tested in an adjuvant setting in high-risk melanomas. Interferons alpha and gamma were found not to be effective in small phase II studies (Elsässer Beile et al. 1989; Landthaler and Braun Falco 1989). Larger studies to assess the therapeutic potential of interferons in high-risk melanomas are still missing.

Another biologic agent with proven activity in metastatic melanoma is IL-2, specific growth factor for T and NK lymphocytes. It induces proliferation of lymphocytes, enhances the expression of IL-2 receptors, and stimulates the development of cytotoxic activity against autologous and allogeneic tumor cells. IL-2 exerts no direct antiproliferative activity on melanoma cells. It was initially reported in vitro to stimulate lymphokine-activated killer (LAK) cells from the leukocytes of patients with melanoma after incubation for 4 days. On reinfusion, these LAK-cells together with varying doses of additional IL-2 administered by continuous intraveneous infusion induced significant disease regression (Rosenberg et al. 1985). Evaluation of a large series of patients treated with high-dose IL-2 intraveneously alone or in combination with LAK cells interferon alpha, tumor necrosis factor alpha, or cyclophosphamide showed response rates between 20% and 35%. The intraveneous application of IL-2 as a single substance revealed to be as effective as the combination with the patients own LAK cells established in vitro with much effort (Rosenberg et al. 1989a). In a subsequent series, continuous infusion of IL-2 was found to produce 18% objective responses in 188 patients with disseminated melanoma, and the results in disseminated melanoma were superior to all other metastasized tumors treated with IL-2 (Dillman et al. 1993). Therefore, IL-2 is one of the most active biologic agents in metastatic melanoma.

The combination of IL-2 with interferon alpha was also investigated in disseminated melanoma. In early series, this combination turned out to be more effective than other combinations tested (Rosenberg et al. 1989a,b). IL-2 combined with interferon alpha revealed additive antitumor effects with objective response rates as high as 36% (Rosenberg et al. 1989). The disadvantage of all IL-2-containing regimens used to be the rather high toxicity of continuous IL-2 infusion, including life-threatening fluid retention, hypotension, and pulmonary edema. Therefore, treatments had to be performed in intensive care units. Later on, subcutaneous application of IL-2 in outpatients was reported with significantly fewer side effects (Atzpodin et al. 1990). It remains still unclear whether subcutaneous application of IL-2 in intermediate doses is as effective as continuous infusion. Trials with low-dose application of IL-2 in combination with interferon alpha showed that it was not effective in disseminated melanoma (Whitehead et al. 1993; Castello et al. 1993). On the other hand, modified dose schedules with high initial doses of IL-2 and subsequent low-dose maintenance therapy by continuous infusion were found to be as effective as previous schedules and revealed considerably less toxicity (Keiholz et al. 1993). Adequate doses and the best route of administration of IL-2 in disseminated melanoma are still to be defined.

Since the antitumor action of interferons is probably due to its antiproliferative effect, it appeared promising to study the efficacy of interferons in combination with cytotoxic drugs. The results of more than 15 clinical trials have already been published; most of them tested the combination of interferon alpha with dacarbazine. More than 500 patients have since been treated with this drug combination in phase II studies. The mean overall response rate was 29% (Table 5). In addition, several studies reported stable diseases in an additional 25%. The toxicity of these types of treatment was significant, but manageable. In three clinical trials, the efficacy of combined treatment with interferon alpha and dacarbazine was compared to monotherapy with dacarbazine. Two of three trials found a significant elevation of response rates and a prolongation of response durations (Falkson et al. 1991; Sertoli et al. 1992), whereas in the third trial only minor advantages in respect to response were observed (Thomson et al. 1992; Table 6). Similarly encouraging results were reported for the combination of interferon alpha with vindesine (Garbe et al. 1992; Smith et al. 1992), but less favorable results were obtained by combining interferon alpha with cisplatin or with vinblastine (Kellokumpu-Lehtinen et al. 1989; Oratz et al. 1989; Schuchter et al. 1989; Gundersen and Flokkmann 1989; Margolin et al. 1990; Richner et al. 1990).

Dacarbazine and cisplatin have likewise been combined with IL-2. Treatment results of this combination seemed to be superior to single-agent

Table 5. Therapeutic results of combined treatment with interferon (IFN)-α and dacarbazine in melanoma patients; meta-analysis of nine clinical trials

Author	Patients (n)	CR (%)	PR (%)	OR (%)	SD (%)
Hersey et al. 1989	74	9	18	27	33
Kerr et al. 1989	17	–	6	6	18
Bajetta et al. 1990	75	8	17	25	–
Breier et al. 1990	17	24	29	53	18
Mulder et al. 1990	31	10	26	36	–
Falcson et al. 1991	30	40	13	53	33
Sertoli et al. 1992	136	7	19	26	–
Thomsen et al. 1992	87	7	14	21	17
Ron et al. 1993	34	18	15	33	–
Total	501	10	19	29	25

CR, complete response; PR, partial response (>50%); OR, overall response; SD, stable disease.

Table 6. Therapeutic results of combined treatment with interferon (IFN)-α and dacarbazine (DTIC) versus dacarbazine alone in metastatic melanoma

Study	Patients (n)	CR + PR (%)	Median duration of response (weeks)
Falcson et al. 1991			
DTIC + IFN-α	27	38	36
DTIC alone	27	17	11
Sertoli et al. 1992			
DTIC + IFN-α	136 (two arms)	26	33
DTIC alone	67	16	11
Thomson et al. 1992			
DTIC + IFN-α	87	21	37
DTIC alone	82	17	41

CR, complete response; PR, partial response (>50%).

therapy with IL-2, but no comparative studies between single-agent therapy and combined schedules have been performed yet (Dillmann et al. 1990; Flaherty et al. 1990; Demschak et al. 1990). Recently, several centers have initiated clinical trials combining cytokines with cytotoxic multidrug regimens, and preliminary reports have been given at the meetings of the American Society for Clinical Oncology. These rather complex therapeutic regimens produced 13%–25% complete remissions and 37%–58% partial remissions among patients with metastatic melanoma (Hamblin et al. 1991; Pyrhonen et al. 1992; Richards et al. 1992a,b; Legha et al. 1992; Table 7). In each of these trials an overall response rate of more than 50% was observed; this is significantly higher than response rates obtained with

Table 7. Therapeutic results of combined treatment with cytokines and polychemotherapy in metastatic melanoma

Regimen	Number	CR + PR (%)	SD (%)
IFN-α + IL-2 + Cispl. + DTIC Hamblin et al. 1991	12	25 + 58	–
IFN-α + DTIC + Bleom. + Vincr. + CCNU Pyrhonen et al. 1992	48	13 + 49	–
IFN-α + IL-2 + Cispl. + BCNU + DTIC + Tam. Richards et al. 1992a	74	15 + 40	25
IFN-α + IL-2 + Cispl. + Vinbl. + DTIC Legha et al. 1992	30	20 + 37	–

CR, complete response; PR, partial response (>50%); SD, stable disease; IFN, interferon; IL, interleukin; Cispl., cisplatin; DTIC, dacarbazine; Bleom., bleomycin; Vincr., vincristine; CCNU, lomustine; BCNU, carmustine; Tam., tamoxifen; Vinbl., vinblastine.

previous cytotoxic drug regimens. In this respect, the introduction of cytokines into cytotoxic treatment regimens seems to substantially improved the therapeutic efficacy of systemic treatment in metastatic melanoma. Unfortunately, these complex regimens are still associated with significant toxicity, and future trials should test combinations and regimens with less adverse reactions.

Intralesional Treatment of Epithelial and Other Skin Cancers

Bowenoid cancers in epidermodysplasia verruciformis were the first epithelial skin cancer lesions to be treated with intralesional interferon injections and were observed to completely disappear after this treatment (Lutzner et al. 1984). Greenway and coworkers were the first to try intralesional treatment of basal cell carcinomas with injections three times a week for 3 weeks (total dose, 13.5 × 10(6) IU interferon alpha). In a series of patients, no evidence of disease was found in any patient by excisional biopsy 2 months after the end of therapy (Greenway et al. 1986). Later, responses of large basal cell carcinomas with intralesional interferon alpha were likewise reported (Grob et al. 1988). Other epithelial skin cancers or precanceroses such as squamous cell carcinomas, solar keratoses, and keratoacanthomas were also found to be resolved by a 3-week treatment with interferon alpha (Wickramasinghe et al. 1989). The responses to intralesional treatment were dose dependent, and lower doses than reported above were found not to be effective (Tank et al. 1989). It was possible to reduce the number of injections by using a sustained-release protamine zinc preparation of interferon alpha-2b and to obtain 80% of histologically proven cures in basal cell carcinomas with three injections and 52% with one single injection (Edwards et al. 1990).

In a larger series of patients, the response rate to 3-week interferon alpha treatment was found to be higher than 80% when investigating the therapeutic results after 1 year (Cornell et al. 1990). Immunohistochemical evaluations of cellular immune reaction in the treated basal cell carcinomas showed an increase of $CD4^+$ helper-inducer T cells and, in addition, of natural killer cells (Mozzanica et al. 1990; Buechner 1991). Immunohistologic changes in the skin lesions suggested that intralesional interferon alpha acts on tumor cells by enhancement of local T cell-mediated immune responses.

Intralesional therapies have also been reported in cutaneous metastases of malignant melanoma. Interferon alpha and interferon beta were both effective in about 40%–60% of injected lesions, with interferon beta showing a somewhat better efficacy (von Wussow et al. 1988; Fierlbeck et al. 1992). Kaposi's sarcoma lesions were likewise treated intralesionally by cytokines. Anecdotal reports described responses to IL-2 (Hauschild et al. 1992) and to GM-CSF (Boente et al. 1993).

Future Prospects

The introduction of cytokines in the treatment of malignant skin tumors significantly enlarged the therapeutic spectrum and clearly improved therapeutic results (Hill et al. 1992). So far, only few cytokines have proven to be active in different malignant skin tumors. Numerous other cytokines have still to be tested for their efficacy in treatment of skin cancers and additional cytokines will probably be introduced in skin cancer treatment in the next few years.

Apart from epithelial skin cancers, few reports have been published on the efficacy of cytokines when administered intralesionally or perilesionally. Interestingly, different cytokines such as interferons alpha and beta, IL-2, and GM-CSF have been described as being effective in different skin tumors. Systematical investigation of their role in intralesional treatment is still lacking for most of the malignant skin tumors. Additional, combined administration of several cytokines or of cytokines and cytotoxic drugs has not yet been examined.

Remarkable progress resulted from combining interferons or IL-2 with other treatment modalities (Wadler 1992). In particular, the combination of cytotoxic drugs and cytokines turned out to be very effective in metastatic melanoma and led to an impressive improvement of treatment results. Additionally, the combination of photochemotherapy with interferon alpha in cutaneous T cell lymphoma produced a very high rate of overall responses, superior to all treatment results described before. So far, optimal doses, optimal routes of cytokine administration, and effective sequential treatment schedules are not based on appropriate experimental and clinical investigations. A rational basis for the design of combination schedules has still to be established. Furthermore, inclusion of additional cytokines with antiproliferative effects or with stimulating activity on host's immune system as well as inclusion of other cytotoxic drugs may further improve results of systemic therapy in skin cancers.

Finally, gene therapy for cancer is currently being tested in clinical trials using lymphocytes or tumor cells modified by the insertion of genes coding for different cytokines (Rosenberg 1992; Ogasawara and Rosenberg 1993; Crowley and Seigler 1993). Cytokines such as IL-2, tumor necrosis factor alpha, interferon gamma, and interferon alpha can enhance the host's antitumor immune response. It is expected that the host's immune system can be stimulated by cytokine-producing tumor cells in order to eradicate cancer cells. A technically feasible clinical application of this approach is the generation of vaccines by introducing such immunostimulatory genes into cancer cells and boosting systemic immune reactions also against the unmodified cells. These trials are at the very beginning in humans and it remains to be seen whether gene therapy for cancer will contribute to the improvement of cancer therapy.

References

Abrams DI, Volberding PA (1986) Alpha interferon therapy of AIDS-associated Kaposi's sarcoma. Semin Oncol 13 [3 Suppl 2]:43–47

Altomare GF, Capella GL, Pigatto PD, Finzi AF (1993) Intramuscular low dose alpha-2B interferon and etretinate for treatment of mycosis fungoides. Int J Dermatol 32:138–141

Atzpodien J, Körfer A, Franks CR, Poliwoda H, Kirchner H (1990) Home therapy with recombinant interleukin-2 and interferon-a-2b in advanced human malignancies. Lancet 335:1509–1512

Bajetta E, Negretti E, Giannotti B et al (1990) Phase II study of interferon-alpha-2a and dacarbazine in advanced melanoma. Am J Clin Oncol 13:405–409

Baumann R, Tauber MG, Opravil M, Hirschel B, Kinloch S, Chave JP, Pletscher M, Luthy R (1991) Combined treatment with zidovudine and lymphoblast interferon-alpha in patients with HIV-related Kaposi's sarcoma. Klin Wochenschr 69: 360–367

Boente P, Sampaio C, Brandao MA, Moreira ED, Badaro R, Jones TC (1993) Local perilesional therapy with rhGM-CSF for Kaposi's sarcoma (letter). Lancet 341:1154

Breier S, Pensel R, Roffe C et al (1990) High dose DTIC with recombinant human interferon alpha-2b (rhifn2b) for the treatment of metastatic malignant melanoma (MMM). Proc Annu Meet Am Soc Clin Oncol 9:A1090

Brockmeyer NH, Mertins L, Daecke C, Goos M (1989) Regression of Kaposi's sarcoma and improvement of performance status by a combined interferon beta and zidovudine therapy in AIDS patients. J Invest Dermatol 92:776

Brunda MJ, Luistro L, Wright RR, Wright RB, Hubbard BR, Murphy M, Wolf SF, Gately MK (1993) Antitumor and antimetastatic activity of interleukin 12 against murine tumors. J Exp Med 178:1223–1230

Brysk MM, Santschi CH, Bell T, Wagner RF Jr, Tyring SK, Rajaraman S (1992) Culture of basal cell carcinoma. J Invest Dermatol 98:45–49
Buechner SA (1991) Intralesional interferon alfa-2b in the treatment of basal cell carcinoma. Immunohistochemical study on cellular immune reaction leading to tumor regression. J Am Acad Dermatol 24:731–734
Bunn PA Jr, Foon KA, Ihde DC, Longo DL, Eddy J, Winkler CF, Veach SR, Zeffren J, Sherwin S, Oldham R (1984) Recombinant leukocyte A interferon: an active agent in advanced cutaneous T-cell lymphomas. Ann Intern Med 101: 484–487
Bunn PA Jr, Ihde DC, Foon KA (1986) The role of recombinant interferon alfa-2a in the therapy of cutaneous T-cell lymphomas. Cancer 57:1689–1695
Castello G, Comella P, Manzo T, Napolitano M, Parziale AP, Galati MG, Daponte A, Casaretti R, Celentano E, Comella G (1993) Immunological and clinical effects of intramuscular rIFN alpha-2a and low dose subcutaneous rIL-2 in patients with advanced malignant melanoma. Melanoma Res 3:43–49
Celerier P, Fleischmann M, Basset Seguin N, Thill L, Bureau B, Litoux P, Dreno B (1993) In vitro induction of basal keratinocyte MY7 antigen expression in cutaneous T-cell lymphoma is associated with response to interferon-alfa therapy. Arch Dermatol 129:1136–1140
Cornell RC, Greenway HY, Tucker SB, Edwards L, Ashworth S, Vance JC, Tanner DJ, Taylor EL, Smiles KA, Peets EA (1990) Intralesional interferon therapy for basal cell carcinoma. J Am Acad Dermatol 23:694–700
Crowley NJ, Seigler HF (1993) Possibilities of immunotherapy and gene therapy for malignant melanoma. Semin Surg Oncol 9:273–278
Davey RT Jr, Davey VJ, Metcalf JA, Zurlo JJ, Kovacs JA, Falloon J, Polis MA, Zunich KM, Masur H, Lane HC (1991) A phase I/II trial of zidovudine, interferon-alpha, and granulocyte-macrophage colony-stimulating factor in the treatment of human immunodeficiency virus type 1 infection. J Infect Dis 164: 43–52
Demchak PA, Mier JW, Robert NJ et al (1990) Interleukin-2 and high-dose cisplatin in patients with metastatic melanoma: a pilot study. J Clin Oncol 9:1821–1830
Dillman RO, Oldham RK, Barth NM et al (1990) Recombinant interleukin-2 and adoptive immunotherapy alternated with dacarbazine therapy in melanoma: a National Biotherapy Study Group trial. J Natl Cancer Inst 82:1345–1349
Dillman RO, Church C, Oldham RK, West WH, Schwartzberg L, Birch R (1993) Inpatient continuous-infusion interleukin-2 in 788 patients with cancer. The National Biotherapy Study Group experience. Cancer 71:2358–2370
Dreno B, Fleischmann M, Valard S, Godefroy W, Bureau B, Stadler JF, Litoux P (1992) Induction of myelo-monocytic My7 antigen (CD13) expression by interferon-alpha in basal cells of cutaneous T-cell lymphomas. Br J Dermatol 126:320–323
Dreno B, Celerier P, Litoux P (1993) Roferon-A in combination with Tigason in cutaneous T-cell lymphomas. Acta Haematol 89 [Suppl 1]:28–32
Dummer R, Muller W, Nestle F, Wiede J, Dues J, Lechner W, Haubitz I, Wolf W, Bill E, Burg G (1991) Formation of neutralizing antibodies against natural interferon-beta, but not against recombinant interferon-gamma during adjuvant therapy for high-rish malignant melanoma patients. Cancer 67:2300–2304
Edwards L, Tucker SB, Perednia D, Smiles KA, Taylor EL, Tanner DJ, Peets E (1990) The effect of an intralesional sustained-release formulation of interferon alfa-2b on basal cell carcinomas. Arch Dermatol 126:1029–1032
Elsässer Beile U, Garbe C, Stadler R, Drews H, Schöpf E (1989) Adjuvante Therapie mit rekombiniertem Interferon alfa-2a beim metastasierten malignen Melanom. Hautarzt 40:266–270

Falkson CI, Falkson G, Falkson HC (1991) Improved results with the addition of recombinant interferon alpha-2b to dacarbazine in treatment of patients with metastatic malignant melanoma. J Clin Oncol 9:1403–1408
Fierlbeck G, d'Hoedt B, Stroebel W, Stutte H, Bogenschütz O, Rassner G (1992) Intraläsionale Therapie von Melanommetastasen mit rekombinantem Interferon-beta. Hautarzt 43:16–21
Fischl MA (1991) Antiretroviral therapy in combination with interferon for AIDS-related Kaposi's sarcoma. Am J Med 90:2S–7S
Fischl M, Lucas S, Gorowski E et al (1986) Interferon alpha-N1 Wellferon (WFN) in Kaposi's sarcoma: single agent or combination with vinblastine (VBL). J Interferon Res 6 [Suppl 1]:4 (abstr)
Fischl MA, Uttamchandani RB, Resnick L, Agarwal R, Fletcher MA, Patrone Reese J, Dearmas L, Chidekel J, McCann M, Myers M (1991) A phase I study of recombinant human interferon-alpha 2a or human lymphoblastoid interferon-alpha n1 and concomitant zidovudine in patients with AIDS-related Kaposi's sarcoma. J Acquir Immune Defic Syndr 4:1–10
Flaherty LE, Redman BG, Chabot GG et al (1990) A phase I-II study of dacarbazine in combination with outpatient interleukin-2 in metastatic malignant melanoma. Cancer 65:2471–2477
Foon KA, Roth MS, Bunn PA Jr (1987) Interferon therapy of non-Hodgkin's lymphoma. Cancer 59 [3 Suppl]:601–604
Ganser A, Brucher W, Brodt HR, Busch W, Brandhorst I, Helm EB, Hoelzer D (1986) Treatment of AIDS-related Kaposi's sarcoma with recombinant gamma-interferon. Onkologie 9:163–166
Garbe C, Krasagakis K (1993) Effects of interferons and cytokines on melanoma cells. J Invest Dermatol 100:239S–244S
Garbe C, Krasagakis K, Zouboulis C, Schröder K, Krüger S, Stadler R, Orfanos CE (1990) Antitumor activities of interferon-alpha, -beta and -gamma on malignant melanoma cells in vitro. Changes of proliferation, melanin synthesis and immunophenotype. J Invest Dermatol 95:231S–237S
Garbe C, Kreuser ED, Zouboulis CC, Stadler R, Orfanos CE (1992) Combined treatment of metastatic melanoma with interferons and cytotoxic drugs. Semin Oncol 19 [Suppl 4]:63–69
Garbe C, Zouboulis ChC, Stadler R et al (1994) Prolongation of life in stage IV melanoma by combined treatment with IFN-a-2a and vindesine (submitted for publication)
Gelmann EP, Preble OT, Steis R, Lane HC, Rook AH, Wesley M, Jacob J, Fauci A, Masur H, Longo D (1985) Human lymphoblastoid interferon treatment of Kaposi's sarcoma in the acquired immune deficiency syndrome. Clinical response and prognostic parameters. Am J Med 78:737–741
Greenway HT, Cornell RC, Tanner DJ, Peets E, Bordin GM, Nagi C (1986) Treatment of basal cell carcinoma with intralesional interferon. J Am Acad Dermatol 15:437–443
Grob JJ, Collet AM, Munoz MH, Bonerandi JJ (1988) Treatment of large basal-cell carcinomas with intralesional interferon-alpha-2a. Lancet 1:878–879
Groopman JE, Gottlieb MS, Goodman J, Mitsuyasu RT, Conant MA, Prince H, Fahey JL, Derezin M, Weinstein WM, Casavante C et al (1984) Recombinant alpha-2 interferon herapy for Kaposi's sarcoma associated with the acquired immunodeficiency syndrome. Ann Intern Med 100:671–676
Gundersen S, Flokkmann A (1989) Interferon in combination with vinblastine in advanced malignant melanoma. A phase I-II study. Cancer 64:1617–1619
Hamblin TJ, Davies B, Sadullah S, Oskam R, Palmer P, Franks CR (1991) A phase II study of the treatment of metastatic malignant melanoma with a combination of

dacarbazine, cisplatin, interleukin-2 (IL-2) and alfa-interferon (IFN). Proc Annu Meet Am Soc Clin Oncol 10:A1029
Hauschild A, Petres Dunsche C (1992) Intraläsionäre Behandlung des klassischen Kaposi-Sarkoms mit Interferon alpha. Hautarzt 43:789–791
Heagy W, Groopman J, Schindler J, Finberg R (1990) Use of IFN-gamma in patients with AIDS. J Acquir Immune Defic Syndr 3:584–590
Hersey P, McLeod RC, Thomson DB (1989) Phase I/II study of tolerability and efficacy of recombinant interferon (Roferon) with dacarbazine (DTIC) in advanced malignant melanoma. J Interferon Res 9 [Suppl 2]:118
Hill AD, Redmond HP, Croke DT, Grace PA, Bouchier Hayes D (1992) Cytokines in tumour therapy. Br J Surg 79:990–997
Johns TG, Mackay IR, Callister KA, Hertzog PJ, Devenish RJ, Linnane AW (1992) Antiproliferative potencies of interferons on melanoma cell lines and xenografts: higher efficacy of interferon beta. J Natl Cancer Inst 84:1185–1190
Keilholz U, Scheibenbogen C, Tilgen W, Bergmann L, Weidmann E, Seither E, Richter M, Brado B, Mitrou PS, Hunstein W (1993) Interferon-alpha and interleukin-2 in the treatment of metastatic melanoma. Comparison of two phase II trials. Cancer 72:607–614
Kellokumpu-Lehtinen P, Nordman E, Toivanen A (1989) Combined interferon and vinblastine treatment of advanced melanoma: evaluation of the treatment results and the effects of treatment on immunological functions. Cancer Immunol Immunother 28:213–217
Kern P, Meigel W, Racz P, Gottesleben A, Dettke T, Dietrich M (1987) Interferon alpha in the treatment of AIDS-associated Kaposi's sarcoma. Onkologie 10:50–52
Kerr R, Pippen P, Mennel R, Jones S (1989) Treatment of metastatic malignant melanoma with a combination of interferon-alpha-2a (IFN-alpha-2a, Roferon) and dacarbazine (DTIC). Proc Annu Meet Am Soc Clin Oncol 8:A1122
Kohn EC, Steis RG, Sausville EA, Veach SR, Stocker JL, Phelps R, Franco S, Longo DL, Bunn PA, Ihde DC (1990) Phase II trial of intermittent high-dose recombinant interferon alfa-2a in mycosis fungoides and the Sezary syndrome. J Clin Oncol 8:155–160
Kovacs JA, Deyton L, Davey R, Falloon J, Zunich K, Lee D, Metcalf JA, Bigley JW, Sawyer LA, Zoon KC et al (1989) Combined zidovudine and interferon-alpha therapy in patients with Kaposi sarcoma and the acquired immunodeficiency syndrome (AIDS). Ann Intern Med 111:280–287
Krasagakis K, Garbe C, Kruger S, Orfanos CE (1991) Effects of interferons on cultured human melanocytes in vitro: interferon-beta but not-alpha or -gamma inhibit proliferation and all interferons significantly modulate the cell phenotype. J Invest Dermatol 97:364–372
Krigel RL, Odajnyk CM, Laubenstein LJ, Ostreicher R, Wernz J, Vilcek J, Pubinstein P, Friedman Kien AE (1985) Therapeutic trial of interferon-gamma in patients with epidemic Kaposi's sarcoma. J Biol Response Mod 4:358–364
Krigel RL, Padavic Shaller KA, Rudolph AR, Poiesz BJ, Comis RL (1989) Exacerbation of epidemic Kaposi's sarcoma with a combination of interleukin-2 and beta-interferon: results of a phase 2 study. J Biol Response Mod 8:359–365
Krown SE, Real FX, Cunningham Rundles S, Myskowski PL, Koziner B, Fein S, Mittelman A, Oettgen HF, Safai B (1983) Preliminary observations on the effect of recombinant leukocyte A interferon in homosexual men with Kaposi's sarcoma. N Engl J Med 308:1071–1076
Krown SE, Real FX, Vadhan Raj S, Cunningham Rundles S, Krim M, Wong G, Oettgen HF (1986) Kaposi's sarcoma and the acquired immune deficiency syndrome. Treatment with recombinant interferon alpha and analysis of prognostic factors. Cancer 57 [8 Suppl]:1662–1665

Krown SE, Gold JW, Niedzwiecki D, Bundow D, Flomenberg N, Gansbacher B, Brew BJ (1990) Interferon-alpha with zidovudine: safety, tolerance, and clinical and virologic effects in patients with Kaposi sarcoma associated with the acquired immunodeficiency syndrome (AIDS). Ann Intern Med 112:812–821

Kuzel TM, Gilyon K, Springer E, Variakojis D, Kaul K, Bunn PA Jr, Evans L, Roenigk HH Jr, Rosen ST (1990) Interferon alfa-2a combined with phototherapy in the treatment of cutaneous T-cell lymphoma. J Natl Cancer Inst 82:203–207

Kuzel TM, Roenigk HH Jr, Samuelson E, Rosen ST (1992) Suppression of anti-interferon alpha-2a antibody formation in patients with mycosis fungoides by exposure to long-wave UV radiation in the A range and methoxsalen ingestion. J Natl Cancer Inst 84:119–121

Landthaler M, Braun Falco O (1989) Adjuvant therapy of high-risk malignant melanoma patients with gamma interferon. J Am Acad Dermatol 20:687–688

Lane HC, Davey RT Jr, Sherwin SA, Masur H, Rook AH, Manischewitz JF, Quinnan GV, Smith PD, Easter ME, Fauci AS (1989) A phase I trial of recombinant human interferon-gamma in patients with Kaposi's sarcoma and the acquired immunodeficiency syndrome (AIDS). J Clin Immunol 9:351–361

Legha S, Plager C, Ring S, Eton O, Talpaz J, Gutterman J, Benjamin RS (1992) A phase II study of biochemotherapy using interleukin-2 (IL-2) + Interferon alfa-2a (IFN) in combination with cisplatin (C) vinblastine (V) and DTIC (D) in patients with metastatic melanoma. Proc Annu Meet Am Soc Clin Oncol 11:A1179

Lollini PL, De Giovanni C, Nicoletti G, Bontadini A, Tazzari PL, Landuzzi L, Scotlandi K, Nanni P (1990) Enhancement of experimental metastatic ability by tumor necrosis factor-alpha alone or in combination with interferon-gamma. Clin Exp Metastasis 8:215–224

Lutzner MA, Blanchet Bardon C, Orth G (1984) Clinical observations, virologic studies, and treatment trials in patients with epidermodysplasia verruciformis, a disease induced by specific human papillomaviruses. J Invest Dermatol 83: 18S–25S

Margolin K, Doroshow J, Akman S et al (1990) Treatment (RX) of advanced melanoma with cis-diamminedichloroplatinum (CDDP) and alpha interferon (alpha IFN). Proc Annu Meet Am Soc Clin Oncol 9:A1074

Meyskens FL Jr, Kopecky K, Samson M, Hersh E, Macdonald J, Jaffe H, Crowley J, Coltman C (1990) Recombinant human interferon gamma: adverse effects in high-risk stage I and II cutaneous malignant melanoma. J Natl Cancer Inst 82:1071

Miles SA, Wang HJ, Cortes E, Carden J, Marcus S, Mitsuyasu RT (1990) Beta-interferon therapy in patients with poor-prognosis Kaposi sarcoma related to the acquired immunodeficiency syndrome (AIDS). A phase II trial with preliminary evidence of antiviral activity and low incidence of opportunistic infections. Ann Intern Med 112:582–589

Mostow EN, Neckel SL, Oberhelman L, Anderson TF, Cooper KD (1993) Complete remissions in psoralen and UV-A (PUVA)-refractory mycosis fungoides-type cutaneous T-cell lymphoma with combined interferon alfa and PUVA. Arch Dermatol 129:747–752

Mozzanica N, Cattaneo A, Boneschi V, Brambilla L, Melotti E, Finzi AF (1990) Immunohistological evaluation of basal cell carcinoma immunoinfiltrate during intralesional treatment with alpha 2-interferon. Arch Dermatol Res 282:311–317

Mulder NH, Schraffordt-Koops H, Sleijfer DT et al (1990) Dacarbazine and alpha-interferon for disseminated malignant melanoma. Proc Annu Meet Am Soc Clin Oncol 9:A1083

Nicolas JF, Balblanc JC, Frappaz A, Chouvet B, Delcombel M, Thivolet J (1989) Treatment of cutaneous T cell lymphoma with intermediate doses of interferon alpha 2a. Dermatologica 179:34–37

Ogasawara M, Rosenberg SA (1993) Enhanced expression of HLA molecules and stimulation of autologous human tumor infiltrating lymphocytes following transduction of melanoma cells with gamma-interferon genes. Cancer Res 53: 3561–3568

Olsen EA, Rosen ST, Vollmer RT, Variakojis D, Roenigk HH Jr, Diab N, Zeffren J (1989) Interferon alfa-2a in the treatment of cutaneous T cell lymphoma. J Am Acad Dermatol 20:395–407

Oratz R, Dugan M, Walsh C et al (1989) Phase II trial of r-alpha 2b-interferon (IFN) and cisplatin (CDDP) in metastatic malignant melanoma (MM). Proc Annu Meet Am Soc Clin Oncol 8:A1123

Otte HG, Herges A, Stadler R (1992) Kombinationstherapie mit Interferon alfa 2a und PUVA bei kutanen T-Zell-Lymphomen. Hautarzt 43:695–699

Plettenberg A, Kern P, Dietrich M, Meigel W (1990) Rekombinantes Interferon alpha 2A in der Behandlung des HIV-assoziierten Kaposi-Sarkoms. Langzeitergebnisse. Med Klin 85:647–652

Pyrhonen S, Hahka Kemppinen M, Muhonen T (1992a) A promising interferon plus four-drug chemotherapy regimen for metastatic melanoma. J Clin Oncol 10: 1919–1926

Pyrhonen S, Kouri M, Holsti LR, Cantell K (1992b) Disease stabilization by leukocyte alpha interferon and survival of patients with metastatic melanoma. Oncology 49:22–26

Real FX, Oettgen HF, Krown SE (1986) Kaposi's sarcoma and the acquired immunodeficiency syndrome: treatment with high and low doses of recombinant leukocyte A interferon. J Clin Oncol 4:544–551

Richards J, Mehta N, Schroeder L, Dordal A (1992a) Sequential chemotherapy/ immunotherapy for metastatic melanoma. Proc Annu Meet Am Soc Clin Oncol 11:A1189

Richards JM, Mehta N, Ramming K, Skosey P (1992b) Sequential chemoimmunotherapy in the treatment of metastatic melanoma. J Clin Oncol 10:1338–1343

Richner J, Cerny T, Joss RA et al (1990) A phase II study of continuous sc alpha-2b interferon (IFN) combined with cisplatin (CDDP) in advanced malignant melanoma (MM). Proc Annu Meet Am Soc Clin Oncol 9:A1085

Rios A, Mansell PW, Newell GR, Reuben JM, Hersh EM, Gutterman JU (1985) Treatment of acquired immunodeficiency syndrome-related Kaposi's sarcoma with lymphoblastoid interferon. J Clin Oncol 3:506–512

Roenigk HH Jr, Kuzel TM, Skoutelis AP, Springer E, Yu G, Caro W, Gilyon K, Variakojis D, Kaul K, Bunn PA Jr et al (1990) Photochemotherapy alone or combined with interferon alpha-2a in the treatment of cutaneous T-cell lymphoma. J Invest Dermatol 95 [Suppl 6]:198S–205S

Ron IG, Inbar MJ, Gutman M, Merimsky O, Chaitchik S (1993) Recombinant interferon alpha-2a in combination with dacarbazine in the treatment of metastatic malignant melanoma: analysis of long-term responding patients. Cancer Immunol Immunother 37:61–66

Rosenberg SA, Lotze MT, Muul LM, Leitman S, Chang AE, Ettinghausen SE, Matory YL, Skibber JM, Shiloni E, Vetto JT, Seipp CA, Simpson C, Reichert CM (1985) Observations on the systemic administration of autologous lymphokine activated killer cells and recombinant interleukin-2 to patients with metastatic cancer. N Engl J Med 313:1485–1492

Rosenberg SA (1992) Gene therapy for cancer. JAMA 268:2416–2419

Rosenberg SA, Lotze MT, Yang JC, Aebersold PM, Linehan WM, Seipp CA, White DE (1989a) Experience with the use of high dose interleukin-2 in the treatment of 652 cancer patients. Ann Surg 210:474–485

Rosenberg SA, Lotze MT, Yang JC, Linehan WM, Seipp C, Calabro S, Karp SE, Sherry RM, Steinberg S, White DE (1989b) Combination therapy with interleukin-

2 and alpha-interferon for the treatment of patients with advanced cancer. J Clin Oncol 7:1863–1874
Ross C, Tingsgaard P, Jorgensen H, Vejlsgaard GL (1993) Interferon treatment of cutaneous T-cell lymphoma. Eur J Haematol 51:63–72
Rozenbaum W, Gharakhanian S, Navarette MS, De Sahb R, Cardon B, Rouzioux C (1990) Long-term follow-up of 120 patients with AIDS-related Kaposi's sarcoma treated with interferon alpha-2a. J Invest Dermatol 95 [Suppl 6]:161S–165S
Sawyer LA, Metcalf JA, Zoon KC, Boone EJ, Kovacs JA, Lane HC, Quinnan GV Jr (1990) Effects of interferon-alpha in patients with AIDS-associated Kaposi's sarcoma are related to blood interferon levels and dosse. Cytokine 2:247–252
Scadden DT, Bering HA, Levine JD, Bresnahan J, Evans L, Epstein C, Groopman JE (1991a) GM-CSF as an alternative to dose modification of the combination zidovudine and interferon-alpha in the treatment of AIDS-associated Kaposi's sarcoma. Am J Clin Oncol 14 [Suppl 1]:S40–44
Scadden DT, Bering HA, Levine JD, Bresnahan J, Evans L, Epstein C, Groopman JE (1991b) Granulocyte-macrophage colony-stimulating factor mitigates the neutropenia of combined interferon alfa and zidovudine treatment of acquired immune deficiency syndrome-associated Kaposi's sarcoma. J Clin Oncol 9:802–808
Schaart FM, Bratzke B, Ruszczak Z, Stadler R, Ehlers G, Orfanos CE (1991) Long-term therapy of HIV-associated Kaposi's sarcoma with recombinant interferon alpha-2a. Br J Dermatol 124:62–68
Schröder K, Garbe C, Waibel M, Reupke H, Detmar M, Dallenbach F, Orfanos CE (1992) Granulozyten-Koloniestimulierender Faktor (G-CSF) in der Behandlung von Patienten mit HIV-assoziiertem mukokutanem Kaposi-Sarkom. Erfolgreicher Einsatz bei virus- bzw. medikamenteninduzierter Leukopenie. Hautarzt 43: 700–706
Schuchter L, McGuire WP, Wohlganger J, Redden T (1989) Sequential treatment of metastatic melanoma with interferon-alpha (IFN) plus cis-platinum (CDDP). Proc Annu Meet Am Soc Clin Oncol 8:A1120
Sertoli MR, Queirolo P, Bajetta E et al (1992) Dacarbazine (DTIC) with or without recombinant interferon alpha-2a at different dosages in the treatment of stage IV melanoma patients. Preliminary results of a randomized trial. Proc Annu Meet Am Soc Clin Oncol 11:A1185
Simoni R, Cavalieri R, Coppola G, Ricciotti L, De Pita O, Criscuolo D, Covelli A, Papa G, Mandelli F (1987) Recombinant leukocyte interferon alfa-2a in the treatment of mycosis fungoides. J Biol Regul Homeost Agents 1:93–99
Smith KA, Green JA, Eccles JM (1992) Interferon alpha 2a and vindesine in the treatment of advanced malignant melanoma. Eur J Cancer 28:438–441
Springer EA, Kuzel TM, Variakojis D, Kaul K, Rosen ST, Roenigk HH Jr (1993) Correlation of clinical responses with immunologic and morphologic characteristics in patients with cutaneous T-cell lymphoma treated with interferon alfa-2a. J Am Acad Dermatol 29:42–46
Stadler R, Garbe C (1991) Disseminated malignant melanoma. New therapeutic approaches. Int J Dermatol 30:239–242
Stadler R, Bratzke B, Schaart F, Orfanos CE (1990) Long-term combined rIFN-alpha-2a and zidovudine therapy for HIV-associated Kaposi's sarcoma: clinical consequences and side effects. J Invest Dermatol 95 [Suppl 6]:170S–175S
Tank B, Habets JM, Naafs B, Damsma O, Stolz E, van Joost T (1989) Intralesional treatment of basal cell carcinoma with low-dose recombinant interferon gamma. J Am Acad Dermatol 21:734–735
Thestrup Pedersen K, Hammer R, Kaltoft K, Sogaard H, Zachariae H (1988) Treatment of mycosis fungoides with recombinant interferon-alpha 2a2 alone and in combination with etretinate. Br J Dermatol 118:811–818

Thomson D, Adena M, McLeod GRC et al (1992) Interferon-2a (IFN) does not improve response or survival when added to dacarbazine (DTIC) in metastatic melanoma: results of a multi-institutional Australian randomized trial QMP8704. Proc Annu Meet Am Soc Clin Oncol 11:A1177

Tura S, Mazza P, Zinzani PL, Ghetti PL, Poletti G, Gherlinzoni F, Montagnani A, Criscuolo D (1987) Alpha recombinant interferon in the treatment of mycosis fungoides (MF). Haematologica 72:337–340

Vegna ML, Papa G, Defazio D, Pisani F, Coppola G, De Pita O, Puddu P, Ferranti G, Simoni R, Mandelli F (1990) Interferon alpha-2a in cutaneous T-cell lymphoma. Eur J Haematol Suppl 52:32–35

Volberding P, Valero R, Rothman J, Gee G (1984) Alpha interferon therapy of Kaposi's sarcoma in AIDS. Ann NY Acad Sci 437:439–446

Volberding PA, Mitsuyasu RT, Golando JP, Spiegel RJ (1987) Treatment of Kaposi's sarcoma with interferon alfa-2b (Intron A). Cancer 59 [Suppl 3]:620–625

Von Wussow P, Block B, Hartmann F, Deicher H (1988) Intralesional interferon-alpha therapy in advanced malignant melanoma. Cancer 61:1071–1074

Wadler S (1992) The role of interferons in the treatment of solid tumors. Cancer 70 [Suppl 4]:949–958

Whitehead RP, Figlin R, Citron ML, Pfile J, Moldawer N, Patel D, Jones G, Levitt D, Zeffren J (1993) A phase II trial of concomitant human interleukin-2 and interferon-alpha-2a in patients with disseminated malignant melanoma. J Immunother 13:117–121

Wickramasinghe L, Hindson TC, Wacks H (1989) Treatment of neoplastic skin lesions with intralesional interferon. J Am Acad Dermatol 20:71–74

Zachariae H, Thestrup Pedersen K (1990) Interferon alpha and etretinate combination treatment of cutaneous T-cell lymphoma. J Invest Dermatol 95 [Suppl 6]:206S–208S

Biochemical Modulation of Cytotoxic Drugs by Cytokines: Molecular Mechanisms in Experimental Oncology

E.D. Kreuser[1], S. Wadler[2], and E. Thiel[2]

[1] Department of Hematology and Oncology, Klinikum Steglitz, Free University of Berlin, Hindenburgdamn 30, 12200 Berlin, Germany
[2] Department of Oncology, Albert Einstein College of Medicine, Montefiore Medical Center, Bronx, New York, USA

Abstract

The combination of cytokines and cytotoxic drugs offers a new approach to increase the therapeutic index in the treatment of neoplastic diseases. There is no consensus on optimal strategies for combining these agents so far. The molecular mechanisms underlying the interaction, however, should be defined in order to design clinical trials based on preclinical rationales. The broad spectrum of cytotoxic drugs whose activity can be enhanced by cytokines argues for multiple levels of drug interaction in vitro: alteration in the cellular drug uptake, modulation of drug target enzymes, and changes in metabolism or disposition of a drug. In vivo interaction between cytokines and cytotoxic agents involves an additional layer of complexity because of the effects of cytokines on the host immune system and on drug-metabolizing enzymes. A major mechanism involved in the synergistic interaction of interferon (IFN) and 5-fluorouracil (5-FU) seems to be the increase of active 5-FU metabolites by IFN. Moreover, IFN can reverse resistance against 5-FU by inhibiting the overexpression of thymidylate synthase. The absence of cytokinetic effects of IFN and FU argues against the recruitment of G_s cells into the cell cycle. Topoisomerase has emerged as a critical intracelluar target of cytotoxic drugs. There is convincing evidence that the synergy between tumor necrosis factor (TNF) and topoisomerase-targeted intercalative (Adriamycin, doxorubicin hydrochloride; m-AMSA, amsacrine; mitoxantrone) and nonintercalative (VM-16, etoposide; VM-26, teniposide) drugs is related to a rapid increase in specific activity of topoisomerase I and II, resulting in enhanced DNA strand breaks and cleavage complex. Furthermore, sensitivity to topoisomerase II targeted drugs can be enhanced by granulocyte colony-stimulating factor (G-CSF) through elevated enzyme activity in tumor cell response to G-CSF. The synergistic interaction between cytokines and cytotoxic agents seems to be sequence dependent. It has recently been demonstrated that newly synthesized metal compounds

Recent Results in Cancer Research, Vol. 139

and IFN are synergistic only after preincubation with cytokines. Cytokines can modulate expression of adhesion receptors on tumor cell lines, thereby influencing their metastatic potential. A considerable number of phase II trials with combination of cytokines and cytotoxic drugs based on these mechanisms have demonstrated promising response rates and tolerable toxicity. Phase III trials are currently in progress to identify enhanced activity combining cytokines and cytotoxic drugs in the treatment of malignancies.

Immunotherapeutic Strategies

In order to improve the therapeutic index, recent strategies in the treatment of malignant tumors have focused on new analogues, various schedules, dose intensification, immunotherapy, and biotherapy as well as biochemical and biologic modulation. Combining cytokines and cytotoxic drugs is the newest approach to increase the therapeutic index (Table 1).

Immunotherapy can be divided into two overlapping categories: active and passive. The goal of active immunotherapy is the stimulation of host

Table 1. Immunotherapeutic strategies with and without cytotoxic drugs in the treatment of neoplasms

Active specific immunotherapy (ASI)
Autologous vaccines
Allogeneic vaccines
ASI and cytotoxic drugs
Passive immunotherapy
Monoclonal antibodies (MAb)
Hybrids
Fragments
Anti-idiotype
Conjugates
Immunotoxins
Radiopharmaceuticals
Cytotoxics
Cytokines
Interferons
Interleukins
Tumor necrosis factor (TNF)
Adoptive immunotherapy
Biological modulation (chemoimmunotherapy)
Cytokine drug/interferon
Cytokine drug/interleukin
Cytokine drug/levamisole
Cytokine drug/TNF
Cytokine drug/growth factors

Modified from Wadler et al. (1991).

antitumor immunity, either cellular or humoral. This can be accomplished in a direct or specific fashion by using tumor vaccines to generate an immune response to tumor-associated antigens (Table 1; Foon 1989). The concept of active, specific immunotherapy (ASI)–using tumor-associated antigens as targets–dates back to the 1960s, when data from animal models demonstrated that specific immunostimulation with killed tumor cells could delay the growth of isogeneic tumors. The rationale for ASI was based on the premise that immunization with unique proteins on the tumor cell surface will elicit a host immune response that results in cytotoxicity for the tumor cells, but spares normal host tissue (Hanna et al. 1991).

Passive immunotherapy relies on the administration of biologically active agents with innate antitumor properties, such as reactivity to monoclonal antibodies and conjugates. In addition, some agents can exert antitumor effects via active and passive mechanisms (Foon 1989).

Nonspecific antitumor immunity can be propagated by immunomodulating compounds such as bacille Calmette-Guérin (BCG), thymosin, and levamisole with or without chemotherapy (Table 1). During the past decade renewed interest in immunotherapy has been stimulated by genetic engineering. This has made highly purified molecules available, including interferons (IFN), interleukins (IL), tumor necrosis factor (TNF), and nonhematopoietic and hematopoietic growth factors (Table 1). Therefore, the term biotherapy encompasses the therapeutic use of any biological substance, but more specifically it connotes the use of products of the mammalian genome. With modern techniques of genetic engineering, the mammalian genome represents the new "medicine cabinet" with cloned and well-defined cytokines (Oldham 1991).

Cytokines work through diverse mechanisms in the biotherapy of cancer. They may: (a) augment the host's defenses through the administration of cells or cytokines, as effectors or mediators of antitumor response; (b) increase the individual's antitumor responses through augmentation or restoration of effector mechanisms; (c) augment the individual's response, using modified tumor cells or vaccines to stimulate a greater response or increase tumor cell sensitivity to an existing biologic response; (d) decrease transformation and/or increase differentiation or maturation of tumor cells; (e) interfere with growth-promoting factors produced by tumor cells; (f) decrease or arrest the tendency of tumor cells to metastasize to other sites; (g) increase the ability of the patient to tolerate damage by cytotoxic drugs; and (h) increase the use of biologic molecules to target and bind to cancer cells, thus increasing antitumor activity of cytotoxic drugs (Oldham 1991).

Among biologic response modifiers, IL-2 is distinguished by its unique capacity to generate a class of tumoricidal lymphocytes, lymphokine-activated killer (LAK) cells. Interest in the potential value of LAK cells in the treatment of human cancers was sparked by the observation that IL-2 and LAK cells can cause objective responses and occasionally complete remissions of advanced cancers (van Haelst-Pisani et al. 1989). The clinical value of adoptive immunotherapy remains unclear, but the IL-2/LAK phenomenon has stimulated basic, clinical, and interdisciplinary research. It seems reasonable to expect that a conseqence of these investigations will be the development of a viable anticancer therapy that relies on augmentation of immune responses already present in the host (van Haelst-Pisani et al. 1989).

Immunotherapeutic Strategies Combined with Cytotoxic Drugs

Since chemotherapy and immunotherapy have reached a plateau in a substantial number of malignant tumors, modulatory strategies which combine both modalities have been developed, partially based on preclinical knowledge of their mechanisms (Tables 2, 3).

Table 2. Modulatory strategies in the treatment of malignant tumors

Biochemical modulators	Biological modulators
Folinic acid	Interferon
Hydroxyurea	Tumor necrosis factor
Dipyridamole	Interleukin
Allopurinol	Growth factors
N-(Phosphonacety)-L-aspartate	Levamisole
Methotrexate	Cyclosporine
Thymidine	
Uridine	
Cisplatin	

Table 3. Cytotoxic drug–cytokine interactions: levels of mechanisms

Tumor cells	Host cells
Cellular modulation	Immunomodulation
Topoisomerase	Natural killer cells
Thymidylate synthese	Monocytes
Thymidine kinase	Macrophages
Pyrimidine phosphorylase	Cytotoxic T lymphocytes
DNA	Pharmacologic modulation
Gene expression	Liver cells
Receptors	
Adhesion receptors	
Growth factor receptors	
Cytokine receptors	
Cell cycle phase	
G_0/G_1 arrest	
G_0/G_1 recruitment	
Effects on tumor cell vasculature	

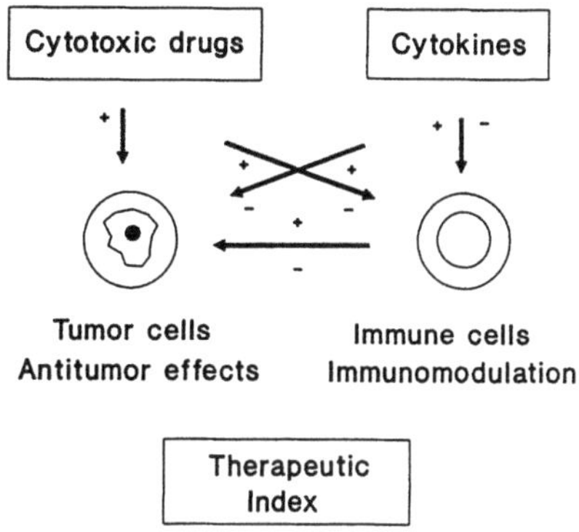

Fig. 1. Interaction of cytokines and cytotoxic drugs

Biochemical modulation refers to the administration of a modulator to manipulate the metabolic pathway of a cytotoxic drug in order to increase cytotoxicity (Martin et al. 1985). Biochemical modulation results from alteration in the cellular uptake, metabolism, or disposition of a drug or its essential cofactors by modulators (Table 2). In contrast, biologic modulation encompasses biochemical modulation, but in addition includes alteration in the host physiology, including immunologic responsiveness, vascularization, or blood flow protective effects on normal host tissue, modulation of receptors, and genomic effects (Table 2). The concept of combining cytokines and cytotoxic drugs to enhance antiproliferative activity is complex (Fig. 1; Table 3). There is convincing evidence of multiple levels of interaction between cytokines and cytotoxic drugs, including a direct modulation of target enzymes of drug metabolism, a modulation of receptors, modulation of cell cycle phases, and modulation of gene expression thereby altering the sensitivity of cytotoxic drugs (Table 3). However, it has clearly been demonstrated in preclinical models that cytokines can act in an indirect pathway in order to enhance the antitumor activity involving the host immune cells (Fig. 1).

Mechanisms of Interactions Between Interferon and Cytotoxic Drugs

IFN constitute one class of biologic modulators that appear capable of circumventing resistance to fluoropyrimidines (Chu et al. 1990; Wadler and Schwartz 1990; Elias and Crissman 1988). Recently, some mechanisms of interaction of 5-fluorouracil (5-FU) and IFN have been elucidated. Preclinical data demonstrated synergy for the combination of 5-FU and IFN (Chu et al. 1990). Several investigators have noted an induction of intratumoral levels of thymidylate synthase within 24 h of 5-FU exposure (Chu et al. 1990; Wadler and Schwartz 1990). Chu et al. (1990) have shown that IFN-γ

can eliminate the acute induction of thymidylate synthase associated with 5-FU exposure, thereby rendering colon cancer cells more sensitive to 5-FU. These investigators demonstrated that the intracellular levels of thymidylate synthase are controlled at a post-transcriptional locus by the efficacy of mRNA translation (Chu et al. 1991). The efficacy of thymidylate synthase mRNA translation appears to be regulated in an autoregulatory fashion by binding of the thymidylate synthase protein product to its own mRNA. Recent evidence suggests that IFN-α can increase levels of active metabolite fluorodeoxyuridylate tenfold, resulting in more thorough inhibition of its target enzyme thymidylate synthase (Elias and Crissman 1988). IFN has also been shown to inhibit thymidine uptake and thymidine kinase activity, thus reducing the salvage pathway of DNA synthesis (Pfeffer and Tamm 1984).

Morever, it has been recently demonstrated that IFN can alter the pharmacokinetics of 5-FU. The administration of IFN-α_{2a} was associated with a dose-dependent decrease in 5-FU clearance. Therefore, the increase in the area under the 5-FU concentration–time curve (AUC) was 1.3-fold and 1.5-fold in patients receiving a higher dose of IFN-α_{2a} (Grem et al. 1991).

The most important putative mechanisms of IFN and FU interactions are as follows:

1. Reduced activity of thymidylate synthase
2. Increased formation of FdUMP
3. Decreased uptake of thymidine to prevent salvage pathway
4. Increase in the area under the 5-FU concentration time curve (AUC)

FdUMP, fluorodeoxyuridine monophosphate

Mechanisms of Interactions Between Tumor Necrosis Factor and Cytotoxic Drugs

Topoisomerase I and II are enzymes that regulate the topological configuration of the DNA (for review, see Wang 1987). Topoisomerase II is an adenosine triphosphate (ATP)-dependent enzyme which catalyzes the breakage and reunion of the duplex DNA, allowing a second segment of DNA to pass through the break site and subsequently change the linking number of covalently closed circular DNA in steps of two (Liu et al. 1980). The activity and amount of the enzyme fluctuates with cell cycle progression; peak activity and maximum content occur during the G_2/M phase (Heck et al. 1988). Topoisomerases have emerged as a critical target of cytotoxic drugs. An increase in cytotoxicity, when actinomycin D was added to lymphotoxin–a cytolytic lymphokine with striking similarity to TNF–was first reported by Eifel et al. (1975). Ostrove and Gifford (1979) noted an increase in [^{3}H]uridine uptake in L929 cells treated with TNF and suggested that the increase in cell killing they noted when TNF and actinomycin D were combined was due to the inhibition of RNA synthesis by the drug. Actinomycin D, besides inhibiting RNA synthesis, has recently been found to interfere with the function of DNA topoisomerase II.

Mammalian topoisomerase II is a common target for a number of intercalative (Adriamycin, doxorubicin hydrochloride; m-AMSA, amsacrine; ellipticine; mitoxantrone) and nonintercalative (VP-16, etoposide; VM-26, teniposide) drugs (Tewey et al. 1984). During the breakage–reunion reaction, topoisomerase II can form a cleavable complex with DNA. These drugs then interfere with the breakage–reunion reaction of topoisomerase II by stabilizing this cleavable complex (De Jong et al. 1990). The formation of the cleavable complex rather than the inhibition of the topoisomerase activity accounts for the cytotoxicity of these drugs (Chen et al. 1984). In addition to the reduced Adriamycin accumulation, part of the resistance in a Adriamycin-resistant human small cell lung carcinoma cell line could be explained by an altered Adriamycin–DNA–topoisomerase II interaction (De Jong et al. 1990).

Recently, it has been shown that rhTNF significantly enhances the cytotoxicity of DNA-targeted cytotoxic drugs in vitro, including Adriamycin, actinomycin, m-AMSA, VM-26, and VP-16, all targeted at DNA topoisomerase II. In contrast, rhTNF had a minimal enhancing effect on the antiproliferative activity of bleomycin, hydroxyurea, and cytosine arabinoside (Ara-C), and no effect on cisplatin, mitomycin, vincristine, and vinblastine, all drugs with dose-related cytotoxic effects on fibrosarcoma cell lines but mechanisms of action which do not appear to involve topoisomerase II (Alexander et al. 1987). Data suggest that the effect is related to the topisomerase-mediated DNA damage caused by these drugs:

1. Topoisomerase I and II are enzymes that regulate the topical configuration of DNA.
2. Topoisomerase II is an ATP-dependent enzyme which catalyzes the breakage and reunion of duplex DNA.
3. Topoisomerase II is a common target for intercalative (doxorubicin, m-AMSA) and nonintercalative drugs (VP-16, VM-26).
4. Topoisomerase II can form a cleavable complex with DNA.
5. Drugs can interfere with the cleavable complex and inhibit DNA synthesis.
6. Adriamycin resistance is associated with low topoisomerase II expression or point mutation.

In combining cytokines and cytotoxic drugs, sequence appears crucial for synergistic antiproliferative interactions (Kreuser et al. 1991, 1992). Hence, pretreatment with rhTNF does not to appear to render tumor cells more vulnerable to subsequent killing by topoisomerase-targeted drugs, but coincident or subsequent treatment with rhTNF augments drug-mediated killing (Alexander et al. 1987). The data may be relevant to the planning of future animal and human trials using rhTNF and topoisomerase-targeted drugs for the treatment of cancer.

Mechanisms of Interactions Between Hematopoietic Growth Factors and Cytotoxic Drugs

Recently, the effects of rhG-CSF on DNA topoisomerase II expression were studied in acute myelogenous leukemia cell lines, which express G-CSF receptors and proliferate in response to exogenous G-CSF (Towatari et al. 1990). G-CSF-stimulated cells demonstrated a significantly increased sensitivity to intercalating and nonintercalating topoisomerase II-targeting drugs, whereas no enhancement of cytotoxicity was observed with alkylating agents (Towatari et al. 1990). The augmented drug sensitivity observed was not due to the increased level of drug transport. Decreased topoisomerase II activity in tumor cells may be expected to induce drug resistance. Therefore, agents that elevate the topoisomerase II activity of tumor cells would be expected as putative modulating agents. Drug sensitivity of G-CSF-treated myeloid leukemia cells is specifically increased against daunorubicin and etoposide, in parallel with the increment of topoisomerase II levels (Kreuser et al. 1992; Towatari et al. 1990). These findings point the way for future clinical trials using G-CSF prior to topoisomerase II inhibitors.

Acute leukemia is a malignant process, characterized by the unrestricted growth and maturational arrest of lymphoid or myeloid precursor cells. Because the proliferation of normal cells of hematopoietic origin is controlled by growth factors, it has been suggested that leukemias may arise by dysregulation of these pathways. Previous studies have shown that autocrine circuits are not involved in the proliferation of acute lymphoblastic leukemia cells in vitro, but that IL-1 and GM-CSF are involved in the proliferation of acute myelogenous leukemia cells (Cohen et al. 1991). Conversely, some cytokines may inhibit the growth of hematopoietic and leukemic cells. GM-CSF, for example, is a growth promotor of acute myeloblastic leukemia colony-forming units (AML-CFU) from patients with AML (Griffin et al. 1989). Recently, Miyauchi et al. (1988, 1989) proposed that blasts in AML are a renewal population maintained by a small subpopulation of stem cells. The balance between self-renewal and differentation in blast stem cells may be an important attribute contributing to treatment outcome.

Ara-C is included in most chemotherapeutic regimens for the treatment of AML. Highly significant changes were seen in the Ara-C survival curves, depending on the growth factors present in the cultures (Miyauchi et al. 1988). Recent in vitro studies have shown that rhGM-CSF triggers the AML blasts to enter the G_1 and S phases of the cell cycle, thereby rendering them more susceptible for subsequent kill by cell cycle-specific drugs (Bhalla et al. 1988; Cannistra et al. 1989). Based on these preclinical data, clinical phase I/II trials were initiated using rhGM-CSF in patients with AML. In vivo recruitment of AML blast cells from G_0 phase into the chemotherapy-sensitive G_1 and S phase was demonstrated in all patients tested following treatment with rhGM-CSF (Bettelheim et al. 1991).

It has been shown that GM-CSF and IL-3 were most effective in increasing the S phase fraction and thereby enhancing the Ara-C-mediated cell kill. In contrast, G-CSF that decreases the G_0 fraction without influencing the percentage of S phase cells does not lead to a significantly increased cell kill by Ara-C (Brach et al. 1990, 1991).

Pretreatment with GM-CSF and IL-3 enhanced the cytotoxic effects of subsequently applied Ara-C approximately tenfold (Hiddemann et al. 1991). Corresponding to these data, a higher fraction of S phase was found after 48-h exposure to GM-CSF and IL-3 and increased incorporation of H-Ara-C into the DNA of leukemic blasts.

Remarkably, intracellular Ara-C-5′triphosphate (Ara-C-TP) formation was not correspondingly enhanced, resulting in a higher Ara-C to Ara-C-TP ratio compared to controls. These results suggest that GM-CSF and IL-3 may not only increase, but also speed up intracellular Ara-C metabolism and phosphorylation (Hiddemann et al. 1991).

In summary, these preclinical data suggest that some molecular mechanisms that lead to synergistic cytotoxicity of hematopoietic growth factors and Ara-C have now been elucidated. Moreover, based on these in vitro data several phase I/II trials were conducted using G(M)-CSF and standard chemotherapy, which demonstrated promising response rates (Hiddemann et al. 1991).

The potential mechanisms of interactions between hematopoietic growth factors and cytotoxic drugs may be summarized as follows:

1. Recruitment of kinetically quiescent AML blasts into the cell cycle by G-CSF and IL-3 render them more susceptible to cytotoxic drugs.
2. GM-CSF and IL-3 enhance the intracellular metabolism of Ara-C and its incorporation into the DNA of leukemic blasts, inducing higher antileukemic activity.
3. Hematopoietic growth factors synergize with inhibitors of DNA synthesis, inducing a more mature phenotype at low doses or enhancing leukemia cell kill at high doses.

Mechanisms of Interactions Between Interleukin and Cytotoxic Drugs

IL-1 is a cytokine with a wide range of biologic properties. Antitumor effects have been demonstrated by various administration routes and in different tumor types (Nakamura et al. 1991). To investigage the combination effects of rhIL-1α and various cytotoxic drugs, mice bearing syngeneic tumors were treated with cytotoxic drugs in combination with rhIL-1α. It was demonstrated that with cisplatin or carboplatin and rhIL-α, a considerable number of animals were completely cured; this was never achieved by the cytotoxic drugs alone (Nakamura et al. 1991). Cytotoxic drugs are considered to be cytotoxic through their direct action against the tumor cells.

On the other hand, IL-1 is a cytokine with multiple antitumor mechanisms, i.e., the enhancement of cytotoxic activities of monocytes, natural killer cells, cytotoxic T lymphocytes, the production of lymphokines such as IL-2 and IFN-τ, which have been demonstrated to have antitumor activites, and the direct cytotoxic action against tumor cells (for review see Nakamura et al. 1991). Therefore, combination therapy with IL-1 and antitumor drugs may be beneficial from both therapeutic and toxological viewpoints to increase the therapeutic index.

Chemoresistant tumor cells may be more susceptible to lysis by activated lymphocytes than chemosensitive counterparts. It has recently been shown that lysability in the doxorubicin-resistant colon carcinoma subline by LAK cells was higher than in the doxorubicin-sensitive cell line (Rivoltini et al. 1990). Any significant role of the multidrug resistance-associated (MDR) glycoprotein (P170) in the susceptibility of colon cancer cells to LAK cells could be excluded. However, LAL susceptibility of human colon cancer cells was dependent on the expression of adhesion molecules and differentiation (Rivoltini et al. 1990). Moreover, it has been shown recently that treating leukemia blasts with cytotoxic drugs significantly augments their LAK susceptibility (Teichmann et al. 1991). These results support a putative benefit of combining cytotoxic drugs and IFN in the treatment of leukemia.

In conclusion, these preclinical data support the concept of combining cytokines and cytotoxic drugs to enhance synergistically their antiproliferative activity. Based on these rationales, clinical trials are in progress to substantiate whether these promising results of basic research can be translated into clinical benefit in the treatment of malignancies.

Acknowledgment. We would like to thank Gabriele Warner for her excellent editorial assistance.

References

Alexander RB, Nelson WG, Coffey DS (1987) Synergistic enhancement by tumor necrosis factor of in vitro cytotoxicity from chemotherapeutic drugs targeted at DNA topoisomerase II. Cancer Res 47:2403–2406

Bettelheim P, Valent P, Andreeff M et al (1991) Recombinant human granulocyte-macrophage colony-stimulating factor in combination with standard induction chemotherapy in de novo acute myeloid leukemia. Blood 77:700–711

Bhalla K, Birkhofer M, Arlin Z et al (1988) Effect of recombinant GM-CSF on the metabolism of cytosine-arabinoside in normal and leukemic human bone marrow cells. Leukemia 2:2810–2814

Brach MA, Riedel D, Mertelsmann RH et al (1990) Synergistic effect of rebombinant human leukemia inhibitory factor (LIF) and 1-β-D arabinofuranosylcytosine (Ara-C) on proto-oncogene expression and induction of differentiation in human U 937 cells. Leukemia 4:646–649

Brach MA, Mertelsmann RH, Herrmann F (1991) Hematopoietins in combination with 1-β-D arabinofuranosylcytosine: a possible strategy for improved treatment of myeloid disorders. Semin Oncol 18 [Suppl J]:16–20

Cannistra SA, Groshek P, Griffin JD (1989) Granulocyte-macrophage colony-stimulating factor enhances the cytotoxic effects of cytosine arabinoside in acute myeloblastic leukemia and in the myeloid blast crisis phase of chronic myeloid leukemia. Leukemia 3:328–334
Chen GL, Yang L, Rowe TC et al (1984) Nonintercalative antitumor drugs interfere with the breakage-reunion reaction of mammalian DNA topoisomerase II. J Biol Chem 259:13560–13566
Chu E, Zinn S, Boarman D et al (1990) The interactions of gamma interferon and 5-fluorouracil in the H630 human colon carcinoma cell line. Cancer Res 50: 5834–5840
Chu E, Koeller DM, Casey JL et al (1991) Autoregulation of human thymidylate synthase messenger RNA translation by thymidylate synthase. Proc Natl Acad Sci USA 88:8977–8981
Cohen A, Grunberger T, Vanek W et al (1991) Constitutive expression and role in growth regulation of interleukin-1 and multiple cytokine receptors in a biphenotypic leukemic cell line. Blood 78:94–102
De Jong S, Zijlstra JG, de Vries EGE et al (1990) Reduced DNA topoisomerase II activity and drug-induced DNA cleavage activity in an Adriamycin-resistant human small cell lung carcinoma cell line. Cancer Res 50:304–309
Eifel PJ, Walker SM, Lucas ZJ (1975) Standardization of a sensitive and rapid assay for lymphotoxin. Cell Immunol 15:208–221
Elias L, Crissman HA (1988) Interferon effects upon the adenocarcinoma 38 and HL-60 cell lines: antiprolifeartie responses and synergistic interactions with halogenated pyrimidine antimetabolites. Cancer Res 48:4868–4873
Foon KA (1989) Biological response modifiers: the new immunotherapy. Cancer Res 49:1621–1639
Grem JL, McAtee N, Murphy RF et al (1991) A pilot study of interferon α-2a in combination with fluorouracil plus high-dose leucovorin in metastatic gastrointestinal carcinoma. J Clin Oncol 9:1811–1820
Griffin JD, Herrmann, YF, Wiper D et al (1989) Effects of recombinant human GM-CSF on proliferation of clonogenic cells in acute myeloblastic leukemia. Blood 67:1448–1453
Hanna MG, Peters LC, Haspel MV et al (1991) Fundamental and applied aspects of successful active specific immunotherapy of cancer. In: Oldham RK (ed) Principles of cancer biotherapy. Dekker, New York, p 253
Heck MMS, Hittelman WN, Earnshaw WC (1988) Differential expression of DNA topoisomerase I and II during the eukaryotic cell cycle. Proc Natl Acad Sci USA 85:1086–1090
Hiddemann W, Kiehl M, Zühlsdorf M et al (1991) Granulocyte-macrophage colony-stimulating factor and interleukin-3 enhance the incorporation of cytosine arabinoside into the DNA of leukemic blasts and the cytotoxic effect on clonogenic cells from patients with acute myeloid leukemia. Semin Oncol 18 [Suppl J]:21–24
Kreuser ED, Keppler BK, Berdel WE et al (1991) Synergistic antitumor interactions between newly synthesized ruthenium complexes and cytokines in human colon carcinoma cell lines. Semin Oncol 18:73–81
Kreuser ED, Schröder JK, Kintzel C et al (1994) Cytokine-mediated VLA modulation can influence the adhesion of human colon cancer cells to extracellular matrix proteins. Eicosanoid 4:16
Liu LF, Liu CC, Alberts BM (1980) Type II DNA topoisomerases: enzymes that can unknot a topologically knotted DNA molecule via a reversible double-strand break. Cell 19:697–707
Martin DS, Stolfi RL, Sawyer RC et al (1985) Application of biochemical modulation with a therapeutically inactive modulating agent in clinical trials of cancer chemotherapy. Cancer Treat Rep 69:421–423

Miyauchi J, Wang C, Kelleher CA et al (1988) The effects of recombinant CSF-1 on the blast cels of acute myeloblastic leukemia in supension culture. J Cell Physiol 135:55–62

Miyauchi J, Kelleher CA, Wang C et al (1989) Growth factors influence the sensitivity of leukemic stem cells to cytosine arabinoside in culture. Blood 73: 1272–1278

Nakamura S, Kashimoto S, Kajikawa F et al (1991) Combination effect of recombinant human inerleukin 1 α with antitumor drugs on syngeneic tumors in mice. Cancer Res 51:215–221

Oldham RK (1991) Cancer biotherapy: general principles. In: Oldham RK (ed) Principles of cancer biotherapy. Dekker, New York, pp 1–21

Ostrove JM, Gifford GE (1979) Stimulation of RNA synthesis in L929 cells by rabbit tumor necrosis factor. Proc Soc Exp Biol Med 160:354–358

Pfeffer LM, Tamm I (1984) Interferon inhibition of thymidine incorporation into DNA through effects on thymidine transport and uptake. J Cell Physiol 121: 431–436

Rivoltini L, Colombo M, Supino R et al (1990) Modulation of multidrug resistance by verapamil of mdrl1 anti-sense oligodeoxynucleotide does not change the high susceptibility to lymphokine-activated killers in mdr-resistant human carcinoma (LoVo) line. Int J Cancer 46:727–732

Teichmann JV, Ludwig WD, Thiel E (1991) Augmentation of the susceptibility of human leukemia to lymphokine-activated killer (LAK) cells by exposure of the leukemic target cells to cytotoxic drugs in vitro and in vivo. Leuk Lymph 5:263–271

Tewey KM, Chen GL, Nelson EM et al (1984) Intercalative antitumor drugs interfere with the breakage-reunion reaction of mammalian DNA topoisomerase II J Biol Chem 259:9182–9187

Towatari M, Ito Y, Morishita Y et al (1990) Enhanced expression of DNA topoisomerase II by recombinant human granulocyte colony-stimulating factor in human leukemia cells. Cancer Res 50:7198–7202

Van Haelst-Pisani CM, Pisani RJ, Kovach JS (1989) Cancer immunotherapy: current status of treatment with interleukin 2 and lymphokine-activated killer cells. Mayo Clin Proc 64:451–465

Wadler S (1991) The role of immunotherapy in colorectal cancer. Semin Oncol 18 [Suppl J]:27–38

Wadler S, Schwartz EL (1990) Antineoplastic activity of the combination of interferon and cytotoxic agents against experimental and human malignancies: a review. Cancer Res 50:3473–3486

Wang JC (1987) Recent studies of DNA topoisomerases. Biochem Biophys Acta 909:1–9

Interleukin-2-Based Immunotherapy and Chemoimmunotherapy in Metastatic Melanoma

U. Keilholz[1], C. Scheibenbogen[1], P. Brossart[1], T. Möhler[1], W. Tilgen[2], and W. Hunstein[1]

[1] Department of Medicine V (Hematology/Oncology), University of Heidelberg, Hospitalstraße 3, 69115 Heidelberg, Germany
[2] Department of Dermatology, University of Heidelberg, Voßstraße 2, 69115 Heidelberg, Germany

Abstract

This report summarizes our experience in the treatment of advanced melanoma with immunotherapy and chemoimmunotherapy. A total of 45 patients initially received immunotherapy with interferon-α (IFNα) and a decrescendo regimen of high-dose interleukin-2 (IL-2). The objective response rate is 31% with an additional 36% of mixed response (MR) and stable disease (SD).

A total of 18 patients failing immunotherapy with IFN-α/IL-2 received subsequent chemotherapy with dacarbacine (DTIC), followed by IFN-α. The response rate for this second-line regimen is 22%. A further 11 patients failing IFN-α/IL-2 received a single dose of DTIC or cisplatinum (CDDP) on day 1, followed by IFN-α/IL-2 according to the same protocol as previously, without chemotherapy. The addition of DTIC or CDDP was fairly well tolerated. Induction of seccondary mediators was not inhibited, suggesting that the immunologic effects mediated by IL-2 are not impaired. A randomized clinical trial is now being performed to compare combined chemoimmunotherapy with immunotherapy alone.

Introduction

There is no established treatment modality for metastatic melanoma with acceptable efficacy. Chemotherapy with dacarbacine (DTIC) or cisplatinum (CDDP) has a response rate between 5% and 30% (Comis 1976; Wagner et al. 1971; Goodnight et al. 1979), but effects on patients survival have not been shown. Combination chemotherapy including cisplatinum has been shown to produce a higher response rate (up to 60%); however, the response duration is usually brief and again there is probably no survival benefit (Nathanson et al. 1981; Luikart et al. 1984).

Recent Results in Cancer Research, Vol. 139

Immunotherapy with interferon-α (IFNα) and interleukin-2 (IL-2) alone resulted in response rates of 5%–25% in phase II studies (MacKie 1991; Rosenberg 1992; Hawkins et al. 1984; Sparano et al. 1993; Robinson et al. 1986; Rosenberg et al. 1985, 1987; Lotze et al. 1986; West et al. 1987). Several phase II studies with a combination of IFN-α and IL-2 using different dosing schedules have shown clinical efficacy, with response rates of up to 35% (Rosenberg et al. 1989; Lee et al. 1989; Bukowski et al. 1990; Bergmann et al. 1990). We have developed a decrescendo IL-2-dosing schedule. A very high initial IL-2 dose increases the induction of high-affinity IL-2 receptors on lymphocytes, enhancing the immunologic efficacy. Subsequent tapering of the IL-2 dose reduces toxicity. The response rate in the first series of 27 patients has been 41% (Keilholz et al. 1993).

Very recently, there have been preliminary reports of phase II studies using a combination of chemotherapy, IFN-α, and IL-2 (Garbe et al. 1992; Oratz et al. 1989; Richner et al. 1990; Schuchter et al. 1989, 1992; Silverman et al. 1991; Falkson et al. 1991; Kirkwood 1991; Margolin et al. 1990; Demchak et al. 1991; Dummer et al. 1991; Richards et al. 1992). Encouraging response rates have been reported with combinations of aggressive chemotherapy and immunotherapy. A moderate dose of CDDP followed by immunotherapy with IFN-α and IL-2 has produced similar response rates of 45%–86% in phase II studies, and in these studies the response duration appears to be longer than with chemotherapy alone. The effect on survival is, however, uncertain.

This report summarizes our experience in the treatment of metastatic melanoma with immunotherapy and chemoimmunotherapy. Patients failing initial immunotherapy with IFN-α/IL-2 subsequently received chemotherapy with DTIC/IFN-α, DTIC/IFN-α/IL-2, or CDDP/IFN-α/*IΛ-2*.

Patients and Methods

Patients with metastatic melanoma have been treated with a modified schedule of IFN-α and IL-2 in our hospital since 1991. This trial has been described in detail elsewhere (Keilholz et al. 1993). The eligibility criteria were histologically proven metastatic malignant melanoma, measurable progressive disease, absence of brain metastases, and a performance status of at least 60% (Karnofsky).

A total of 10 million U IFNα/m^2 was given s.c. on days 1–5, and a decrescendo regimen of IL-2 was used: 1 mg/m^2 every 6 h, followed by 1 mg/m^2 every 12 h, 1 mg/m^2 every 24 h, and 0.25 mg/m^2 every 24 h $\times$ 3. Treatment was repeated after 4 weeks. In case of partial response (PR), additional cycles were administered as long as antitumor responses were observed. In the case of progression, mixed response (MR), or stable disease (SD) after three treatment cycles, subsequent chemotherapy with 850 mg DTIC/m^2 on day 1, followed by 3 million U IFN-α/day on days 2–6 as described by Tilgen et al. (1993) was offered to these patients. This treatment was repeated every 3–4 weeks in the absence of disease progression.

In a pilot study in preparation for a randomized trial comparing chemoimmunotherapy and immunotherapy, 11 patients not responding to the standard IFN-α/IL-2 regimen received a single dose of 850 mg DTIC/m^2 or 100 mg CDDP/m^2 on day 1, followed by IFN-α/IL-2 according to the same protocol as previously, without chemotherapy. In cases of at least SD, this regimen was repeated twice after 4–6 weeks. Toxicity, induction of secondary cytokines, and tumor response were monitored and compared with immunotherapy alone. The trials had been approved by the University of Heidelberg Ethics Committee.

Results

A total of 45 patients were eligible to receive immunotherapy with IFN-α and IL-2. The results are summarized in Table 1. The toxicity of this regimen was moderate and is reported in detail elsewhere (Keilholz et al. 1993). We observed three complete remissions (CR), 11 PR, three MR, 13 SD, and 15 cases of progressive disease (PD). The current objective response rate is 31%, with an additional 36% of MR and SD.

Eighteen patients who had failed IFN-α/IL-2 (MR, SD, or PD after immunotherapy) received DTIC/IFN-α (Table 2). The response rate for this second-line regimen is 22%. The toxicity of this regimen is low, as described elsewhere (Tilgen et al. 1993).

Eleven further patients failing IFN-α/IL-2 were included in a pilot study evaluating the addition of cytostatic agents to immunotherapy; four patients received immunotherapy and a combination of DTIC and immunotherapy, five patients received immunotherapy and a combination of CDDP and

Table 1. Results of initial immunotherapy with interferon-α (IFN-α) and interleukin-2 (IL-2)

	Patients	
	(*n*)	(%)
Total	45	100
CR	3	7
PR	11	24
MR	3	7
SD	13	29
PD	15	31

CR, complete remission; PR, partial response; MR, mixed response; SD, stable disease; PD, progressive disease.

Table 2. Results of second-line protocols

	All patients		Response to previous IFN-α/IL-2	
	(*n*)	(%)	SD (*n*)	PD (*n*)
DTIC/IFN-α as second-line treatment				
CR	2	11	1	1
PR	2	11	1	1
SD/MR	5	28	2	3
PD	9	50	2	7
Total	18	100	6	12
Addition of DTIC or CDDP as secone-line treatment				
CR	0	0	0	0
PR	2	18	1	1
SD/MR	2	18	1	1
PD	7	64	0	7
Total	11	100	2	9

DTIC, dacarbacine; IFN, interferon; IL, interleukin; CR, complete remission; PR, partial response; SD, stable disease; MR, mixed response; PD, progressive disease; CDDP, cisplatinum.

immunotherapy, and two patients received all three protocols. The most prominent subjective toxicities were malaise, a flu-like syndrome, nausea, vomiting, and diarrhea. With the exception of nausea and vomiting, which occurred more frequently during chemoimmunotherapy, there was no difference noted in toxicities between the three forms of treatment. Objective toxicities included liver toxicity, renal toxicity, hematologic toxicity, and arterial hypotension. Renal and hematologic toxicity were more pronounced with the addition of chemotherapy. The most prominent toxicity was grade III renal toxicity in three patients receiving CDDP and immunotherapy. In all patients, however, the serum creatinine returned to normal within 4 weeks after discontinuation of treatment. No permanent toxicities were observed. Table 3 shows the serum concentrations of IFN-γ, tumor necrosis factor alpha (TNF-α), and sCD25 in patients receiving immunotherapy alone versus chemoimmunotherapy. The maximum value of the respective mediator has been chosen for comparison, and no significant differences were noted between the three different treatment protocols.

Two of 11 patients showed signs of tumor regression after the addition of DTIC to immunotherapy, and two further patients after the addition of CDDP to immunotherapy. Two of these patients (one with CDDP, one with DTIC) fullfilled the criteria for a PR (Table 2).

Table 3. Induction of secondary mediators by interleukin-2 (IL-2)

	IFN-α/IL-2	+ DTIC	+ CDDP
IFN-γ (pg/ml)	4.5 ± 3.3	5.9 ± 3.4	1.9 ± 0.9
TNF-α (pg/ml)	61 ± 34	91 ± 48	81 ± 21
sCD25 (U/l)	13.0 ± 2.1	18.2 ± 3.9	17.8 ± 10.8

Mean ± SD of the maximum values. The maximum was observed after 18 h of IL-2 infusion for IFN-γ, after 42 h for TNF-α, and at the end of treatment of sCD25. IFN, interferon; TNF, tumor necrosis factor; DTIC, dacarbacine; CDDP, cisplatinum.

In 29 patients, who had failed the standard IFN-α/IL-2 regimen, the response rate to second-line chemotherapy was 21% (Table 2). Thus, the overall response fate of the whole patient cohort is approximately 50%. The overall median survival is 17 months.

Discussion

Various phase II studies with a combination of IFN-α and IL-2 using different dosing schedules have been performed, showing response rates between 0% and 35% (Rosenberg et al. 1989; Lee et al. 1989; Bukowski et al. 1990; Bergmann et al. 1990). With our IL-2-dosing schedule (Keilholz et al. 1993), we were able for the first time to separate efficacy and toxicity of IL-2, achieving an improved response rate with a less toxic schedule as compared to the widely used continous high-dose intravenous infusion of IL-2 as proposed by West et al. (1987). In the current series of patients with higher tumor burden than the original cohort, we were able to maintain the response rate in the range of 30%.

The addition of chemotherapy to immunotherapy offers the possibility of higher response rates, but also adds considerable toxicity. We therefore evaluated a different approach: sequential immunotherapy and chemotherapy. A response rate of 21% was observed, adding up to a total response rate of 52%. The sequential approach is well tolerated and does not subject patients responsive to immunotherapy alone to the additional toxicity of chemotherapy.

However, the combination of chemotherapy and immunotherapy may offer certain advantages, leading to improved responses. The pharmacokinetics and pharmacodynamics of cytostatic agents as well as cytokines may be altered. Damage to tumor cells may improve antigen presentation by macrophages, and CDDP may synergize with IL-2 in the activation of macrophages. The question of whether chemotherapy impairs the effects of IL-2 has not been systematically adressed. It has been shown that DTIC and CDDP do not abolish the IL-2-mediated cellular responses (e.g., lymphocytosis, LAK activity) in the peripheral blood (Redman et al. 1991). A direct comparison between two patient groups or within a group of patients has, however, not yet been published. According to our observations, the addition of a single dose of DTIC or CDDP was found to be fairly well tolerated. More importantly, induction of secondary mediators was not inhibited, suggesting that this moderate form of chemotherapy does not impair the immunologic effects mediated by IL-2. A randomized clinical trial is necessary (and currently being performed) to compare first-line combined chemoimmunotherapy to immunotherapy alone.

Acknowledgements. The authors greatly appreciate the help of Anita Jochim, who performed the cytokine measurements, and Anne-Marie Geueke for data collection.

References

Bergmann L, Weidmann E, PS Mitrou, Runne U, Keilholz U, Bartsch HH et al (1990) Interleukin-2 in combination with interferon-alpha in disseminated malignant melanoma and advanced renal cell carcinoma. A phase I/II study. Onkologie 13:137–140

Bukowski RM, Murthy S, Sergi J, Budd GT, McKeever S, Medendorp SV et al (1990) Phase I trial of continuous infusion recombinant interleukin-2 and intermittant recombinant interferon.a2a: clinical effects. J Biol Response Mod 9:538–545

Comis RL (1976) DTIC (NSC-45388) in malignant melanoma: a perspective. Cancer Treat Rep 64:1123

Demchak PA, Mier JW, Robert NJ, O'Brien K, Gould JA, Atkins MB (1991) Interleukin-2 and high dose cisplatin in patients with metastatic melanoma: a pilot study. J Clin Oncol 9:1821–1830

Dummer R, Becker JC, Kalhammer U, Michaelis A, Ostmeier H, Tschammler A, Hartmann AA, Burg G (1991) Combined chemo- and immunotherapy using dacarbazine and continuous infusion of interleukin 2 in metastatic malignant melanoma. Results of a phase II clinical trial. Eur J Dermatol 1:201–205

Falkson C, Falkson G, Falkson HC (1991) Improved results with the addition of interferon alpha-2b to dacarbazine in the treatment of patients with metastatic malignant melanoma. J CLin Oncol 9:1403–1408

Garbe C, Kreuser E-D, Zouboulis CC, Stadler R, Orfanos E (1992) Combined treatment of metastatic melanoma with interferons and cytotoxic drugs. Semin Oncol 19:63–69

Goodnight JE Jr, Moseley HS, Eiber FR et al (1979) cis-Dichlorodiammineplatinum (II) alone and combined with DTIC for treatment of disseminated malignant melanoma. Cancer Treat Rep 63:2005

Hawkins MJ, McCune CS, Speyer JL et al (1984) Recombinant alpha-2 interferon (IFN-alpha 2) (SCH-30500) in patients with metastatic malignant melanoma (MMM): an ECOG pilot study. Proceedings of the American Society of Clinical Oncology, 20th annual meeting, 6–8 May, Toronto, Canada, p 51

Keilholz U, Scheibenbogen C, Tilgen W, Bergmann L, Weidmann E, Seither E, Richter M, Brado B, Mitrou PS, Hunstein W (1993) Interferon-alpha and interleukin-2 in the treatment of metastatic melanoma: comparison of two phase II trials. Cancer 72:607–614

Kirkwood JM (1991) Studies of Interferons in the therapy of melanoma. Semin Oncol 18:83–90
Lee KH, Talpaz M, Rothberg JM, Murray JL, Papadopoulos N, Plager C et al (1989) Concomitant administration of recombinant human interleukin-2 and recombinant interferon 2A in cancer patients: a phase 1 study. J Clin Oncol 7:1726–1732
Lotze MT, Chang AE, Seipp CA et al (1986) High-dose recombinant Interleukin-2 in the treatment of patients with disseminated cancer: responses, treatment, related morbidity and histologic findings. J Am Med Assoc 256:3117–3124
Luikart SD, Kennealey GT, Kirkwood JM (1984) Randomized phase III trial of vinblastine, bleomycin, and cis-dichlorodiammine-platinum versus dacarbazine in malignant melanoma. J Clin Oncol 2:164
MacKie R, (1991) Recombinant interleukin-2 and other types of treatment of advanced malignant melanoma. Curr Opinion Oncol 3:345–348
Margolin K, Doroshow J, Akman S et al (1990) Treatment (RX) of advanced melanoma with cis-diamminedichloroplatinum (CDDP) and alpha interferon (alpha IFN). Proc Am Soc Clin Oncol 9:1074
Nathanson L, Kaufman SD, Carey RW (1981) Vinblastine infusion, bleomycin, and cis-dichlorodiammine-platinum chemotherapy in metastatic melanoma. Cancer 48:1290
Oratz R, Dugan M, Walsh C et al (1989) Phase II trial of r-alpha 2b-interferon (IFN) and cisplatin (CDDP) in metastatic malignant melanoma (MM). Proc Am Soc Clin Oncol 8:1123
Redman BG, Flaherty L, Chou TH, Nakeff A, Pillote K, Kaplan J (1981) Sequential dacarbazine/cisplatin and interleukin-2 in metastatic melanoma: immunological effects of therapy. J Immunother 10:147–151
Richards JM, Mehta N, Ramming K, Skosey P (1992) Sequential chemoimmunotherapy in the treatment of metastatic melanoma. J Clin Oncol 10:1338–1343
Richner J, Cerny T, Joss RA et al (1990) A phase II study of continuous sc alpha-2b interferon (IFN) combined with cisplatin (CDDP) in advanced malignant melanoma (MM). Proc Am Soc Clin Oncol 9:1085
Robinson WA, Mughal TI, Thomas MR et al (1986) Treatment of metastatic malignant melanoma with recombinant interferon-Alpha-2. Immunobiol 172:275–282
Rosenberg SA (1992) The immunotherapy and gene therapy of cancer. J Clin Oncol 10:180–199
Rosenberg SA, Lotze MT, Muul LM et al (1985) Observations on the systemic administration of autologous lymphokine-activated killer cells and recombinant Interleukin-2 to patients with metastatic cancer. N Engl J Med 313:1485
Rosenberg SA, Lotze MT, Muul LM et al (1987) A progress report on the treatment of 157 patients with advanced cancer using lymphokine-activated killer cells and interleukin-2 or high dose interleukin-2 alone. N Engl J Med 316:889–905
Rosenberg SA, Lotze MT, Yang JC, Linehan WM, Seipp C, Calabro S et al (1989) Combination therapy with interleukin-2 and alpha-interferon for the treatment of patients with advanced cancer. J Clin Oncol 7:1863–1874
Schuchter L, McGuire WP, Wohlganger J et al (1989) Sequential treatment of metastatic melanoma with interferon-alpha (IFN) plus cisplatinum (CDDP). Proc Am Soc Clin Oncol 8:1120
Schuchter LM, Wohlganger JA, Fishman EK, MacDermott ML, McGuire WP (1992) Sequential chemotherapy and immunotherapy for the treatment of metastatic melanoma. J Immunotherapy 12:272–276
Silverman P, Creger RJ, Spitzer TR et al (1991) Phase II trial of cisplatin and interferon-alpha-2b in advanced malignant melanoma, breast carcinoma, and non-small cell lung carcinoma. Proc Am Soc Clin Oncol 10:1041

Sparano JA, Fisher RI, Sunderland M et al (1993) Randomized phase III trial of treatment with high-dose interleukin-2 alone or in combination with interferon alfa-2a in patients with advanced melanoma. J Clin Oncol 11:1969–1977

Tilgen W, Zirott U, Keilholz U, Longére G, Scheibenbogen C, Petzoldt D (1993) Combined modality therapy of metastatic melanoma: the "Heidelberg approach." Melanom Res 3 [Suppl 1]:51

Wagner DE, Ramirez G, Weiss AJ (1971) Combination phase I-II study of imidazole carboxamid (NSC 45388). Oncology 26:310

West WH, Tauer KW, Yanelli JR, Marshall GD, Orr DW, Thurman GB, Oldham RK (1987) Constant infusion recombinant interleukin-2 in adoptive immunotherapy of advanced cancer. N Engl J Med 316:898–905

Combination Therapy of Cutaneous T Cell Lymphoma with Interferon Alpha-2a and Photochemotherapy

R. Stadler and H.G. Otte

Department of Dermatology, Minden Medical Center, Teaching Unit of the University of Münster, Portastraße 7-9, 32423 Minden, Germany

Abstract

The efficacy of a combination treatment with interferon alpha-2a and photochemotherapy was investigated in 16 patients with cutaneous T cell lymphoma. During the initial treatment, interferon alpha-2a was given subcutaneously at maximum dose of 9 million IU. Simultaneously, photochemotherapy with a maximum single dose of 3.0 J/cm^2 was applied. After a complete or partial remission had been achieved, the dose of interferon was continued as permanent treatment at 3–9 million IU a week. Photochemotherapy was maintained twice a week for a minimum of 2 months and then stopped depending on the course of the disease. The combination treatment was well tolerated and all patients responded to the initial therapy. Three patients were withdrawn at an early stage of therapy, as they developed erythrodermia after photochemotherapy. The permanent treatment led to a complete remission in ten out of 13 patients and to a partial remission in three patients. During the follow-up period (now 10–40 months), therapy was stopped in four patients because of progression and in one patient because of newly diagnosed Hodgkin's disease. In another three patients, who developed local recurrences, a repetition of the initial treatment schedule was necessary to keep them in remission.

Introduction

Cutaneous T cell lymphoma (CTCL) represent a heterogenous group of malignant T cell proliferations of the skin, for which a standarized therapy does not yet exist (Table 1).

Therapeutic measures, such as photochemotherapy, radiotherapy with fast electrons, and topically applied cytostatic drugs which only reach the skin to a relevant degree, are often not able to prevent the systemic spreading of

Recent Results in Cancer Research, Vol. 139

Table 1. Patients' characteristics

Patient no.	Sex	Age[a] (years)	Length of illness[b] (months)	Stage	Type	Previous therapy
1	m	72	14	III	MF	PC therapy, retinoids
2	m	82	2	IVa	MF	
3	m	58	4	IIb	MF	Oral glucocorticoids
4	m	67	120	IIb	MF	PC therapy
5	m	58	84	IIa	MF	
6	m	57	120	IIa	MF	PC therapy, local X-ray
7	m	68	24	Ib	Pagetoid reticulosis	PC therapy
8	m	62	120	IIb	MF	UVB rays, PC therapy, cignolin
9	m	73	5	III	MF	
10	m	59	6	IIb	Pleomorph	
11	f	63	6	IIb	Pleomorph	
12	m	64	36	Ib	MF	UVB rays
13	f	24	3	Ia	MF	Local glucocorticoids
14	m	62	36	IIb	MF	Local glucocorticoids
15	m	35	9	Ia	MF	PC therapy
16	m	65	48	Ia	MF	

MF, mycosis fungoides; pleomorph, pleomorphic T cell lymphoma; PC therapy, photochemotherapy.
[a] Average, 61 years.
[b] Average, 40 months.

the disease (Roenigh et al. 1990). A systemic chemotherapy can only have a short-term positive effect on the course of the disease (Holloway et al. 1992; Roenigh et al. 1990). Besides, because of its side effects this therapy can only be applied in a restricted way.

In the last 10 years numerous studies have shown the efficacy of interferon with CTCL (Bunn et al. 1984; Bunn and Norris 1990; Dreno et al. 1989; Simoni et al. 1987; Stadler et al. 1989; Vonderheid et al. 1987). In most of the studies human, recombined interferon alpha was given at a medium dose of 18–36 million IU systemically (Bunn and Norris 1990; Simoni et al. 1987). The degree of response ranged from 45% to 85%, depending on the patients (Bunn and Norris 1990; Simoni et al. 1987). There are only a few studies with small numbers of patients pertaining to the efficacy of low doses of interferon alpha (Bunn and Norris 1990; Dreno et al. 1989; Vonderheid et al. 1987). As the duration of remission with interferon montherapy, depending on the choice of patients, only lasted between 5.5 and 10 months and as the percentage of complete remissions was low (15%–40%), new possible therapeutic methods were searched for (Bunn and Norris 1990; Kuzel et al. 1990; Roenigh et al. 1990).

In present studies pertaining to a small amount of patients, interferons in combination with retinoids have shown a degree of response ranging from 66% to 80%, and the percentage of complete remissions ranged between 20% and 50% (Braathen and McFadden 1989; Bunn and Norris 1990; Threstrup-Pedersen et al. 1988).

While mainly the early stages of the CTCL can be sucessfully but not curatively treated with photochemotherapy alone (Gilchrest et al. 1976; Roenigh et al. 1990), the few currently available studies regarding a combination of interferon and photochemtherapy reported that the degree of response was about 90%, with a high rate of complete remissions (80%) (Kuzel et al. 1990; Roenigh et al. 1990).

Because of the encouraging therapeutic results, we treated 16 patients suffering from CTCL, stages Ia–IVa, with a combination of interferon alpha-2a and photochemotherapy (temporary results in Otte et al. 1992).

Patients

The 16 patients, two women and 14 men, aged between 24 and 82 years, were diagnosed as suffering from CTCL on account of the clinical, histological, and immunohistological pictures; 13 patients had CTCL of the mycosis fungoides type, two had a pleomorphic T cell lymphoma, and one patient had a pagetoid reticulosis type Ketron-Goodman.

The duration of the illness, including the premycotic stages, ranged between 2 months and 10 years (average, 40 months). Therapeutic attempts with partial X-ray treatment, photochemotherapy, ultraviolet rays, retinoids, local or systemic glucocorticoids, or with cignolin, sometimes in combination, were used in some of the patients (Table 1).

The division into stages of CTCL was done according to the classification into four stages proposed by Bunn and Lamberg (1973; Table 2). In order to assess their respective stages, all the patients underwent comprehensive staging tests. A HTLV I/II infection was precluded by serological means (enzyme-linked immunosorbent assay, ELISA). According to the test results, three patients were assigned to stage Ia, two to stage Ib, two to stage IIa, six to stage IIb, two to stage III, and one patient to stage IVa (Table 1). Indications of a Sézary syndrome were not diagnosed in any of the patients.

Therapy Schedule

In the initial phase, after low dose had been given, interferon alpha-2a was administered three times a week at a maximum dose of 9 million IU subcutaneously, according to the clinical picture. If the response was not

Table 2. Therapy results

Patient no.	Therapy result after initial therapy	Therapy result with conser vative therapy	Length of therapy success[a] (months)	Reason for stopping therapy or additional therapy
1	PR			Stopped, erythrodermia
2	PR	CR	32+	Repeated initial therapy after 10 months
3	PR	CR	36+	
4	PR	CR	40+	Repeated initial therapy after 21 months
5	PR			Stopped, erythrodermia
6	PR	CR	13	Stopped, Hodgkin's disease
7	PR	CR	20	Stopped, progression
8	PR	PR	25	Repeated initial therapy after 17 months/stopped, progression
9	PR			Stopped, erythrodermia
10	PR	PR	6	Stopped, progression
11	PR	PR	3	Stopped, progression
12	CR	CR	28+	
13	PR	CR	23+	
14	CR	CR	19+	Repeated initial therapy after 11 months
15	PR	CR	13	
16	PR	CR	10	

PR, partial remission; CR, complete remission.
[a] Average, 20.6 months.

sufficient, in some cases a maximum daily dose of 9 million IU, on average a total dose of 140 million IU, was administered.

Simultaneously, photochemotherapy with 0.6 mg 8-methoxypsoralen/kg was carried out four times a week. As the sensitizing properties to light were known about a therapy with interferon (Roenigh et al. 1990), photochemotherapy was started with a dose of $0.25\,J/cm^2$, which was raised individually according to tolerance.

The maximum single dose was $3.0\,J/cm^2$. The total dose of the photochemotherapy ranged between 7.1 and $130\,J/cm^2$, on average $30.4\,J/cm^2$ (Table 3).

Additional therapeutic measures, such as glucocorticoids or X-ray therapy, were only necessary in three patients (Table 3). All the other patients only needed nursing. To the end of the initial phase, the therapy lasted between 30 and 84 days (average, 51 days).

The subsequent conservative therapy was carried out with interferon alpha-2a at a dose between 3 and 9 million IU administered in two to three injections a week. The photochemotherapy was continued for at least 2

Table 3. Detailed data regarding initial therapy

Patient no.	IFN alpha maximum dose (mio. IU)	IFN alpha total dose (mio. IU)	Photochemo-therapy max. dose (J/cm^2)	Photochemo-herapy total dose (J/cm^2)	Length of therapy (days)	Additional therapy
1	3	99	1, 2	17, 9	75	Topical steroids
2	3	15	0, 7	7, 1	36	
3	9	138	1, 5	28, 2	57	X-ray therapy
4	9	108	2	30, 6	31	
5	3	35	1	13, 8	31	
6	3	71	1	9, 2	48	
7	9	138	1, 25	27, 3	36	
8	9	416	2, 5	62, 9	78	X-ray therapy
9	9	119	1	14, 6	56	
10	6	89	1	17, 4	42	
11	9	146	1, 5	20, 2	42	
12	9	148	1, 5	22, 3	48	
13	9	93	1, 75	23, 5	30	
14	9	147	1	31, 8	41	
15	9	165	3	130, 0	84	
16	9	310	2	40, 0	76	
Average	7.3	139.8	1.5	30.4	50.7	

IFN, interferon.

months (average, 8 months), 2 days a week, and was then stopped if the clinical picture was stable.

Results

The therapeutic success was assessed according to the clinical and cellular picture. Complete healing of all the pathological changes of the skin was assessed as a complete remission; improvement of more than 50% of the previously affected areas was assessed as a partial remission.

After the initial therapy two patients had reached a complete remission and 11 patients had reached a partial remission. Three patients who had at first also shown some improvement later developed an increasing reddening of the integument under photochemotherapy. Thus, the therapy had to be stopped early. As a result, all the patients had responded to the combination therapy initially.

The conservative therapy led to a complete remission in ten patients and to a partial remission in three patients (Figs. 1–3).

During the follow-up period of 10–40 months (average, 20.6 months), four patients developed progression and the combination therapy had to be stopped. Two of these had a pleomorphic T cell lymphoma, which is distinguished by a higher grade of malignancy. One patient developed Hodgkin's disease and underwent polychemotherapy.

In another three patients with local recurrences, a repetition of the initial therapy again led to a complete remission in two cases and to a partial remission in one case (Table 2).

All the patients tolerated the combination therapy with interferon alpha-2a and photochemotherapy well. Slight parainfluenzal side effects of the interferon therapy, especially during the initial phase, could be controlled by prior administration of paracetamol. When receiving a daily dose of 9 million IU interferon alpha-2a, one patient had sleep disturbances and nightmares. Nightly administration of a hypnotic put an end to these disturbances. When the interferon dose was reduced to 3 million IU, sleep disturbances no longer occurred.

A regular check of the laboratory parameters showed on average an 8% drop in the haemoglobin level, a 35% drop in the leukocyte count, and an 18% drop in the thrombocyte value. Alterations of the kidney retention levels or of the transaminases were only observed in individual patients. Regarding the gamma glutamyltransferase (GT), an average increase of 15% was observed, and regarding glutamate pyruvate transaminase (GPT), an increase of 20%. A consistent tendency for the whole group of patients regarding all the other laboratory parameters which were regularly checked was not found. It was not necessary to reduce the dose or to stop the therapy because of the above-mentioned side effects.

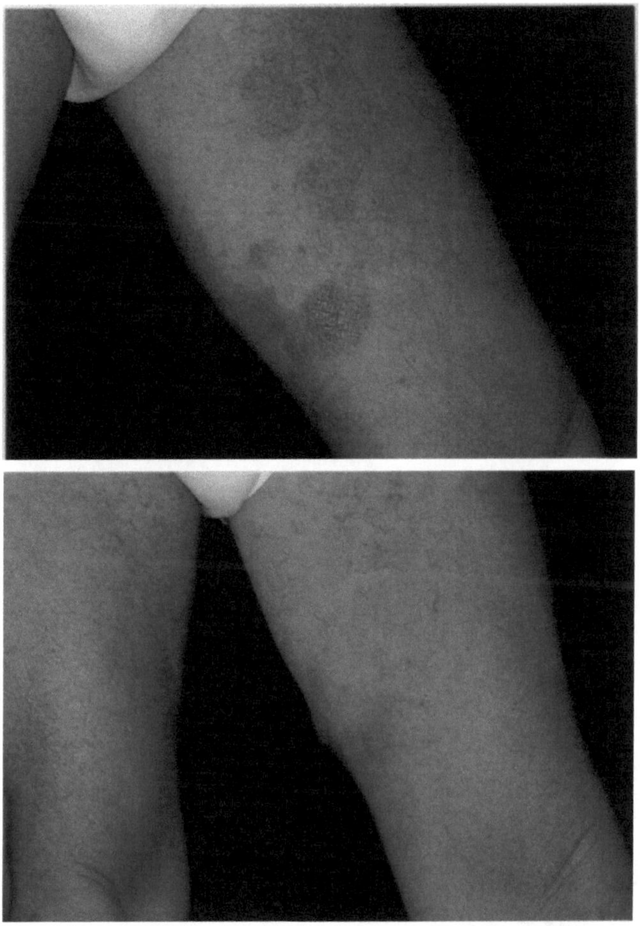

a

b

Fig. 1a,b. Patient no. 10 with pleomorphic T cell lymphoma. **a** Before therapy. **b** Eleven weeks after start of therapy

All the patients tolerated photochemotherapy, apart from occasional nausea after taking the 8-methoxypsoralen tablets, which could be avoided by reducing the dose without any complications. As stated before, after an intially good response to the combination therapy, three patients developed increasing reddening and infiltration of the skin after the photochemotherapy. Thus, we had to refrain from continuing their therapy.

Discussion

Good response to combination therapy with interferon alpha-2a and photochemotherapy by patients with CTCL was confirmed in this study. At

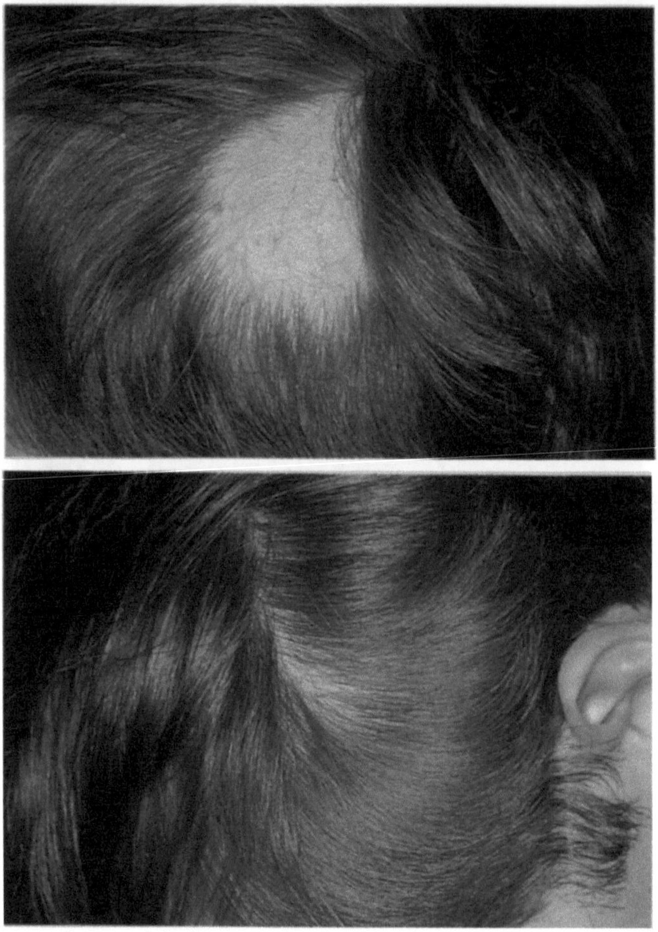

a

b

Fig. 2a,b. Patient no. 13. **a** Clear alopecia mucinosa before therapy. **b** Complete remission after 6 months of therapy

least initially, an improvement or a symptom-less stage of CTCL was achieved by all the patients with a combination of a maximum dose of 9 million IU interferon alpha-2a and a photochemotherapy. We think that the response of the more malignant pleomorphic T cell lymphomas is noteworthy. With 76% complete remissions, a better result than stated for a single interferon therapy was achieved (Brunn et al. 1984); 80% complete remissions, as reported in studies regarding combined interferon and photochemotherapy, was not achieved (Brunn and Norris 1990; Kuzel et al. 1990; Roenigh et al. 1990). This difference might be explained by the varying therapy schedules of other authors, which include lower interferon doses and a shorter application of photochemotherapy. Because of this, the cumulative interferon doses and photochemotherapy doses are lower com-

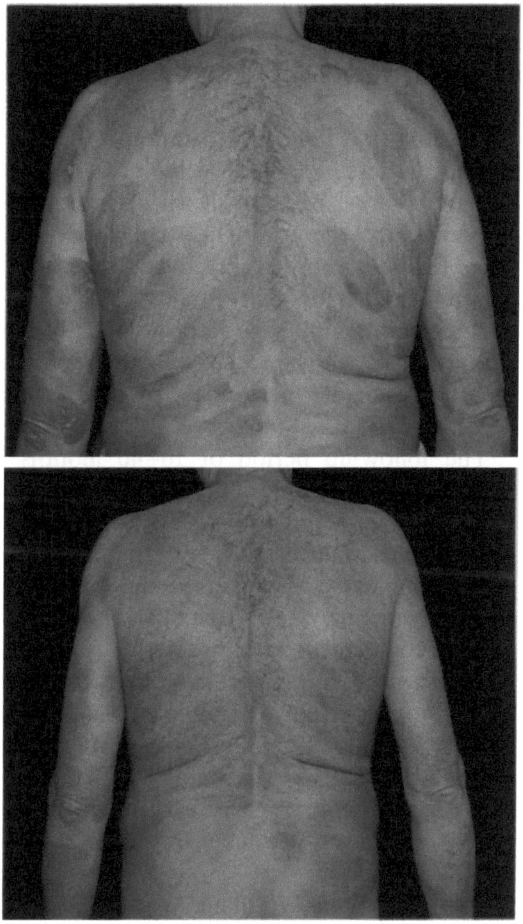

a

b

Fig. 3a,b. Patient no. 14. **a** Before therapy. **b** After 2 months of therapy

pared to Kuzel et al. (1990). This difference, however, cannot yet be reliably assessed because of the low number of patients.

On average it took 51 days to achieve remission; this corresponds to our results of 1–2 months stated in other studies.

On the whole, the side effects of combination therapy in our patients were minor. At the beginning of the interferon therapy, most of the patients complained of having a temperature and parainfluenzal symptoms, which were relieved by paracetamol. During the course of the treatment, most of the patients got used to the interferon therapy, and paracetamol was no longer necessary. Only one patient suffered from sleep disturbances with nightmares, which was treated sucessfully by administering a hypnotic. Serious side effects on the blood and on the so-called hepathic and renal values necessitating a reduction of the dose did not occur with the stated, relatively low interferon dose. In contrast, other studies which described treatment with higher doses of interferon had to adjust the doses more frequently.

Sensitivity to light with interferon therapy (Roenigh et al. 1990), which makes it necessary to reduce the dose of photochemotherapy, was found in all our patients. Because of this, it was possible to use lower single doses of photochemotherapy. The total dose of photochemotherapy to achieve remission was considerably lower than the total dose with photochemotherapy alone (Roenigh et al. 1990). Only in three patients (19%) did photochemotherapy have to be stopped because of increased reddening and infiltration of the skin, as defined by photosensibilization. Other authors reported a similar percentage in their respective studies (Roenigh et al. 1990).

The follow-up period of 10–40 months is too short to make a final assessment on the long-term effects of the combination therapy.

Up to now, only four patients have showed disease progression, and two of them were diagnosed as suffering from a more malignant pleomorphic T cell lymphoma; it therefore seems that after a remission, low-dose monotherapy with interferon alpha-2a is sufficient to control CTCL, except for the more malignant variants.

In summary, this study shows that combination therapy with an interferon alpha-2a dose of up to 9 million IU and photochemotherapy followed by a conservative therapy of 3–9 million IU interferon alpha-2a a week is a well-tolerated and effective therapy for CTCL. Further studies with longer follow-up periods are necessary in order to assess the importance of this therapy regarding treatment of CTCL.

Acknowledgment. We thank W. Schäfer for taking the photographs.

References

Braathen LR, McFadden N (1989) Successful treatment of mycosis fungoides with the combination of etretinate and human recombinant interferon alpha-2a. J Dermatol Treat 1:29–32

Bunn PA Jr, Foon KA, Ihde DC et al (1984) Recombinant leukocyte A interferon: an active agent in advanced cutaneous T-cell lymphomas. Ann Intern Med 101:484–487

Bunn PA, Lamberg SI (1979) Report of the committee on staging and classification of cutaneous T-cell lymphomas. Cancer Treat Rep 63:725–728

Bunn PA, Norris DA (1990) The role of interferons and monoclonal antibodys in cutaneous T-cell lymphomas. J Invest Dermatol 95:209S–212S

Dreno B, Godefroy WY, Fleischmann M, Bureau B, Litoux P (1989) Low-dose recombinant interferon-alpha in the treatment of cutaneous T-cell lymphomas. Br J Dermatol 121:543–544

Gilchrest BA, Parish JA, Tannenbaum LR, Haynes Fitzpatrick TB (1976) Oral methoxsalen photochemotherapy of mycosis fungoides. Cancer 38:683–698

Holloway KB, Flowers FP, Ramos-Caro FA (1992) Therapeutic alternatives in cutaneous T-cell lymphoma. J Am Acad Dermatol 27:367–378

Kuzel TM, Gilyon K, Springer E, Variakojis D, Kaul K, Bunn PA, Evans L, Roenigk HH, Rosen ST (1990) Interferon alpha-2a combined with photochemotherapy in the treatment of cutaneous T-cell lymphoma. J Natl Cancer Inst 82(3):203–207

Otte HG, Herges A, Stadler R (1992) Kombinationstherapie mit Interferon alfa 2a und PUVA bei kutanen T-Zell-Lymphomen. Hautarzt 43:695–699

Roenigh HH, Kuzel TM, Skoutelis AP, Springer E, Yu G, Caro W, Gilyon K, Vaiakojis D, Kaul K, Bunn PA, Evans L, Rosen ST (1990) Photochemotherapy alone or combined with interferon alpha-2a in the treatment of cutaneous T-cell lymphoma. J Invest Dermatol 95:198S–205S

Simoni R, Cavalieri R, Coppola G, Ricciotti L, De Pita O, Criscuolo D, Covelli A, Papa G, Mandelli F (1987) Recombinant leukocyte interferon alpha-2a in the treatment of mycosis fungoides. J Biol Regul Homeost Agents 1:93–99

Stadler R, Mayer-Da-Silva A, Bratzke B, Garbe C, Orfanos C (1989) Interferons in dermatology. J Am Acad Dermatol 20:650–656

Threstrup-Pedersen K, Hammer R, Kaltoft K, Sogaard H, Zachariae H (1988) Treatment of mycosis fungoides with recombinant interferon alpha-2a alone an in combination with etretinate. Br J Dermatol 118:811–818

Vonderheid EC, Thompson R, Smiles KA, Lattanand A (1987) Recombinant interferon alpha-2b in plaque-phase mycosis fungoides. Arch Dermatol 123: 757–763

Systemic Treatment for Cutaneous Lymphomas

V. Mielke, G. Staib, and W. Sterry

Department of Dermatology, University of Ulm, Oberer Eselsberg 40, 89070 Ulm, Germany

Abstract

Primary malignant T cell lymphomas of the skin form a heterogenous group. Relevant classifications were recently made to separate different entities by various criteria. This is of great importance, because one should only rely on those therapeutical trials in which patients were included according such classifications. In this paper, we will mainly focus on therapeutic modalities for mycosis fungoides, which is the most frequent cutaneous T cell lymphoma and which may serve as a model disease. In principle, local (e.g., psoralens and ultraviolet A, PUVA) and systemic therapies (e, g., interferon-α_{2a}) can be applied. Very recently, we were able to demonstrate that even in initial stages of mycosis fungoides, the T cell clone is not restricted to the skin, but rather is present in low amounts in the peripheral blood. Therefore, systermic therapeutic modalities alone or in combination with local strategies (interferon-α_2a and acitretin/PUVA and interferon-α_2a) should be more effective, which will be proven by currently running clinical trials.

Introduction

Based on the concept that primary malignant T cell lymphomas of the skin form a heterogenous group, relevant classifications were recently made by various criteria in order to separate all the different entities and not to use the single term cutaneous T cell lymphoma (CTCL) for all the diseases (Sterry et al. 1992; Willemze et al. 1994). This is of great importance before discussing therapy, because one should only rely on those therapeutical trials in which patients were included according to the classifications mentioned above. In the following, therapeutic modalities will be mainly focused on a single cutanous T cell lymphoma, the mycosis fungoides, which is the most frequent one and which may serve as a model disease.

Recent Results in Cancer Research, Vol. 139

At present it is well established that almost from the beginning mycosis fungoides is characterized by monoclonal CD4+ T cell proliferations (Staib et al., submitted). After individually different time intervals the skin lesions sequentially develop from patches via plaques into tumors, before lymph nodes and internal organs become involved macroscopically.

Local Therapy

During the last few decades a broad spectrum of different local therapies have been established for treatment of patients with mycosis fungoides. The rationale for this was based on the concept that the tumor initially is restricted to the skin and that only a very minor population of tumor cells will recirculate to the blood and/or to regional lymph nodes in order to reach the skin again for a second or third time (skin-homing T cells). Therefore, local treatments should be effective, at the same time, sparing the patient severe systemic side effects.

In 1974, PUVA therapy (8-methoxy-psoralene plus ultraviolet A) was introduced and the efficacy, especially in early stages of mycosis fungoides (Ia and Ib), was demonstrated in several studies (Abel et al. 1987; Hönigsmann et al. 1984). PUVA has been considered as the gold standard of therapy for patients with mycosis fungoides. Moreover, other local therapies such as the application of nitrogen mustard and corticosteroids as well as electron beam radiation and X-ray therapy have been used as local agents with the intention of curing the disease (Holloway et al. 1992; Kaye et al. 1989).

The major problem of all local therapeutic modalities is that the disease may reoccur and eventually progress into phases of higher malignancy. This could be due to the fact that the use of the local drug or agent is restricted only to those skin regions where the disease is visible to the clinician or detectable by histology. The hypothesis that subclinical lesions are present is further supported by clinical experience that, after starting PUVA therapy, additional skin lesions show up. Moreover, a relapse may originate from specific anatomic regions, where local therapeutic modalities cannot act sufficiently (perianal, genital, and axillary region). Very often, after local therapy for a long time with partial or complete clinical remission, the disease reoccurs or is most advanced in these regions.

Systemic Therapy

To overcome disadvantages of local therapies, many groups have started to treat patients with mycosis fungoides with combination therapies, including systemically active principles. In most of these regimens one local therapeutic modality (PUVA, UVB, etc.) is combined with a systemic drug (retinoids,

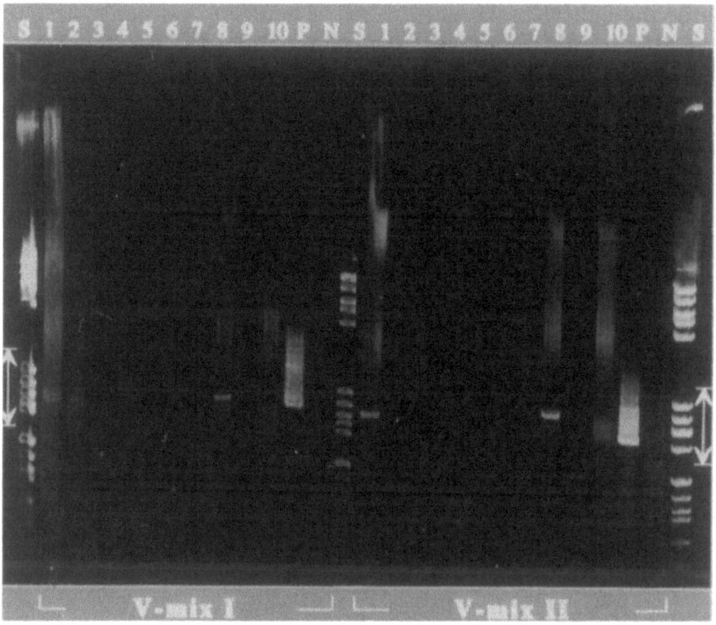

Fig. 1. Polymerase chain reaction (PCR) of the T cell receptor (TCR) gamma chain gene in mononuclear cells of peripheral blood in patients with cutaneous T cell lymphomas. Amplification products were separated by temperature gradient gel electrophoresis (TGGE). Silver staining. A single band (*lanes 1, 8,* and P) represents a clonal amplification product (approximately 280bp). *S*, DNA standard (Boehringer V). *1*, mycosis fungoides (MF), plaque stage; *8*, MF, tumor stage; *P*, positive control (HUT-78); *N*, negative control

interferons, etc.). An additional reason for using combination therapies has been derived from modern in vitro studies. We have recently demonstrated that even in initial peripheral T cell lymphomas of the mycosis fungoides type, the T cell clone is not restricted to skin lesions, but rather is constantly present and detectable in the peripheral blood, something which is normally overlooked in the analysis of blood smears. However, using polymerase chain reaction for the T cell receptor gamma chain gene with specific primers for all V and J regions, initial blood involvement can be detected (Fig. 1).

Psoralens and Ultraviolet A with Retinoids

Vitamin A analogues (retinoids) are effective in the treatment of mycosis fungoides (Holloway et al. 1992). In 11 of 25 CTCL patients, a partial response was observed, whereas complete remissions were only achieved in three patients (Kessler et al. 1987). Therefore, retinoids were mostly used in combination therapies such as etretinate and PUVA (RePUVA). Using this combination, the response rate was improved. Moreover, the number of PUVA treatments as well as the total UVA dose required was decreased (Thomsen et al. 1989)

Psoralens and Ultraviolet A with interferon-α_{2a}

Interferon-α_{2a} as an antiviral and antitumor agent was introduced in the therapy of CTCL in the late 1970s. Efficacy together with tolerable side effects (mild fever, fatigue, malaise, weight loss, etc.) were demonstrated in several studies. A review by Bunn and Norris (1990) reveals that the overall response rate appears to be about 60% and the complete response rate approxinately 19%. More recently, interferon α_{2a} was predominantly used in combination therapies. Mostow and coworkers have found that in PUVA-refractory mycosis fungoides the addition of interferon α_{2a} to PUVA could lead to complete clinical remissions. Moreover, total UVA dosages and time of therapy could be decreased (Mostow et al. 1993). however, neither prospective, randomized studies nor dose-finding studies have been performed to address the question of which combination therapy is most efficient.

As a consequence, a prospective multicenter study was started last year by the EORTC Cutaneous Lymphoma Study Group to investigate the difference of therapeutic efficacy between PUVA/interferon α_{2a} (3 times/week and 3 × 9 million IU/week) and interferon α_{2a}/acitretin (3 × 9 million IU/week and 50 mg/day) in patients with initial peripheral T cell lymphomas of mycosis fungoides type and of pleomorphic T cell lymphoma type. Only patients in stages I and II can be included in this study. A second multicenter study will probably answer the question of whether the additional low-dose application of interferon α_{2a} prolongs the disease-free time interval after complete remission is achieved.

Extracorporeal Photophoresis

Currently, it is not clear, whether the efficacy of PUCA therapy is limited to the skin or whether PUVA has an additional effect on circulating blood cells. In order to further enhance the action on white circulating blood cells, in 1987 Edelson and coworkers developed extracorporeal photophoresis. Two hours after oral application of 8-methoxypsoralen (8-MOP) the patients undergo leukopheresis. The buffy coat lymphocytes are then exposed to UVA. Thereafter, the photoirradiated cells are reinfused into the patient. In the original multicenter clinical trial about two thirds of patients (n = 37) showed a clinical response, including nine patients with complete remission (Edelson et al. 1987). Extracorporeal photophoresis is now considered by these authors to be the standard therapy of erythrodermic and/or leukemic CTCL Disadvantages are that extracorporeal photophoresis is not available in all medical centers and that this therapy is time consuming and relatively expensive.

Chemotherapy

In advanced stages of mycosis fungoides with or without involvement of internal organs, single chemotherapeutic agents, e.g., cyclophosphamide, chlorambucil, methotrexate, cisplatin, or polychemotherapies (COP) e.g., cyclophosyhamide, oncovin (vincristine), and prednisone are mainly used to control the disease, but it has never been demonstrated that these regimens were followed by complete remissions for a long time (Hoppe et al. 1990).

References

Abel EA, Sendagorta E, Hoppe RT, Hu CH (1987) PUVA treatment of eryghrodermic and plaque-type mycosis fungoides. Arch Dermatol 123:897–901

Bunn PA, Norris DA (1990) The therapeutic role of interferons and monoclonal antibodies in cutaneous T-cell lymphomas. J Invest Dermatol 95 [Suppl]:209s–212s

Edelson R, Berger C, Gasparro F (1987) Treatment of cutaneous T-cell lymphoma by extracorporeal photochemotherapy. N Engl J Med 316:297–303

Holloway KB, Flowers FP, Ramos-Caro FA (1992) Therapeutic alternatives in cutaneous T-cell lymphoma. J Am Acad Dermatol 27:367–378

Hönigsmann H, Brenner W, Ruaschmeier W, Konrad K, Wolff K (1984) Photochemotherapy for cutaneous T cell lymphoma. J Am Acad Dermatol 10:238–245

Hoppe RT, Cox RS, Fuks Z (1990) Electron-beam therapy for mycosis fungoides: the Stanford University experience. Cancer Treat Rep 63: 691–700

Kaye FJ, Bunn PA, Steinberg SM, Stocker JL, Ihde DC, Fischmann AB, Glatstein EJ, Schechter GP, Phelps RM, Foss FM, Parlette HL, Anderson MJ, Suaville EA (1989) A randomized trial comparing combination electron-beam radiation and chemotherapy with topical therapy in the initial treatment of mycosis fungoides. N Engl J Med 321:1784–1790

Kessler JF, Jones SE, Levine N (1987) Isotretinoin and cutaneous helper T-cell lymphoma (mycosis fungoides). Arch Dermatol 123:201–204

Mostow EN, Neckel SL, Oberhelmann L, Anderson TF, Cooper KD (1993) Complete remissions in psoralen and UV-A (PUVA)-refractory mycosis fungoides-type cutaneous T-cell lymphoma with combined interferon alpha and PUVA. Arch Dermatol 129:747–752

Staib G, Mielke V, Griesser H, Menke M, Duller B, Sterry W. PCR-analysis of T-cell receptor gamma genes for differentiation of cutaneous T-cell lymphomas and reactive T-cell dominated skin diseases. Br J Dermatol (submitted)

Sterry W, Siebel A, Mielke V (1992) HTLV-1-negative pleomorphic T cell lymphoma of the skin: clinicopathologic correlations and natural history of 15 patients. Br J Dermatol 126:456–462

Thomsen K, Hammar H, Molin L (1989) Retinoids plus PUVA (RePUVA) and PUVA in mycosis fungoides, plaque stage. Acta Derm Venereol (Stockh) 69: 536–538

Willemze R, Beljaards RC, Rijlaarsdam U (1994) Classification of primary cutaneous large cell lymphomas. Dermatol Clin 12/2:361–373

Extracorporeal Photopheresis – A New Approach for the Treatment of Cutaneous T Cell Lymphomas

H.P.M. Gollnick, M. Owsianowski, J. Ramaker, S.C. Chun, and C.E. Orfanos

Department of Dermatology, University Medical Center Steglitz, The Free University of Berlin, Hindenburgdamm 30, 12200 Berlin, Germany

Abstract

Extracorporeal photochemotherapy (extracorporeal photopheresis, ECP) is going to become a new alternative in the treatment of cutaneous T cell lymphomas (CTCL), autoimmune disorders, and transplant rejections. After the first promising results in the treatment of CTCL reported in 1987 by Edelson et al. increasing numbers of CTCL patients in a growing number of ECP centers throughout the United States, Europe, and Japan have been successfully treated. Today, it seems that in particular Sézary's syndrome and the erythrodermic variant of mycosis fungoides (MF) respond very well to ECP. Compared to historical controls of MF with lymph node involvement, the median survival of the ECP-treated patients increased from 30 months to up to 60 months. It is our experience that the tumor stage of MF, however, cannot be treated with ECP alone, but is successfully controlled by combination regimens, for example with recombinant interferon alpha. CTCL patients heavily pretreated by polychemotherapy and severe endogenous or iatrogenic immunsuppression do not respond sufficiently and are not good candidates for ECP.

The adverse reactions under ECP are well controlled and very low in number. In particular, general immunosuppression by ECP has not been reported so far.

Introduction

Presently the treatment behavior in cutaneous T cell lymphoma (CTCL) in dermatology is changing. This is particularly true for patients in the T_2 and T_3 stage, with and without lymph node involvement, and T_4 erythrodermic CTCL, with or without leukemic phase (erythrodermic form of mycosis fungoides and Sézary's syndrome). New treatment combinations have

Recent Results in Cancer Research, Vol. 139

been tried and successfully carried out (Holloway et al. 1992). Recombinant interferon alpha (rIFN-α), for example, is very effective in combination with photochemotherapy (psoralens and ultraviolet A, PUVA) or combined with retinoids (isotretinoin/etretinate). These treatment procedures are fairly nonaggressive when compared to classical chemotherapy with cytotoxic and cytostatic drugs (COP/CHOP/COP-BLAM with and without granulocyte-macrophage colony-stimulating factor, GM-CSF). Many centers still perform minimally aggressive chemotherapy with the Knospe scheme with or without a combination of spotted radiotherapy or topical carmustine (BCNU) and mustard nitrogen. Since the first preliminary results with extracorporeal photopheresis (ECP) were reported by Edelson et al. in 1987, this therapeutic concept had a meteoric career. ECP centers in dermatologic departments and departments of other branches of medicine have increased in number in the United States up to 60 and in Europe up to 30, with more that ten in Germany alone (Edelson et al. 1987, 1991).

Background of Mechanisms of Action

In short, the mechanisms of action behind ECP are deduced from experimental evidence in which it has been shown that the intravenous exposure of the immune system, in particular in mice, with syngeneic cells from in vitro manipulated autoreactive clones of T cells can induce autoimmune diseases. In particular, in the model of experimental encephalomyelitis it was shown that when cells which were in vitro lethally damaged but not totally destroyed (preserved T cell receptor, TCR) were reinjected into syngeneic mice, the animal become resistant to the induction of the disease by repeated infusion of viable autoreactive T cells (Ben-Nun et al. 1981; Bergar et al. 1990; Marks et al. 1990; Perez et al. 1989). There is increasing evidence that by extracorporeal photoirradiation of a buffy coat made of leukocytes and plasma loaden with 8-methoxypsoralen (8-MOP) and activation by UVA, the cells will become stimulated in an immunoreaction after reintroduction to the patient's immune system against the malignant clone of T cells. This is followed by an improved ability of the host's immune system to fight, for instance, against lymphoma cells or other pathological clones, as in T cell-autoimmune diseases (Gasparro et al. 1990; Khavari et al. 1988; Marks et al. 1990).

Technical Procedure

Presently, the procedure of ECP is done in the following way: 8-MOP is taken orally 30–120 min (depending on the galenic formulation of the drug) before starting the procedure. A new method is to inject liquid 8-MOP into the buffy coat bag in order to guarantee exact plasma levels (Knobler 1987).

The patient is placed beside the photopheresis machine either in bed or on a chair as for dialysis, depending on his or her general condition. Venous access is performed mostly in the cubital veins. Blood is taken at about 20–40 ml/min, depending on the patient's blood pressure, and is centrifugated and samples of the buffy coat (leukocytes and plasma) are taken in a separate bag. The average amount of plasma sampled is 300 ml per treatment. Six centrifugation cycles are necessary to sample about 240 ml leukocytes, i.e., six cycles, 40 ml each. The erythrocyte fraction is immediately reinfused after every centrifugation cycle. Immediately after the first leukocytes have passed into the buffy coat bag, irradiation by an UVA source is started and the leukocytes, together with the plasma, are circulated through a specially constructed plastic tube placed between two rows of UVA lamps. The irradiation time is about 3–4 h, depending on the hematocrit. A loss of UV energy must be calculated based on the additional number of erythrocytes in the buffy coat. The average irradiation dose of a peripheral mononuclear blood cell is about 2 J/cm^2. Depending on the form of venous access, the patient is either detached from the machine immediately after centrifugation (sampling period) or remains in bed continuously beside the machine until irradiation has been finished. Thereafter, the buffy coat with the irradiated cells and plasma components is reinfused over a period of about 45–60 min. The same procedure is repeated on the next day. Two treatment sessions constitute one treatment cycle, which is normally repeated again after 4 weeks. Depending on the type of CTCL, disease progression, combined treatment regimens, or treatment during remission, the intervals between cycles can be reduced to 2 weeks or prolonged to 6–8 weeks.

Overall Results

During the last 5 years, some reports appeared on the successful outcome of CTCL with photopheresis (Armus et al. 1990; Edelson et al. 1987; Heald et al. 1992; Knobler 1987; Zic et al. 1992). The most impressive study is the one from 19987 in which it was shown that 27 out of 37 CTCL patients with otherwise resistant CTCL responded with an average of 64% decrease in the cutaneous involvement after 22 ± 10 weeks (Edelson et al. 1987). Eight of ten patients with lymph node involvement belonged to the responder group, 24 out of 29 had an exfoliative type of CTCL erythroderma, and 20 out of 28 had a disease which was formerly refractory to standard chemotherapy regimens. In an update it was reported that the median survival time of the patients from the erythroderma group was 62 months, which is about twice as long as was reported with other CTCL treatment modalities (Edelson et al. 1991; Green et al. 1981; Weinstock and Horm 1988). On the other hand, 25% of the CTCL patient showed a limited response only, and adjunctive therapies have therefore been tried. For example, Heald et al. noticed additional improvement by the addition of low-dose oral methotrexate in those patients not responding to photopheresis alone. The dose selected was similar to that which is used in psoriatic erythroderma (approximately 15 mg/week). Another adjunctive therapy is the use of recombinant interferon alpha three times a week or every other day, or spotted local radiotherapy of tumors (Rook et al. 1991). Furthermore, there is strong evidence that follow-up therapy with photopheresis every 4 weeks can help to prolong or maintain the remission after electron beam therapy (Edelson et al. 1991; Heald et al. 1992). Our own experience in more than 20 patients with advanced stages of CTCL (T3 and T4) show that Sézary's syndrome and the erythrodermic phase of MF responded well to monotherapy of ECP. In tumor stages of MF, however, it is appropriate to combine from the beginning ECP with interferon alpha, which acts additively or synergistically to ECP (Vowels et al. 1992). The overall results of the studies reported so far and our own results are presented in Table 1.

Selection of Cutaneous T Cell Lymphoma Patients

As long as the mechanisms of action in ECP are not fully understood, indications and selection of cases depend to a great extent on personal experience and written reports. However, there is a consensus that one selection criterium is important, namely a competent immune system which can respond with an specific immune reaction to a modified malignant cell reintroduced after photopheresis to the body. Therefore, as was discussed in depth at the third Meeting of the European Society of Extracorporeal Photochemotherapy in September in Berlin, patients should only be included in a photopheresis scheme if an appropriate immune response can be evaluated before starting. This should be done by flow cytometry to get information about the leukocyte subpopulations and the number of CD8 cells

Table 1. Results of extracorporeal photopheresis[a] in cutaneous T cell lymphoma

Reference	Patients (*n*)	TMN	CR	PR	SD	PRO
Edelson et al. (1987)	37	≥T3	9	13	5	10
Heald et al. (1992)	19	≥T3	5	10	4	–
Armus et al. (1990)	8	≥T2/T3	3	4	–	1[a]
Heald et al. (1992)	29	≥T3	6	6	5	?
Zic et al. (1992)	20	≥T2	5	6	4	?[a]
Berlin-Steglitz Medical Center (unpublished)	17	≥T3	3	6	3	5[a]

CR, complete remission; PR, partial remission; SD, stable disease; PRO, progressive disease.
[a] With adjunctive treatment in some cases (inferferon alpha, local radiotherapy, methotrexate).

(suppressor/cytotoxic subset), the CD45RO (suppressor/inducer subset, and the number of NK cells. Multitest Merieux provides information about the recall antigen profile; if possible, in vitro tests should also be performed, i.e., stimulation of peripheral blood monoclonal cells (PBMC) in vitro with phytohemagglutinin (PHA), pokeweed mitogen (PWM), and concanavalin A (ConA). On the other hand, it has been shown that Sézary patients with low or not detectable CD8 cells by flow cytometry before therapy can respond, giving concrete evidence that in particular cases only a few cells are necessary for the transmission of a specific clone-directed immune response. Furthermore, it was the consensus that concurrent strong immunosuppressive medication, with the exception of low-dose methotrexate or chlorambucil, should be avoided. Finally, it was recommended that drugs are used which probably work synergistically or which bring additive effects, e.g., alpha interferon. These effects may be the release of tumor necrosis factor (TNF) alpha, increase of NK cell activity, antiproliferative effects, immunomodulation, and enhancement of tumor-infiltrating lymphocytes after photopheresis (Rook et al. 1991; Vowels et al. 1992).

Adverse Effects

It is rather surprising that in thousands of ECP treatment sessions only a very small number of major adverse effects have been reported. These were in particular concurrent staphylococcal infection in two cases due to immunoincompetence of CTCL patients and lack of supervision. Patients with recurrent herpes simplex infection have shown a flare up immediately after treatment, in two cases a generalized eczema herpeticatum-like rash. In some patients hypotension can be seen during the sampling period, which in most cases is only temporary and can be managed without difficulties. From publications and data on file (Therakos Ltd.), there is now evidence that during or immediately after a procedure no patient has died as a result of a technical complication of ECP. Other adverse effects are local pain at the venous access, hematomas due to heparinization, and local phlebitis. A general immunosuppression is not induced, as far as we know from all reports in the literature and from our own experience. For example, follow-up of the reaction of PBMC to PHA stimulation and measurement of different cytokines in vitro showed and increase in major cell mediators such as gamma interferon, GM-CSF, and interleukin-6 secretion of the cells paralleled by the general improvement of the patient's condition.

The Future of Extracorporeal Photopheresis in Cutaneous T Cell Lymphoma Patients

Up to now all reports on ECP in CTCL so far reflect noncontrolled studies, because only ECP response data and data on the remission time are compared to historical ones (Green et al. 1981; Weinstock and Horm 1988). Therefore, further evidence for the reliability of ECP can only be obtained from controlled studies presently going on. The European Society of Extracorporeal Photochemotherapy has initiated two studies: one will compare ECP combined with interferon alpha with ECP and spotted radiotherapy in T2/T3 with and without lymph node involvement; the other will investigate ECP and Weinstein's scheme followed by ECP during maintenance.

Other indications for ECP not discussed in this context are diseases in which autoreactive T cell clones are most preferentially responsible for the development of diseases such as chronic graft versus host disease and transplant rejections (heart, kidney) (Bolwell et al. 1990), progressive systemic sclerosis (Rook et al. 1992), cutaneous lupus erythematosus (Knobler et al. 1992), and pemphigus vulgaris (Gollnick et al. 1993).

References

Armus S, Keyes B, Cahill C, Berger C, Crater D, Scarborough D, Klainer A, Bisaccia E (1990) Photopheresis for the treatment of cutaneous T cell-lymphoma. J Am Acad Dermatol 23:898–902

Ben-Nun A, Wekerle H, Cohen IR (1981) Vaccination against autoimmune encephalomyelitis with T-lymphocyte line cells reactive against myelin basic protein. Nature 292:60–61

Berger CL, Perez MI, Laroche L, Edelson R (1990) Inhibition of autoimmune disease in a murine model of systemic lupus erythematosus induced by exposure to syngeneic photoinactivated lymphocytes. J Invest Dermatol 94:52–57

Bolwell B, Fishleder A, Lichtin A, Koo A, Camisa C, Green R, Barna B (1990) Photopheresis in the treatment of chronic graft vs host disease (cGVHD). 32nd Annual Meeting of the American Society of Hematologists, 2106A

Edelson R, Berger C, Gasparro F, Jegasothy B, Heald P, Wintroub B, Vonderheid E, Knobler R, Wolff K, Plewig G, McKiernan G, Christiansen I, Oster M, Honigsmann H, Wilford H, Kokoschka E, Rehle T, Perez M, Stingl G, Laroche L (1987) Treatment of cutaneous T-cell lymphoma by extracorporeal photochemotherapy. N Engl J Med 316:297–303

Edelson RL, Heald P, Perez M, Rook A (1991) Photopheresis update. Prog Dermatol 25(3):1–6

Gasparro FP, Dall'Amico R, O'Malley M, Heald PW, Edelson RL (1990) Cell membrane DNA: a new target for psoralen photoadduct formation. Photochem Photobiol 52:315–321

Gollnick HPM, Owsianowski M, Taube KM, Orfanos CE (1993) Unresponsive severe generalized pemphigus vulgaris successfully controlled by extracorporeal photophoresis. J Am Acad Dermatol 28:122–124

Green SB, Byar DP, Lamberg SI (1981) Prognostic variables in mycosis fungoides. Cancer 47:2671–2677

Heald P, Perez M, Christensen I, Dobbs N, McKiernan G, Edelson RL (1989) Photopheresis therapy of cutaneous T-cell lymphoma: the Yale-New Haven Hospital experience. Yale J Biol Med 62/6:629–638

Heald P, Rook A, Perez M, Wintroub B, Knobler R, Jegasothy B, Gasparro F, Berger C, Edelson R (1992) Treatment of erythrodermic cutaneous T-cell lymphoma with extracorporeal photochemotherapy. J Am Acad Dermatol 27:427–433

Holloway KB, Franklin FP, Ramos-Caro FA (1992) Therapeutic alternatives in cutaneous T-cell lymphoma. J Am Acad Dermatol 27:367–378

Khavari PA, Edelson RL, Lider O, Gasparro FP, Weiner HL, Cohen IR (1988) Specific vaccination against photoinactivated cloned T-cells. Clin Res 36:662 A

Knobler RM (1987) Photopheresis–extracorporeal irradiation of 8-MOP containing blood–a new therapeutic modality. Blut 54:247–250

Knobler RM, Graninger W, Graninger W, Lindmaier A, Trautinger F, Smolen JS (1992) Extracorporeal photochemotherapy for the treatment of systemic lupus erythematosus. Arthritis Rheum 35:319–324

Marks DI, Rockman SP, Oziemski MA et al (1990) Mechanisms of lymphocytotoxicity induced by extracorporeal photochemotherapy for cutaneous T-cell lymphoma. J Clin Invest 86:2080–2085

Perez M, Edelson R, Laroche L, Berger C (1989) Inhibition of antiskin allograft immunity by infusions with syngeneic photoinactivated effector lymphocytes. J Invest Dermatol 92:669–676

Rook AH, Freundlich B, Jegasothy BV, Perez MI, Barr WG, Jimenez SA, Rietschel RL, Wintroub B, Kahaleh MB, Varga J, Heald PW, Steen V, Massa MC, Murphy GF, Perniciaro C, Istfan M, Ballas SK, Edelson RL (1992) Treatment of systemic sclerosis with extracorporeal photochemotherapy. Arch Dermatol 128:337–346

Rook AH, Prystowsky MB, Cassin M, Boufal M, Lessin SR (1991) Combined therapy for Sézary syndrome with extracorporeal photochemotherapy and low-dose interferon alpha therapy. Arch Dermatol 127:1535–1540

Vowels BR, Cassin M, Boufal H, Walsh LJ, Rook AH (1992) Extracorporeal photochemotherapy induces the production of tumor necrosis factor-α by monocytes: implications for the treatment of cutaneous T-cell lymphoma and systemic sclerosis. J Invest Dermatol 98:686–692

Weinstock MA, Horm JW (1988) Population-based estimate of survival and determinants of prognosis with mycosis fungoides. Cancer 260:42–46

Zic J, Arzubiaga C, Salhany KE, Parker RA, Wilson D, Stricklin GP, Greer J, King LE (1992) Extracorporeal photophoresis for treatment of cutaneous T-cell lymphoma. J Am Acad Dermatol 1992:729–736

Laser Therapy of Skin Tumors

M. Landthaler, R.-M. Szeimies, and U. Hohenleutner

Department of Dermatology, University of Regensburg, 93042 Regensburg, Germany

Abstract

Malignant skin tumors can be treated by CO_2 laser excision or vaporization, neodymium: yttrium aluminum garnet (Nd:YAG) laser coagulation, and systemic or topical photodynamic therapy (PDT). Possible indications for CO_2 laser vaporization include superficial basal cell carcinomas, actinic keratoses, Bowen's disease, actinic cheilitis, and leukoplakias. The Nd:YAG laser may be used for coagulation of basal cell carcinomas, squamous cell carcinomas, Kaposi's sarcoma, and metastatic skin tumors. Systemic and topical PDT is still an experimental modality and is mostly applied for treatment of basal cell carcinomas. However, laser treatment of skin tumors is not yet considered as standard therapy and should be confined to selected patients. Further clinical studies are necessary to determine the role of laser therapy in this special indication.

Introduction

Although laser therapy of tumors is well established in many medical specialities, treatment of skin tumors with lasers is not yet a routine method.

Malignant skin tumors can be treated by laser excision, laser coagulation, laser vaporization, or photodynamic therapy (PDT). The most commonly applied lasers are the CO_2 laser, the neodymium: yttrium aluminum garnet (Nd:YAG) laser, and the dye laser as well as incoherent light sources for PDT (Landthaler 1992).

The CO_2 laser is a continuous wave light source emitting in the infrared at 10.600 nm. The radiation of this laser is strongly absorbed by tissue water, independently of the presence of chromophores. A focal small spot size and a high output power generate high-power densities, resulting in vaporization

Recent Results in Cancer Research, Vol. 139

and cutting of tissue. With a defocused laser beam it is possible to vaporize tissue.

CO_2 laser excision of skin tumors has the following advantages compared to scalpel surgery (Dover et al. 1990):

1. Hemostasis and reduced postoperative swelling due to the fact that blood and lymph vessels up to a diameter of 0.5 mm are sealed
2. Hemostasis in highly vascular tissues and in anticoagulated patients
3. Decreased postoperative pain resulting from the sealing of nerve endings
4. No interaction with pacemakers or electronic monitoring systems
5. Surgery in infected surgical sites is possible

The Nd:YAG laser also emits in the infrared with a wavelength of 1060 nm. Since Nd:YAG laser radiation is relatively poorly absorbed in tissue, it penetrates deeply into the skin, resulting in coagulation up to a depth of 6 mm. The depth of coagulation can be controlled by variation of laser power and exposure time (Landthaler et al. 1984).

Photodynamic therapy is an experimental modality using red light in conjunction with a systemic or topical photosensitizer. Photosensitizers have a longer retention time in malignant tumors compared with normal tissue. Irradiation with red light at a wavelength of 630 nm results in photochemical generation of cytotoxic oxygen species within the tumor. Targets of PDT may be proliferating tumor cells as well as tumor vasculature. Hematoporphyrin derivative (HpD) is a synthetic derivative of hemoglobin and a mixture of porphyrins. It can be used systemically by intravenous administration. One of the major side effects of systemic application is severe photosensitization of the skin lasting up to 6 weeks after injection (Wieman et al. 1988; Gomer 1988).

5-Aminolaevulinic acid (ALA) is a precursor of protoporphyrin IX (Pp IX) in the biosynthetic pathway of heme. Since epidermal and tumor cells can synthesize Pp IX when exposed to an adequate concentration of exogeneous ALA, the substance can be used for topical photodynamic therapy (Kennedy et al. 1990). Light sources for PDT are argon pumped-dye lasers (wavelength, 630 nm), gold vapor lasers (wavelength, 628 nm) but also incoherent light sources with a wavelength between 600 and 700 nm (Szeimies et al. 1994).

Clinical Applications

Most studies regarding laser therapy of skin tumors deal with patients with basal cell carcinomas.

In 1981, Bailin et al. described a CO_2 laser modification of Mohs surgery, and Wheeland et al. (1987) in 1987 the combination of CO_2 laser vaporization and curettage of superficial basal cell carcinomas (BCC). Despite excellent results, Wheeland et al. did not advocate this form of treatment for all types of BCC and especially not for BCC in high-risk locations such as the central face.

Another approach to laser therapy of BCC is coagulation by means of the Nd:YAG laser. Due to the limited depth of coagulation, only fairly superficial and moderately sized tumors should be treated. In a study of our own (Landthaler 1992), 172 epithelial skin tumors in 50 patients were treated; 85% of these tumors were BCC. In all cases a 3-year follow-up was possible, and the 3-year cure rate was 85%. These preliminary data demonstrate that the Nd:YAG laser qualifies for therapy of epithelial tumors, but the recurrence rate of 15% was unacceptably high. The advantages of Nd:YAG laser therapy are that the procedure is on an outpatient basis, in most cases only one treatment was necessary, there was low risk of bleeding or infection, and there was no need for postoperative dressings. The greatest disadvantages were the lack of histological control, delayed wound healing, and the lack of long-term results. Improvements in cure rate are possible by extending safety margins and deeper coagulation by increasing laser power and exposure time, but this may result in worse cosmetic results. Indications for Nd:YAG laser coagulation are tumors in older patients, multiple superficial tumors, and tumors in damaged skin. However, since cryotherapy is suited for these indications as well and yields better cosmetic results, the Nd:YAG laser in our experience cannot be considered as a routine method.

As early as 1981, Dougherty reported the use of systemic photodynamic therapy for cutaneous and subcutaneous malignancies. Many studies have since been published demonstrating that cutaneous and subcutaneous tumors do respond to systemic photodynamic therapy, but most of these studies lack sufficient patient numbers and important data such as type of BCC, localization, tumor thickness, histologic data, and long-term follow-up (see references in Landthaler 1992). Systemic photodynamic therapy may be of advantage especially with multiple tumors as well as in patients with nevoid BCC syndrome. Tse et al. (1983) described systemic PDT of 40 BCC in three patients; 33 lesions (82.5%) showed complete response on biopsy findings. Within a follow-up of 12–14 months the recurrence rate was 10.8%. Especially thicker ulcerated and crusted lesions did not respond to PDT.

To avoid side effects of systemic PDT, skin tumors can be treated by topical PDT. Santoro et al. treated 292 BCC with a tumor thickness less than 2 mm in 50 patients by topical PDT using Tetraphenylporphinsulfonate (TPPS) photosensitizer in a 2% solution. Recurrence rate was 10.6% (Santoro et al. 1990). Kennedy and coworkers (1990) treated 80 BCC with a topical application of 20% ALA oil-in-water emulsion; 90% of the treated tumors showed a complete response. Although these two studies clearly demonstrate that BCC do respond to topical PDT, this procedure has still to be considered as an experimental therapy and further research is necessary.

Since in most of the reports describing laser treatment of BCC patients with squamous cell carcinomas (SCC) were included, it is obvious that SCC can be treated with the same procedures as BCC, but one has to keep in mind the fact that SCC have the potential to become invasive and to metastasize (Landthaler 1992).

Superficial skin tumors such as Bowen's disease and actinic cheilitis can be treated by CO_2 laser vaporization or topical PDT. Leukoplakias of the oral mucosa can be treated by means of CO_2 laser vaporization or Nd:YAG laser coagulation, but before treatment of oral leukoplakias biopsies are mandatory to avoid inadequate treatment of invasive carcinoma (references in Landthaler 1992). Smaller superficial nodules of Kaposi's sarcoma can be cogulated by means of the argon laser, and more nodular and thicker lesions by the Nd:YAG laser. Recently, five cases of AIDS-related Kaposi's sarcoma with diffuse superficial and nodular oral lesions treated with HpD and systemic PDT were reported. Dramatic, early, partial and complete responses were observed (Schweitzer and Visscher 1990).

Since the CO_2 laser is capable of sealing blood and lymph vessels, it was hoped that this laser could be of benefit in oncologic surgery by preventing dissemination of tumor cells during surgical procedures. However, recently, a retrospective study of patients with malignant melanoma who underwent surgical treatment by scalpel or CO_2 laser excision, respectively, was conducted. It did not prove the benefit of CO_2 laser with respect to recurrence rate and survival of patients (Bilik et al. 1987). Additionally, it must be kept in mind that skin graft take is impaired after CO_2 laser excision and that biologically active material can be transported to deep tissue layers during laser cutting (Lejeune et al. 1980; Frenz et al. 1988). Therefore, in our opinion neither the Nd:YAG-laser nor the CO_2 laser have a definite place in therapy of primary malignant melanomas.

Nd:YAG laser coagulation or CO_2 laser excision may be helpful in selected patients as a palliative therapy in metastatic skin tumors. This is also true for PDT, especially in patients with erysipelas carcinomatosum following breast cancer (Landthaler 1992).

Conclusion

Without doubt, lasers can be used in selected patients for therapy of malignant skin tumors, with some advantages compared to conventional therapeutic modalities, but this treatment modality cannot be considered as standard therapy of skin tumors.

Laser application may be of advantage in:

1. Multiple superficial tumors
2. Older patients refusing scalpel surgery
3. Patients with pacemakers and bleeding tendency
4. Tumors in specific locations such as the oral mucosa or the genital area
5. Palliative treatment.

Future clinical studies are necessary to determine definitely the role of laser therapy for skin tumors.

References

Bailin PL, Ratz JL, Lutz-Nagey L (1981) CO_2 laser modification of Mohs' surgery. J Dermatol Surg Oncol 7:621–623

Bilik R, Kahanovich S, Rubin M et al (1987) Morbidity and recurrence rates after surgical treatment of malignant melanoma by scalpel versus CO_2 laser beam. Surg Gynecol Obstet 165:333–338

Dougherty T (1981) Photoradiation therapy for cutaneous and subcutaneous malignancies. J Invest Dermatol 77:122–124

Dover JS, Arndt KA, Geronemus RG, Olbricht SM, Noe JM, Stern RS (1990) Illustrated cutaneous laser surgery. A practitioner's guide. Appleton and Lange, Norwalk

Frenz M, Mathezloic F, Stoffel MHS et al (1988) Transport of biologically active material in laser cutting. Lasers Surg Med 8:562–566

Gomer CJ (1988) Photodynamic therapy in the treatment of malignancies. Semin Hematol 26:27–34

Kennedy JC, Pottier RH, Pross DC (1990) Photodynamic therapy with endogeneous protoporphyrin IX: basic principles and present clinical experience. J Photochem Photobiol 6:143–148

Landthaler M (1992) Premalignant and malignant skin lesions. In: Achauer BM, Vanderkam VM, Berns MW (eds) Lasers in plastic surgery and dermatology. Thieme, Stuttgart, pp 34–44

Landthaler M, Brunner R, Haina D et al (1984) Der Neodym-YAG-Laser in der Dermatologie. Munch Med Wochenschr 126:1108–1112

Lejeune FJ, van Hoof G, Gerard A (1980) Impairment of skin graft take after CO_2 laser surgery in melanoma patients. Br J Surg 67:318–320

Santoro O, Bandieramonte G, Melloni E et al (1990) Photodynamic therapy by topical meso-tetraphenylporphine-sulfonate tetrasodium salt administration in superficial basal cell carcinomas. Cancer Res 50:4501–4503

Schweitzer VG, Visscher D (1990) Photodynamic therapy for treatment of AIDS-related oral Kaposi's sarcoma. Otolaryngol Head Neck Surg 102:639–649

Szeimies RM, Hein R, Bäumler W et al (1994) A possible new incoherent lamp for photodynamic treatment of superficial skin lesions. Acta Derm Venereol (Stockh) 74:117–119

Tse DT, Dutton JJ, Weingeist TW et al (1983) HPD photoradiation for ocular melanoma and basal cell nevus syndrome. Lasers Surg Med 3:168 (abstract)

Wheeland RG, Bailin PL, Ratz JL, Roenigk RK (1987) Carbon dioxide laser vaporization and curettage in the treatment of large or multiple superficial basal cell carcinomas. J Dermatol Surg Oncol 13:119–125

Wieman TJ, Mang TS, Fingar VH et al (1988) Effect of photodynamic therapy on blood flow in normal and tumor vessels. Surgery 104:512–517

Management of Human Immunodeficiency Virus-Associated Malignancies

M.A. Conant

University of California Medical Center, San Francisco, California, USA

Abstract

A number of malignancies which have been seen with other immunodeficiency diseases have appeared in patients immunosuppressed by the human immunodeficiency virus (HIV) infection. These include Kaposi's sarcoma, lymphomas, superficially spreading basal cell carcinomas, and squamous cell carcinomas. The fact that Kaposi's sarcoma is the most common of these malignancies and is seen almost exclusively among homosexual men remains an enigma.

The dermatological treatment of Kaposi's sarcoma includes observation, surgical excision, radiation therapy, interlesional chemotherapy, and topical liquid nitrogen. When the disease becomes more aggressive, systemic chemotherapy, using a combination of chemotherapeutic agents, will often slow disease progression. It is essential that the chemotherapy be given in a dose that will slow the course of the malignancy, but will not further immunosuppress the patient.

The treatment of lymphomas in HIV-infected patients has been less than satisfactory, with a high mortality rate. Aggressive therapy of these lymphomas using combination therapy has been the most successful in increasing survival.

Malignancies with Known Human Immunodeficiency Virus Association

The first harbinger of the acquired immunodeficiency syndrome (AIDS) epidemic was the recognition by physicians in New York and San Francisco that a rare cutaneous malignancy, Kaposi's sarcoma, was being seen with astonishing frequency amongst 30-year-old homosexual men. In the first year of the epidemic, more than half of all of the cases of AIDS were attributed to Kaposi's sarcoma (Centers for Disease Control 1981). Soon,

Recent Results in Cancer Research, Vol. 139

non-Hodgkin's B cell lymphoma was recognized as a second AIDS-associated malignancy (Ziegler et al. 1982). Over time, two other malignancies, superficial spreading basal cell carcinoma and squamous cell carcinoma emerged as HIV associated malignancies. Three other malignancies have also been seen in HIV-positive individuals: malignant melanoma, Hodgkin's disease, and Sezary's disease.

The epidemiology of Kaposi's sarcoma has strongly suggested that this rare and unusual condition may not be a true sarcoma, but indeed may represent a vascular hyperplasia which manifests itself in immunodeficient individuals (Tappero et al. 1993). In the United States, Kaposi's sarcoma is seen almost exclusively in homosexual men. If a male acquires HIV infection from a blood transfusion or from intravenous drug use, his chance of developing Kaposi's sarcoma is only 2%, whereas a male who becomes HIV infected from having sex with another man has a 15%–30% chance of developing Kaposi's sarcoma. Furthermore, the incidence of Kaposi's sarcoma in HIV-infected men has declined steadily and progressively from 1981 until the present time. In the early 1980s, Kaposi's sarcoma constituted 35%2–350% of all of the initial AIDS diagnoses. Today, Kaposi's sarcoma constitutes only 12%–17% of initial AIDS diagnoses. Finally, Kaposi's sarcoma is being seen with increased frequency in HIV-negative homosexual men who were sexually active in the late 1970s and early 1980s. I have cared for one such patient, who showed no evidence of Kaposi's sacoma until he was immunosuppressed so that he could receive a pancreas and kidney transplant. Shortly after his immunosuppression, lesions of Kaposi's sarcoma developed at sites of trauma, where staples had been placed into his abdominal wound. When his immunosuppressive therapy was reduced, his lesion of Kaposi's sarcoma partially involuted, but did not completely disappear.

All of these observations lead to the hypothesis that Kaposi's sarcoma is caused by some infectious agent or some environmental substance that was transmitted among homosexual men in the 1970s and early 1980s. This agent, in the presence of a normal immune system, does not produce disease; however, if the patient becomes immunosuppressed as a result of HIV infection or some other source of immunosuppression, the lesions of Kaposi's sarcoma appear. This hypothesis does of course provide the hope that if the causative agent could be identified, a direct and effective treatment for Kaposi's sarcoma might be developed.

Lymphomas are seen with increased frequency in individuals who are profoundly immunosuppressed. Since many of these lymphomas appear to be B cell lymphomas, which have been associated with chronic Epstein-Barr virus infection, it appears that these lymphomas, like Kaposi' sarcoma, are the direct result of an infectious agent which produces an opportunistic malignancy as a result of HIV-induced immunosuppression. While the incidence of B cell lymphomas is extremely low, the prevalence of this condition is increasing due to the increased survival of HIV-infected patients as a result of aggressive physician/patient management, antiretroviral intervention, and prophylaxis against opportunistic infections. As we become more and more successful in preventing the opportunistic infections which are killing our patients, we will unfortunately see larger numbers of patients presenting with non-Hodgkin's lymphomas.

Studies have not yet established a direct correlation between superficially spreading body basal cell skin cancers and HIV infection. Clinicians seeing large numbers of HIV-infected patients, however, have identified these malignancies as a common cutaneous problem and one which appears to occur at much greater frequency that is seen in age- and race-matched immunocompetent individuals. It is of interest that most of these malignancies present as superficially spreading body basal cell skin cancers and not nodular ulcerative basal cell skin cancers of the face and sun-exposed areas.

Finally, squamous cell carcinoma is being seen with increased frequency particularly in the anogenital area (Melbye et al. 1993). The frequency of this malignancy is almost certainly due to the high incidence of human papillomavirus (HPV) infection common amongst homosexual men (Palefsky et al. 1993). Often, these malignancies will present as a small perianal papule confused by the patient with a preexisting wart. Excisional biopsy will show evidence of human papillomaviral infection as well as squamous cell carcinoma in situ. These malignancies should be managed aggressively, since recurrences are frequent and metastases are common.

Human papilloma infection of the vulva and cervix of HIV-infected women is also extremely common (Bensaid-Mrejen and Barau 1993). Invasive squamous cell carcinoma of the cervix is already being seen with increased frequency withing HIV-infected women in the northeastern part of the United States. These cancers are extremely aggressive and often the woman dies of metastatic carcinoma of the cervix before succumbing to her underlying HIV disease.

Squamous cell carcinoma of the glabrous skin of the body is also seen with increased frequency in HIV-infected individuals. Wide surgical excision or aggressive ablative therapy is essential, since these cancers are very aggressive and tend to recur with astonishing rapidity.

Suspected Human Immunodeficiency Virus-Associated Malignancies

Malignant melanoma has been reported to occur more frequently in HIV-infected individuals. This association has certainly not been well established, and it may well be that the association has been that of two common conditions occurring in the same population of patients. Further, homosexual men, particularly those who are infected with HIV, often choose to use their spare time and extra income to vacation in locations such as the Caribbean and the Hawaiian Islands and may be at greater risk of malignant melanoma simply because of lifestyle rather than their immune status.

Hodgkin's disease has also been seen with increased frequency in HIV-infected individuals (Hessol et al. 1993). Again, it is not certain whether this is a nonlinked association of two common problems occurring in young men simultaneously or whether Hodgkin's disease is causally related to HIV infection.

Finally, Sezary's syndrome has been seen in a few individuals infected with both HTLV-I and HIV. It is thought that the coinfection with two related retroviruses may lead to an acceleration of one or both of the disease processes because of the influence of enhancing genes from the coinfecting virus.

Treatment of Kaposi's Sarcoma

The treatment of Kaposi's sarcoma depends on a number of clinical considerations. These include the patient's CD4 count, the total number of lesions, the duration of each of the lesions, the rate of new lesion formation, and the location of individual lesions.

Many patients will develop Kaposi's sarcoma early in the course of their disease, even with CD4 counts as high as 800–1200. Generally, these patients will have a slowly progressive course characterized by periods when there are bursts of new lesions and periods of remission when new lesion formation is rare. As the CD4 count drops, the rate of new lesion formation increases, and when the CD4 count drops below 200 the rate of new lesion formation may become considerable and may require systemic chemotherapy for control. Other patients are seen who do not develop lesions of Kaposi's sarcoma until late in the course of their disease, often after they have developed other AIDS-defining infections, such as *Pneumocystis carinii* pneumonia. These patients will often experience only one or two lesions of Kaposi's sarcoma and the condition will not constitute a major cause of morbidity or a major cosmetic problem. As a rule, the higher the CD4 count, the slower the progression of the Kaposi's sarcoma and the greater response to any therapeutic modality chosen by the clinician.

The total number of Kaposi's lesions will, of course, determine the optimal treatment program. Patients with only one or two lesions in sites that are not conspicuous may elect to have no treatment at all. Patients with extensive lesions on the face, where they are a source of tremendous emotional pain, or on the lower legs or thighs, where they can cause significant physical pain, will need aggressive therapy. It should be remembered that lesions of Kaposi's sarcoma appear in waves. The clinician who is confronted with a patient who has suddenly developed ten or 15 new lesions should not be stampeded into a program of systemic chemotherapy based on the erroneous assumption that ten or 15 more lesions will soon follow. It is common for the patient to develop a burst of new lesions and then go many weeks to months with only one or two additional lesions.

The duration of the lesion will also determine treatment. Newly formed lesions respond dramatically to intralesional vinblastine, topical liquid nitrogen application, and radiation therapy, whereas older lesions will only flatten in response to these treatment modalities, but a slate gray macular pigmentation will remain. A physician managing a patient with Kaposi's sarcoma should urge the patient to present at the clinic as soon as a new lesion is seen, so that lesion can be treated at the earliest possible date.

The rate of new lesion formation will ultimately decide whether the patient needs to consider systemic chemotherapy or one of the newer experimental interventions. Patients who are developing only a few lesions each month can generally be managed with interlesional chemotherapy, liquid nitrogen, or radiation therapy. In those patients where ten or 15 new lesions are appearing each month, the clinician and the patient should discuss the judicious use of systemic chemotherapy.

Finally, the location of the lesion will often dictate therapy. One small lesion on the cheek can be well managed with interlesional vinblastine. A lesion of the same size occurring on the conjunctiva of the lower lid is best handled with radiation therapy. A lesion on the plantar surface of the foot responds well to liquid nitrogen or a combination of liquid nitrogen and vinblastine, whereas multiple coalescing lesions of the lower extremity are best managed by occlusive stockings and extended-field radiation therapy.

The clinician should not forget that even if the patient is receiving systemic chemotherapy, there is still a place for interlesional treatment, especially with those lesions causing undo emotional pain for the patient, such as lesions on the face or lesions which are visible when the patient goes to the beach or the gymnasium. Indeed, interlesional therapy is even more effective in the patient with Kaposi's sarcoma who is receiving concomitant chemotherapy.

Treatment Modalities

The treatment of Kaposi's sarcoma can be divided into the local management of individual lesions, systemic chemotherapy, and experimental treatments. The local management can be accomplished with five commonly used techniques (Tappero et al. 1993): observation, intralesional vinblastine, liquid nitrogen, excision, and radiation therapy. A single individual lesion can simply be observed. It should be remembered, however, that the presence of even one lesion can cause tremendous emotional stress for many patients. While the clinician may not think that one lesion of Kaposi's sarcoma in the mons pubis is of any great consequence, since few people will actually see the lesion, the physical presence of the lesion is viewed by the patient as an invasion of his body and patients are often profoundly grateful if the physician will treat the lesion to either eradicate it or reduce its size.

In my hands interlesional vinblastine injected into the lesion every 2 weeks is the single mose effective treatment modality that I have found. The vinblastine is diluted to 0.2 mg per cc and 0.05 cc is injected at each site every 2 weeks until the lesion is no longer palpable or completely eradicated. Injections should be spaced at 5 mm intervals, so that small lesions may need only one injection where larger lesions may need four or five injections. The needle should be placed perpendicular to the skin and the clinician should remember that the greatest pathology resides in the upper two thirds of the dermis. We generally inject 2 cc (40 injection sites) every 2 weeks.

Patients are undressed and placed in a prone position and 40 lesions are injected. Two weeks later, the patient returns and is undressed and placed in the supine position, when 40 additional lesions are injected. In this way, all lesions can be treated in a reasonable time and the amount of blood to which the practitioner is exposed is kept to a minimum. An individual lesion usually requires three to five treatments. Lesions that are treated shortly after their appearance will be totally eradicated. Lesions which are older, and where there has already been extensive hemosiderosis into the surrounding dermis, will flatten and assume a slate gray pigmentation, but total eradication of the lesion will not be possible. Treatment should continue until the lesion is no longer palpable.

Liquid nitrogen is a fast an effective way of treating lesions and often gives a favorable cosmetic result. Aggressive use of liquid nitrogen can result in a central white scar, which is accentuated by the violaceous or gray appearance of the Kaposi's sarcoma, giving a bulls eye appearance. The combination of liquid nitrogen and interlesional vinblastine can be used with great facility on the palmar surfaces of the hands and the plantar surfaces of the feet. The direct injection of the lesion on the bottom of the foot results in tremendous pain. Those lesions can be lightly frozen with liquid nitrogen and then, just at the moment that the thaw occurs, the needle can be introduced with very little pain and then the interlesional Velban (vinblastine sulfate) can be injected into the lesion.

Excision of lesions is an obvious treatment modality. This is usually used to establish the initial diagnosis with an excisional biopsy. In my experience, the single instance where excisional therapy is the treatment of choice is in the occasional patient who develops an exophytic nodule of Kaposi's sarcoma, usually on the lower extremity. In these cases, marsupialization of the lesion, which is then allowed to heal by secondary intention, often gives an excellent cosmetic result.

Radiation therapy can be used to treat individual lesions of Kaposi's sarcoma. This modality is particularly useful in managing Kaposi's sarcoma lesions that are located on the eyelids or the conjunctiva. Kaposi's sarcoma in the mouth should be managed with intralesional vinblastine rather than radiation therapy, because of the severe xerostomia that often follows radiation treatment of the oral mucosa. Extended-field radiation therapy of large lesions of Kaposi's sarcoma of the feet, lower legs, or thighs is often the treatment of choice. Many radiation therapists choose to treat single lesions of Kaposi's sarcoma with 800 rad radiation given at a single visit. This approach is generally extremely effective and requires less patient time and less utilization of resources.

The systemic management of Kaposi's sarcoma is generally achieved using either single-agent vinblastine or a combination of vinblastine and vincristine or a combination of Adriamycin (doxorubicin hydrochloride), bleomycin, and vincristine or with oral VP-16. These treatments can result in profound toxicities and should be administered only by a trained chemotherapist or oncologist. The principles of AIDS systemic chemotherapy should be to use the lowest possible dose of chemotherapeutic agents, which will slow down the progression of the Kaposi's sarcoma. This is contrary to the principles of cancer chemotherapy. In the cancer patient, the oncologist attempts to eliminate all of the viable cancer cells. This requires pushing the chemotherapy up to the threshold of toxicity. If this approach is used in the HIV patient, profound immunosuppression will occur, opportunistic infections will appear, and the patient's life expectancy will be shortened. The principle of systemic chemotherapy of the HIV-positive patient is to slow down the progression of the disease in an effort to give the patient as much quality time as possible and hopefully to prolong his life until more effective forms of treatment can be found.

Interferon alpha has been used with limited success in treatment of patients with Kaposi's sarcoma (Kovacs et al. 1989). In some series, up to 50% of patients treated with interferon alpha with a dose of 10 million units a day (3–30 million) have shown partial or complete resolution of index lesions. Unfortunately, the treatment is of greatest efficacy when the patient's CD4 count is above 400. This is of course the group where disease progression is usually slow and patients respond to other more conservative treatment modalities. In my experience I have seen resolution of index lesions while the patient is being treated with systemic interferon alpha with the simultaneous appearance of new lesions of Kaposi's sarcoma at another location. This, coupled with the fact that some patients show a dramatic response to systemic treatment will interferon alpha and others show little or no response at all, suggests that there are different populations of Kaposi's sarcoma cells in the same and in different patients which appear to be more or less sensitive to interferon alpha therapy. Interferon alpha has been shown to have antiviral, antiproliferative, and immunomodulating characteristics. Which of these mechanisms of action are responsible for the benefits seen in Kaposi's sarcoma in the interferon alpha patient is not clear.

Experimental Treatments

Many new experimental treatments are being investigated. One such treatment is the combination of a cancer chemotherapeutic agent, 5-fluorouracil, and purified bovine collagen to produce a sustained release preparation which would require only one injection of each individual lesion (Conant et al. 1993). Early results with this technique have shown that it is well tolerated; however, the response to the purified bovine collagen with the 5-fluorouracil was no better than the response to the collagen alone. This suggests that trauma to the lesion with a subsequent inflammatory response may be all that is necessary to see partial or complete resolution of Kaposi's sarcoma lesions.

Liposomal daunorubicin is being used experimentally to treat Kaposi's sarcoma (Jablonski et al. 1993). Liposomes containing daunorubicin target the lesions of Kaposi's sarcoma. This results in a higher concentration of medication at the tumor site and sparing of noninvolved tissue. Good results were reported at the Ninth International AIDS Meeting in Berlin; however, experience in the clinic would suggest that in some patients this treatment loses its efficacy after 6–8 months.

Finally, the artificial expansion of natural killer T cells is being investigated as a treatment for Kaposi's sarcoma (Moody et al. 1993). In this treatment, patients are leukapheresed each month and their CD8 natural killer cells are harvested. These cells are then grown in vitro using phytohemagglutinin and interleukin-2 (IL-2) as T cell growth promoters. At the end of 2 or 3 weeks, the cells are reinfused into the patient and IL-2 is given daily for 5 days to continue T cell stimulation. The procedure has been well tolerated by patients, but it is still too early to assess its benefit as a treatment for Kaposi's sarcoma.

Treatment of Lymphomas

The treatment of lymphomas in HIV-infected patients has been less than satisfactory,with a high mortality rate. In non-HIV-infected patients a 90% remission rate with a 2-year survival rate of 60% has been achieved. In HIV-positive patients, the complete response rate has generally been less that 50% and 2-year survival has been considerably lower because of the appearance of HIV-associated opportunistic infections. Aggressive therapy with cyclophosphamide doxorubicin, vincristine, and prednisone (CHOP) has been the mainstay of treatment. Recently, better results have been achieved by using recombinant granulocyte-macrophage colony-stimulating factor (GM-CSF). This combination allows for the use of high-dose cancer chemotherapeutic agents in individuals with poor hematologic reserve (Kaplan et al. 1991).

Treatment of Basal Cell and Squamous Cell Carcinoma

Patients with patches of eczema which have been persistent for weeks to months should have these areas examined closely and biopsies should be taken. Frequently, superficial body basal cell carcinomas are found at such sides. These tumors can be easily removed with conservative curettement and desiccation.

The treatment of squamous cell carcinoma should be aggressive, since these malignancies frequently recur. In our hands wide surgical incision with meticulous follow-up has been the most successful form of treatment. Since squamous cell carcinoma is extremely common in patients with vulva, cervical, and anal HPV, careful follow-up of the HIV-infected patient with HPV disease is essential. Regular vaginal and anal examinations are essential if squamous cell carcinoma in situ is to be discovered and removed before invasive or metastatic disease occurs.

Great strides have been made in the past few years in extending the lives of HIV-infected people. In the early 1980s, an individual with a diagnosis of AIDS generally died within 6–9 months. Today, 12 years later, that same individual can look forward to living at least 40 months. The reason for this increased longevity is due to a variety of factors, including natural selection, patient empowerment, aggressive physician management, antiretroviral therapy, and prophylaxis against opportunistic infections. Unfortunately, as we conquer each of the AIDS-associated conditions which previously resulted in the deaths of our patients, newer opportunistic infections and malignancies have appeared as the major causes of morbidity and mortality. In my clinic in 1990, *Mycobactrium avium intercellulare* was the single most common cause of hospitalization and death. Just 2 years later, we have seen only one case of *Mycobacterium avium intercellulare* in an individual who we prophylaxed against that condition with clarithromycin. Now more than 40% of our patients are developing cytomegaloviral infection, which has replaced *Mycobactrium avium intercellulare* as the major cause of morbidity and death.

Hopefully, we will soon have prophylactic treatments that will prevent the development of cytomegaloviral infection. Unfortunately, when this occurs opportunistic malignancies such as squamous cell carcinomas, basal cell carcinomas, and lymphomas will be seen with increasing frequency in the long-term surviving HIV patients.

References

Bensaid-Mrejen D, Barau G (1993) A screening and treatment unit for HPV infections in HIV infected women: advantages. Poster PO-B14-1649. IXth international conference on AIDS, Berlin, 6–11 June 1993

Centers for Disease Control (1981) Follow-up on Kaposi's sarcoma's and Pneumocystis pneumonia. MMWR 30:409–410

Conant M, Illeman M, Michaud A, Irey D, Orenberg E (1993) Treatment of Kaposi's sarcoma with interlesional MPT 5003 FU (fluorouracil) therapeutic implants. Poster PO-B12-1602. IXth international conference on AIDS, Berlin, 6–11 June 1993

Hessol NA, Buchbinder SP, Katz MH et al (1993) Increased incidence of Hodgkin disease in homosexual men with HIV infection. Poster PO-C12-2885. IXth international conference on AIDS, Berlin, 6–11 June 1993

Jablonski H, Szelenyi H, Armbrecht C, Mauss S, Niederau C, Strohmeyer G (1993) Liposomal doxorubicin-a new formulation for the treatment of Kapsoi's sarcoma: a study on safety and efficacy in AIDS patients. Poster PO-B-12-1573. IXth international conference on AIDS, Berlin, 6–11 June 1993

Kaplan L, Kahn J, Crowes SL et al (1991) Clinical and virologic effects of recombinant human granulocyte macrophage colony stimulating factor in patients receiving chemotherapy for human immunodeficiency virus associated non-Hodgkin's lymphma: results of a randomized trial. J Clin Oncol 9:929–940

Kovacs JA, Deyton L, Davey R et al (1989) Combined zidovudine and interferon alpha therapy patients with Kaposi's sarcoma and the acquired immune deficiency syndrome. Ann Intern Med 111:280–287

Melbye M, Cote T, Biggar RJ et al (1993) High incidence of anal cancer among AIDS patients. Poster PO-B14-1636 IXth international conference on AIDS, Berlin, 6–11 June 1993

Moody DJ, Kremer AB, Kahn J, Okarma TB (1993) Impact of CD8 cellular therapy with concomitant IL-2 adminstration on the peripheral blood lymphocyte composition in AIDS patients with Kaposi's sarcoma. Poster PO-B28-2162. IXth international conference on AIDS, Berlin, 6–11 June 1993

Palefsky JM, Holly EA, Ahn DK (1993) Progression of anal cytologic changes in men with group IV HIV disease. Poster WS-B17-6. IXth international conference on AIDS, Berlin, 6–11 June 1993

Tappero JW, Conant MA, Wolfe SF et al (1993) Kaposi's sarcoma. JAAD 28: 371–395

Ziegler JL, Miner RC, Rosenbaum EL (1982) Outbreak of Burkitts-like lymphomas in homosexual men. Lancet 2:631–633

Subject Index

FSC
www.fsc.org
MIX
Papier aus verantwortungsvollen Quellen
Paper from responsible sources
FSC® C105338

If you have any concerns about our products,
you can contact us on
ProductSafety@springernature.com

In case Publisher is established outside the EU,
the EU authorized representative is:
Springer Nature Customer Service Center GmbH
Europaplatz 3, 69115 Heidelberg, Germany

Printed by Libri Plureos GmbH
in Hamburg, Germany